Directory of Psychological Tests in the Sport and Exercise Sciences

Second Edition

Andrew C. Ostrow, Ph.D.
Editor
West Virginia University

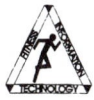 Fitness Information Technology, Inc., Publishers
P. O. Box 4425, University Avenue
Morgantown, WV 26504-4425

Library of Congress Card Catalog Number: 96-86376

ISBN: 1-885693-06-0

Cover Design: Pegasus
Copyeditor: Sandra R. Woods
Production Editor: Craig Hines
Printed by: BookCrafters

Printed in the United States of America
10 9 8 7 6 5 4 3 2 1

Fitness Information Technology, Inc.
P. O. Box 4425, University Avenue
Morgantown, WV 26504-4425 USA
(800)-477-4348
(304)-599-3482 (phone/fax)
E:mail: fit@access.mountain.net

In memory of G. Lawrence Rarick,

Professor Emeritus

University of California, Berkeley—

my mentor, friend, and colleague

About the Editor

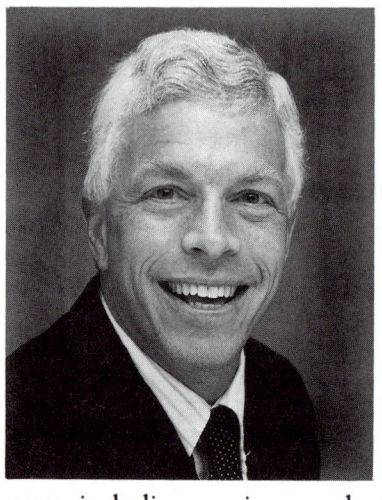

Andrew C. Ostrow completed the Ph.D. degree at the University of California, Berkeley. Currently, he is Professor and Program Coordinator for the Sport Behavior Program, School of Physical Education, at West Virginia University. He also has served as an adjunct professor in the Department of Psychology. Dr. Ostrow has numerous publications and presentations in the sport psychology field. He has taught undergraduate and graduate courses in the psychology of sport for the last 23 years, including a unique graduate course ("Sport Psychometrics") on psychological assessment in sport. He has directed a number of theses and dissertations focusing on the development of sport-specific psychological tests, including two published tests that appear in this directory.

Dr. Ostrow is the author and editor of two textbooks related to the psychological aspects of aging and physical activity. He is a member of the American Psychological Association and the Association for the Advancement of Applied Sport Psychology.

Dr. Ostrow is married and has two daughters. He enjoys traveling, wine, running, competing in racquet sports, and losing to his wife in golf.

Table of Contents

*New test (second edition of book).

Preface

The *Directory of Psychological Tests in the Sport and Exercise Sciences* summarizes information on 314 psychological scales, questionnaires, and inventories* specific to sport and exercise settings, that have been reported in the refereed, international scientific literature since the first International Congress of Sport Psychology was held in Rome, Italy more than 30 years ago. There has been an increasing emphasis by researchers and clinicians on the use of sport- or exercise-specific psychological tests. The use of these objective, self-report psychological tests continues to be the dominant mode of psychological assessment evident in the scientific literature pertinent to sport and exercise settings.

As sport- and exercise-specific psychological tests have become more widely used in research investigations and applied services, it is important that students, teachers, researchers, clinicians, and other professionals have quick access to information on these tests. I felt that a user-friendly directory was needed that provided interested individuals with information on the contents, psychometric properties, and availability of sport- and exercise-specific psychological tests. To this end, I have spent the last 8 years locating and summarizing information on sport- or exercise-specific psychological tests that have been reported in the international scientific literature.

When I began to search the research literature in 1988, I was uncertain as to how many of these tests I would uncover. To my surprise, I located over 200 sport- or exercise-specific psychological tests of which 175 tests were summarized in the first edition of the directory that was published in 1990.

In this second edition, I report on 314 tests that meet the criteria that I will describe later. Of these 314 psychological tests, 141 are new tests that did not appear in the first edition of the directory. (Two tests reported in the first edition were deleted from the second edition as requested by the test authors.) This represents an increase of approximately 80% in the number of new tests that are reported in the second edition. The vast majority of these new tests have appeared in the research literature during the last 5 years. A significant portion of these new tests are exercise-specific psychological tests that are applicable for use in exercise and rehabilitation settings.

The second edition also contains expanded reference lists for each test. Reference sources that evaluate the psychometric characteristics of

*To simplify the language used throughout the directory, the term *test* (rather than scale, questionnaire, or inventory) will be used to describe these psychological instruments.

the test are highlighted. In addition, I have spent countless hours on the Internet attempting to update the mailing addresses and phone/fax numbers of principal test authors. The second edition also contains e–mail addresses where available.

Almost all of the psychological tests reported in this directory were developed and are being used for research purposes, rather than for diagnosis or evaluation. Some of the tests are undergoing continued development. The majority of tests are not commercially published; rather, test users need to contact the author or source publisher to obtain a copy of the latest version of the test. It is important that the test user determine if a test is copyrighted and then contact the copyright holder for permission to use the test.

The second edition contains 20 chapters organized principally by psychological constructs such as aggression, anxiety, leadership, and motivation. The back of the directory contains subject, test title, test acronym, and test author indices to help the reader quickly locate the psychological test(s) of interest. Within each chapter are found test summaries that are organized alphabetically by the title of the test. Each test summary follows a similar format and highlights the purposes, foci, psychometric properties, norms, availability, and references pertinent to the test.

The directory does not attempt to review or evaluate the sport- and exercise-specific psychological tests presented. I have encouraged test authors whose work is cited in this directory to keep me apprised of revisions to their tests. In addition, new test authors (or authors of tests I have excluded inadvertently from the directory) are encouraged to forward to me copies of refereed publications that describe their sport- or exercise-specific psychological tests.

In the first edition, I indicated that a book was needed that would provide reviews by distinguished test authors of the tests cited in the directory. I am pleased to announce that Dr. Joan Duda, Professor, Purdue University, has agreed to serve as editor of a textbook titled *Advances in Sport and Exercise Psychology Measurement* that will be published shortly by Fitness Information Technology, Inc. This book includes over 50 contributing authors who will address psychological measurement issues in sport and exercise settings, and make recommendations for future research in this area.

In the first edition of the directory, I had cautioned the reader that self-report paper-and-pencil psychological tests, although extremely prominent in the psychology and sport psychology literature, are not the only means of assessment available. In fact, the standardized test is often only one of a battery of psychological assessment approaches taken. However, given the prominence of sport- and exercise-specific tests reported in the literature, I felt that a directory of this nature would serve as a useful reference book.

Oscar Buros, founder and editor of the widely acclaimed Mental Measurements Yearbook series, was cited (Conoley & Kramer, 1989) regarding the benefits of a comprehensive directory of psychological tests. I believe his observations relative to the value of such a directory are reflected in the *Directory of Psychological Tests in the Sport and Exercise Sciences:*

1. To impel psychological test authors and publishers to promote higher standards for test construction and validation;
2. To make test users more aware of the strengths and limitations of psychological tests;
3. To stimulate comprehensive reviews of psychological tests;
4. To make consumers and the public more aware of appropriate test selection and use.

I was very pleased by the positive comments I received from numerous readers and by the favorable reviews of the first edition of the directory that were published in a number of academic journals. It is my intent to make this project a life-long endeavor.

Andrew C. Ostrow, Ph.D.
West Virginia University

Reference

Conoley, J. C., & Kramer, J. J. (Eds.) (1989). *The tenth mental measurements yearbook*. Lincoln, NE: The University of Nebraska Press.

Acknowledgments

Although I researched and wrote a preliminary summary for each of the 314 tests that appear in the directory, the content and quality of the book reside primarily with each of the several hundred test authors who devoted countless hours to developing and validating these sport- or exercise-specific psychological tests. I am particularly grateful to those test authors who updated the initial test summaries I sent them and/or who provided me with additional references related to their tests.

I am also grateful to Dr. Stuart Biddle, University of Exeter, England, who while as president of FEPSAC (the European Federation of Sport Psychology) assisted me in conducting a survey of the FEPSAC membership to ensure that the European community was well represented in this book and to further enhance the international appeal of the directory. A special thank you to Dr. Dana Brooks, Dean of the School of Physical Education at West Virginia University. Dana has provided me with the encouragement and freedom to pursue this time-consuming project. I am also thankful to my research assistants, particularly Melissa Bailey and Ty Cook, and to graduate students who enrolled in the sport psychometrics class I teach at West Virginia University; these students, from time to time, surprised me by reporting on a psychological test that I had not previously uncovered. I am also grateful to Kelli Caseman and Judy Vincie, who helped me prepare the final manuscript; to Sandra Woods, my copy editor; and to Craig Hines, who served as production editor for the book. Most importantly, I am also grateful to my wife, Lynne, and daughters, Jennifer and Olivia, whose patience, encouragement, and love made the task of serving as editor of this directory more enjoyable.

I would be remiss if I did not conclude by paying a special tribute to Dr. G. Lawrence Rarick, Professor Emeritus, University of California, Berkeley, who passed away while I was completing the final draft of this book. Larry was a renowned scholar in the motor development field. More importantly, he was a mentor to numerous graduate students during his career. Larry was my advisor when I completed the Ph.D. at the University of California, Berkeley, 25 years ago. He had the remarkable ability to serve multiple roles, as a mentor and friend, as an individual who stood for academic excellence, and as someone who was committed to the personal and social development of graduate students. He has had a profound influence on my career as a college professor. The second edition of this book was written in memory of G. Lawrence Rarick.

How the Directory Was Developed

I was not able to rely on computer-based literature searches to locate the tests reported in the directory. For the most part, I located the principal reference source describing each psychological test by meticulously scanning the methodology section of every published research investigation appearing in more than 45 journals and conference proceedings over a 30-year period. Needless to say, the reader may feel that there are more exciting ways to spend one's time.

I delimited the literature search based on the following parameters:

1. Only reference sources that were refereed, that were written in the English language, and that appeared in the international scientific literature from 1965 to 1995 were evaluated.

2. The principal focus of psychological tests selected centered on the domains of sport, exercise, or related nonutilitarian physical activity. Tests related to areas such as sport pedagogy or leisure behavior were not considered.

3. Psychological tests were delimited to self-report paper-and-pencil tests that reported evidence of subject reliability and/or test validity. Tests not providing evidence for reliability or validity in the primary source evaluated were not included in the directory.

4. Behavioral observation scales, surveys, psychophysiological tests, motor behavior tasks, and developmental and neuropsychological tests were excluded from the directory.

5. Tests frequently used by sport psychology researchers that were not initially conceived as sport or exercise specific, such as the Test of Attentional and Interpersonal Style or the Profile of Mood States, were excluded from the directory. Tests that merely represented slight modifications of these more global tests were also excluded.

Based on these criteria, I searched for sport- or exercise-specific psychological tests in the following reference sources:

Periodicals
Adapted Physical Activity Quarterly (1984*–1992)
Annals of Sports Medicine (1982*–1986; 1988)
Australian Journal of Physical Education (1967–1986; 1988–1992)
Australian Journal of Sport Sciences (1981–1983)
British Journal of Physical Education (1989–1994)

British Journal of Sports Medicine (1979–1982; 1984–1987; 1989–1992)
Canadian Journal of Applied Physiology (1976*–1994)
Carnegie Research Reports (1967–1985)
Exercise and Sport Sciences Reviews (1973*–1995)
Human Movement Science (1982*–1992)
International Journal of Physical Education (1980–1995)
International Journal of Sport Psychology (1970*–1995)
International Journal of Sports Medicine (1984–1987; 1989–1991)
International Review of Sport Sociology (1966–1980; 1990–1993)
Journal of Applied Sport Psychology (1989*–1995)
Journal of Human Movement Studies (1975*–1991)
Journal of Motor Behavior (1969*–1992, 1995)
Journal of Sport & Exercise Psychology (1979*–1995)
Journal of Sport and Social Issues (1988–1992, 1995)
Journal of Sport Behavior (1978*–1995)
Journal of Sports Medicine and Physical Fitness (1978; 1982–1992)
Journal of Sports Sciences (1984–1995)
Medicine and Science in Sport and Exercise (1975–1980; 1982–1989)
Motor Skills: Theory in to Practice (1976*–1982)
Perceptual and Motor Skills (1965–1995)
Physical Education Review (1988–1991, 1994)
Physical Educator (1965–1989, 1991–1993, 1995)
Quest (1965–1995)
Research Quarterly for Exercise and Sport (1965–1995)
Scandinavian Journal of Sport Sciences (1980–1989)
Sociology of Sport Journal (1984*–1995)
Soviet Sports Review (1988–1991)
Sports Medicine (1984*–1992)
The Academy Paper (1990, 1992)
The Physician and Sportsmedicine (1979–1992)
The Sport Psychologist (1987*–1995)

Conference Proceedings
American Alliance for Health, Physical Education, Recreation, and Dance annual conference (1969; 1973–1974; 1980; 1984–1987)

Association for the Advancement of Applied Sport Psychology annual conference (1986*–1989; 1990, 1991, 1993, plus *Journal of Applied Sport Psychology* supplement issues 1994, 1995)

*Represents the first year of publication of the periodical.

British Proceedings of Sport Psychology (1975)

Canadian Society for Psychomotor Learning and Sport Psychology annual convention (1969*–1975; 1977–1979; 1982–1989)

National Association for Physical Education in Higher Education proceedings (1979–1985)

North American Society for the Psychology of Sport and Physical Activity annual convention (1973*; 1975; 1977–1984; 1988–1989; 1991,1992 plus *Journal of Sport & Exercise Psychology* supplements, 1993–1995)

North American Society for the Sociology of Sport annual convention (1981) *Proceedings of the International Symposium on Psychological Assessment in Sport* (1975)

Proceedings of the World Congress of Sport Psychology (1969; 1973; 1989, 1993)

The limited holdings of the several university libraries I visited placed constraints on my ability to access every journal issue since 1965. However, I reviewed every issue of the more prominent journals in sport psychology (such as the *Journal of Sport & Exercise Psychology* and the *International Journal of Sport Psychology*) since their inception. In addition to these journals and conference proceedings, I also examined several edited books in sport psychology.

In preparing the first edition of the book, I first relied on six experts, who were also authors of tests in the directory, to comment on the organizational structure and content validity of the summaries reported prior to forwarding these summaries to test authors. In the preparing the second edition of the directory, I first developed the initial draft of each test summary. Where a test had been reported as revised in the literature, I updated the test summary, and I identify in this edition the most recent source for the test.

Each test summary that I had developed was then forwarded to the appropriate principal test author for review. The test authors were asked to critique, update, and/or revise the summary of their test(s) that I had developed. I also included as a guide a draft copy of the summary I had prepared of the Exercise Motivations Inventory by David Markland and Lew Hardy. All test authors were asked to furnish me with copies of research articles that reported psychometric information on the latest versions of their tests. The authors were also asked to examine and update the reference lists I had prepared pertinent to their tests. I also asked the authors to alert me to new sport-

*Represents the first annual conference in which proceedings were published.

or exercise-specific psychological tests that they or their colleagues had developed.

I indicated to each principal test author that if a response was not received by a designated date, it would be assumed that the test author was satisfied with the test summary I had developed. A total of 135 test summaries (43.00%) were returned, of which 76 (or 56.30%) of the returned summaries were new test summaries that had not appeared in the first edition. The test authors typically did not make major revisions to the initial summaries. In several cases, authors either re-wrote the summaries I had prepared or forwarded to me manuscripts that were recently accepted for publication that provided updated revisions to their test(s). The test authors were particularly helpful in providing additional psychometric references related to their tests. Six envelopes containing test summaries were returned as undeliverable.

It should be noted that I have not attempted to incorporate the psychometric information reported by all listed references in preparing each final test summary. Indeed, this task is well beyond the resources that are currently available for this project. I have relied extensively on the contributing test authors to keep me apprised of the latest psychometric data they or others have gathered documenting the integrity of their tests. It should be noted, however, that for the vast majority of tests reported in the directory, there have not been follow-up psychometric studies conducted. This poses a serious limitation for the test user.

I have spent countless hours using the Internet and other sources in an attempt to update the mailing address, phone and fax numbers, and e-mail address of each principal author (noted in the "Availability" section of each test summary). I relied extensively on the use of gopher search procedures, on WhoWhere (http://www.whowhere.com/), on the web sites of colleges and universities throughout the world, and on a print-out of e-mail addresses provided by the Exercise and Sports Psychology list service (sportpsy) operated by Dr. Michael L. Sachs at Temple University. I also relied on the *Directory of Graduate Programs in Applied Sport Psychology* (1995), Michael L. Sachs, Kevin L. Burke, and Lois A. Butcher, editors (Fitness Information Technology, Inc., publisher) for current address, phone/fax number, and e-mail address information. In this way, users of the directory can readily contact test authors regarding the availability of their tests.

I also hope that test users will continue to apprise test authors of the findings emanating from the use of these tests. In this way, psychological measurement in the sport and exercise sciences is advanced further.

How To Use the Directory

The organization format is identical for each test described in the directory. Each test summary is intended to provide the reader with quick access to concise information about a test rather than to serve as a test review or critique. The test summaries do not contain all information required by the reader to administer, score, and interpret test results. Users are encouraged to contact test authors for additional information.

The format for each test summary is as follows:

Test Title: Presents the test title and acronym exactly as cited in the source. Parentheses surrounding the acronym indicate that this is the acronym used by the test authors. Brackets surrounding the title or acronym signify that I assigned a title or acronym. An asterisk appearing before a test title signifies that this test did not appear in the first edition of the directory.

Test author(s): Originally listed test authors as their names appeared in the source. Subsequently, these names were retained or modified based on correspondence with the principal author listed in the source.

Source: Cites the refereed publication or refereed professional presentation in which the most recent version of the test is described.

Purpose: Describes the general objective(s) and intent of the self-report assessment.

Description: Briefly describes the nature of subscales, presents examples of test items, and indicates the measurement scale used to evaluate test item responses.

Construction: Describes sequentially the procedures used to develop the test, prior to computing estimates of reliability and validity. Indicates how items were selected initially and subsequently modified. Also indicates the procedures followed during item analyses and in the establishment of content validity.

Reliability: Presents estimates of internal consistency and/or test stability based on data cited in the source.

Validity: Presents evidence for concurrent, predictive, and/or construct validity based on data cited in the source.

Norms: Indicates if test norms are presented in the source. Otherwise, presents a description of the sample(s) upon which the descriptive and/or psychometric data were based.

Availability: Indicates the name, address, and office phone and fax numbers of the principal author of the test. E-mail addresses are also provided where available, which is a new feature of the second edition. A double asterisk indicates that the principal test author returned the test summary developed by the editor; the reader should recognize that these authors have the most up-to-date addresses, phone/fax numbers, and e-mail addresses reported in the directory.

References: Indicates references that have utilized the test instrument. An asterisk indicates that the reference centered on further examination of the psychometric properties of the test instrument.

Chapter 1

Achievement Orientation

Tests in this chapter measure achievement orientations of sport participants in terms of competitiveness, the desire to win, striving for goals, task versus ego orientation, motives to approach/avoid success and to avoid failure, and perceptions of motivational climate and effort.

* New test (second edition of book)

1 Achievement Motivation In Physical Education Test (AMPET)

Tamotsu Nishida

Source: Nishida, T. (1988). Reliability and factor structure of the Achievement Motivation in Physical Education Test. *Journal of Sport &Exercise Psychology, 10,* 418-430.

Purpose: To assess achievement motivation for learning in physical education.

Description: The AMPET contains seven 8-item subscales: Learning strategy (LS), overcoming obstacles (OO), diligence and seriousness (DS), competence of motor ability (CMA), value of learning (VL), anxiety about stress-causing situations (ASCS), and failure anxiety (FA). Participants' responses to each item are assessed using a 5-point Likert scale. The AMPET also contains an 8-item lie scale to check response accuracy.

Construction: Original items of the AMPET were developed based on research and theories related to factors that constitute motivation/will to win in sport, and behavioral characteristics associated with individuals at various levels of achievement motivation. Item and factor analyses (see Nishida, 1987) reduced the original pool of items from 83 to 64. Principal component factor analysis supported seven principal factors essential for measuring achievement motivation for learning in physical education. These factors correspond to the subscales above.

Reliability: Alpha reliability coefficients for each subscale ranged from .80 (FA) to .92 (CMA) among 3,220 Japanese elementary school children, from .82 (FA) to .94 (CMA) among 3,346 Japanese junior high school students, and from .84 (FA) to .95 (CMA and ASCS) among 3,489 Japanese high school students. Test-retest reliability coefficients across a 5-week interval ranged from .71 (FA) to .85 (CMA) among these elementary school students (n=115), from .65 (VL) to .88 (CMA) among a junior high school student subsample (n=120), and from .68 (DS) to .80 (CMA) among the high school students (n=137). Acceptable internal consistency and test-retest reliability coefficients were also reported for two derived composite subscales: the tendency to achieve success and the tendency to avoid failure.

4

Validity: The construct validity of the AMPET was examined through factor analysis of these Japanese students' responses to the test. The analysis confirmed the seven factor structure for all samples combined. Similar factor structures emerged when factor analyses were conducted separately by grade level and by gender.

Norms: Psychometric data (including item descriptive statistics) were presented for the 10,055 Japanese students noted above. (See Nishida, 1989, for additional information on normative data).

**Availability: Contact Tamotsu Nishida, Research Center of Health, Physical Fitness and Sports, Nagoya University, Furo-cho, Chikusa-ku, Nagoya, 464-01 Japan. (Phone # 052-789-3952; FAX # 052-789-3957; E-mail: a40453a@nucc.cc.nagoya-u.ac.jp)

References

Nishida, T. (1987). A new test for achievement motivation for learning in physical education: Construction of a questionnaire and a preliminary study on typology of the motivation. *Nagoya Journal of Health, Physical Fitness and Sports, 10*, 47-60.

*Nishida, T. (1989). A study on standardization of the Achievement Motivation in Physical Education Test. *Japanese Journal of Physical Education, 34*, 45-62.

*Nishida, T. (1991). Achievement motivation for learning in physical education class: A cross-cultural study in four countries. *Perceptual and Motor Skills, 72*, 1183-1186.

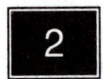

[Approach-Avoidance Motivations Scale For Sports] [AAMSS]
Brent S. Rushall and Randy G. Fox

Source: Rushall, B. S., & Fox, R. G. (1980). An Approach-avoidance Motivations Scale for sports. *Canadian Journal of Applied Sport Sciences, 5*, 39-43.

Purpose: To assess an individual's motives to approach success and to avoid failure in competitive sports.

Description: The scale contains 23 items focusing on approach or avoidance orientations to competition, training, and the sporting experience. Participants respond on a 4-point ordinal scale.

Construction: Gjesme and Nygard's general Achievement Motives Scale (30 items) was modified to be specific to sport situations. Six items were added that related to specific competition and training circumstances. An assessment of test-retest reliability across 3 days ($n=29$ physical education majors), as well as the establishment of content validity by 12 experts in the psychology of sport and in psychology, resulted in the retention of 28 items with at least 64% agreement.

Reliability: An additional evaluation of test-retest reliability ($n=23$ varsity team members) over a 4-day interval indicated at least 64% agreement for each of the 28 items.

Validity: Multiple regression analyses were conducted to examine the extent to which derived factor scores of the scale were predictive of improvement in swimming performance among athletes participating in the 1977 Canadian Winter Swimming Championships. Among 90 male elite swimmers, 4.39% of the variance in improved swimming performance was accounted for by four factors of the scale. For 86 female elite swimmers, three factors accounted for 9% of the variance in improved swimming performance.

Norms: Not cited. Psychometric data were reported for 176 male and female elite swimmers and 23 varsity athletes.

Availability: Contact Brent S. Rushall, Department of Exercise and Nutritional Sciences, San Diego State University, San Diego, CA 92182-0171. (Phone # 619-594-4094; FAX # 619-594-6553; E-mail: brushall@mail.sdsu.edu)

References

Henschen, K. P., Horvat, M., & Roswal, G. (1992). Psychological profiles of the United States Wheelchair Basketball Team. *International Journal of Sport Psychology, 23,* 128-137.

Whitehead, J., & Edwards, S. (1984). A-state and achievement motivation in volleyball [Abstract]. *Journal of Sports Sciences, 2,* 202-203.

3 [Athletic Achievement Motivation Test] [AAMT]
Luc M. Lefebvre

Source: Lefebvre L. (1978). Achievement motivation and causal attribution in male and female athletes. In U. Simri (Ed.), *Proceedings of the International Symposium on Psychological Assessment in Sport* (pp. 163-170). Netanya, Israel: Wingate Institute for Physical Education and Sport.

Purpose: To assess the achievement motives of elite athletes.

Description: The test assesses four areas: intrinsic motivation, risk preference, positive fear of failure, and fear of success. Participants respond to each item on a 7-point dimensional scale.

Construction: Items were constructed from the interview statements of 40 elite Belgian athletes, as well as from different achievement motivation questionnaires. A content analysis was performed yielding four sets of internally valid items.

Reliability: Split-half internal consistency (*n*=30) was reported as acceptable for each area, as well as for the entire test.

Validity: Not discussed.

Norms: Not presented. Psychometric data were reported for 30 elite Belgian athletes (15 males and 15 females) who were candidates for the 1976 Olympic games. Athletes represented track, swimming, and gymnastics.

Availability: Unknown.

4 *Competitive Motive Inventory (CMI)
Ye Ping

Source: Ping, Y. (1993). Competitive motives as predictors of cognitive trait anxiety in university athletes. *International Journal of Sport Psychology, 24,* 259-263.

Purpose: To assess the competitive motives that exist among athletes engaged in a variety of sports.

Description: The CMI contains 38 items and five subscales: Desire for Victory; High Ability Demonstration; Social Approval; Enjoyment; and Self Challenge. Participants respond to each item using a 4-point Likert scale with the anchorings 1 *(strongly disagree)* to 4 *(strongly agree)*.

Construction: The CMI was developed using some items from a previous inventory developed in Japan, from a review of the literature, and from open-ended responses of individuals in an exploratory investigation.

Reliability: Cronbach alpha internal consistency coefficients (*N*=406) ranged from .58 (Self Challenge) to .81 (Desire for Victory).

Validity: Exploratory principal components factor analysis (*N*=406) with varimax rotation led to the retention of the six-factor solution accounting for 46.1% of the variance.

Norms: Not cited. Psychometric data were reported for 406 (254 males; 152 females) athletes attending a university in Japan.

Availability: Last known address: Jinnaka-cho 1-18-12, Toyota City, Aichi-ken 471 Japan.

5 | Competitive Orientation Inventory (COI)
Robin S. Vealey

Source: Vealey, R. S. (1986). Conceptualization of sport-confidence and competitive orientation: Preliminary investigation and instrument development. *Journal of Sport Psychology, 8,* 221-246.

Purpose: To assess individual differences in the tendency to strive toward achieving a sport-related goal.

Description: The COI employs a matrix format of 16 cells. One dimension of the matrix (rows) represents different levels of performance in

8

sport (e.g., very good, below average), whereas a second dimension establishes different outcomes (e.g., easy win, close loss). Participants are asked to complete the matrix by assigning a number from 0 *(very unsatisfying situation)* to 10 *(very satisfying situation)* to each cell in the matrix. Two scores are derived--an outcome orientation score and a performance orientation score.*

Construction: A major consideration in the development of the COI was the need for a format in which the participant would be forced to weigh the values of wanting to win versus performing well. To this end, a matrix format was selected. A total of 99 high school students and 101 college students were administered the COI and the Crowne-Marlowe Social Desirability Scale in a noncompetitive situation. Participants' responses to each cell were treated as a test item. Adequate variability between and within cells was found. No relationship was found between participants' responses to the COI and the Marlowe-Crowne Social Desirability Scale. These findings were replicated with independent samples of high school (n=103) and college (n=96) athletes.

Reliability: Internal consistency coefficients were not computed, because the COI is not an additive scale. Test-retest reliability coefficients among a sample of high school (n=109) and college (n=110) athletes were .69 (1-day interval), .69 (1-week interval), and .69 (1-month interval) for the COI-performance score. For COI-outcome, test-retest reliability coefficients were .69 (1 day), .69 (1 week), and .63 (1 month).

Validity: Concurrent validity coefficients were reported between the responses of 199 high school and college athletes to the COI (performance orientation) and their corresponding responses to the physical self-presentation confidence subscale of the Physical Self-Efficacy Scale (r=.17). COI-performance was inversely related to external locus of control (r=-.29), and COI-outcome was positively correlated to external locus of control when Rotter's Internal-External Control Scale was employed. COI-performance and COI-outcome were not found to be related to subjects' responses to the SCAT, CSAI-2, or the perceived physical ability subscale of the Physical Self-Efficacy Scale.

Construct validity was established by demonstrating among elite gymnasts (n=48) that both COI-performance and COI-outcome were correlated with participants' pre- and postcompetitive state sport-confidence

---

*Vealey (1988) indicated that the COI-outcome and COI-performance subscales are highly correlated and recommended adoption of a COI composite score that has similar psychometric properties

levels. COI responses were also found to influence athletes' attributional patterns and COI-performance scores were related to their self-perceptions of performance.

Norms: Preliminary normative data were presented (Vealey, 1988) for 262 high school athletes, 156 athletes ages 12-14 years, 226 college athletes, and 48 elite gymnasts.

**Availability: Contact Robin S. Vealey, Department of Physical Education, Health, and Sport Studies, Phillips Hall, Miami University, Oxford, OH 45056. (Phone # 513-529-2720; FAX # 513-529-5006; E-mail: rsvealey@miamiu.muohio.edu)

References

Gill, D.L. & Dzewaltowski, D. A. (1988). Competitive orientations among intercollegiate athletes. Is winning the only thing? *The Sports Psychologist, 2*, 212-221.

*Gill, D. L., Kelley, B. C., Martin, J. J., & Caruso, C. M. (1991). A comparison of competitive-orientation measures. *Journal of Sport & Exercise Psychology, 13*, 266-280.

Kelley, B. C., Gill, D. L., & Hoffman, S. J. (1989). Competitive sport orientation as a function of religious orientation, athletic experience, and gender [Abstract]. *Psychology of motor behavior and sport* (p. 124). Kent, OH: Proceedings of the North American Society for the Psychology of Sport and Physical Activity annual convention.

*Martin, J. J., & Gill, D. L. (1991). The relationship among competitive orientation, sport-confidence, self-efficacy, anxiety, and performance. *Journal of Sport & Exercise Psychology, 13*, 149-159.

Vealey, R. S. (1988). Achievement goals of adolescent figure skaters: Impact on self-confidence, anxiety, and performance. *Journal of Adolescent Research, 3*, 227-243.

*Vealey, R. S. (1988). Sport-confidence and competitive orientation: An addendum on scoring procedures and gender differences. *Journal of Sport & Exercise Psychology, 10*, 471-478.

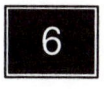 **6**

[Competitiveness/Coachability Questionnaire] [CCQ]
Ardan O. Dunleavy

Source: Dunleavy, A. O. (1980). Competitiveness and coachability of male varsity swimmers as assessed by peer and coach ratings: A generalizability study with forecasting. *Abstracts: American Alliance for Health, Physical Education, Recreation, and Dance* (p. 68). Annual convention, Detroit, MI.

Purpose: To assess competitiveness and coachability among male college varsity swimmers.

Description: The CCQ contains 20 items; 10 items assess competitiveness, and 10 items assess coachability.

Construction: Not discussed.

Reliability: Alpha internal consistency coefficients of .67 and .91 were reported for the competitiveness and coachability subscales, respectively ($n=20$).

Validity: Not discussed.

Norms: Not cited. Psychometric data were based on 20 male college varsity swimmers.

Availability: Last known address: Ardan Dunleavy, Department of Kinesiological Studies, Texas Christian University, Fort Worth, TX 76129.

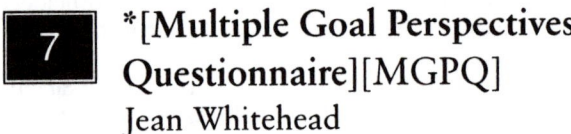

7   *[Multiple Goal Perspectives Questionnaire][MGPQ]
Jean Whitehead

Source: Whitehead, J. (1992). Toward the assessment of multiple goal perspectives in children's sport [Abstract]. *Proceedings of the Olympic Scientific Congress* (Volume 2). p. 14.

Purpose: To assess multiple goal perspectives among children participating in sport.

Description: The MGPQ asks children to record a critical incident when they felt successful in sport. They are then asked to record the extent to which their feelings on that occasion corresponded with three subscale pairs containing a total of 26 Likert-type items: victory-ability, mastery-breakthrough, social approval-teamwork.

Construction: Participants ($N=890$) completed the Achievement

Orientation Questionnaire (Ewing, 1988), and they added further items to those listed. A longer, 50-item questionnaire that included newer dimensions was completed by 1,198 children. Exploratory factor analyses of age and gender subgroups produced 13-16 factors; however, a 6-factor structure was viewed by the author as most relevant.

Reliability: Cronbach alpha coefficients (*N*=986) ranged from .48 (mastery) to .76 (teamwork) (J. Whitehead, personal communication, January 11, 1993). Subsequent revision (*N*=56) yielded coefficients ranging from .78 (ability) to .86 (teamwork) with a new response format (J. Whitehead, personal communication, April 10, 1996).

Validity: Confirmatory factor analyses (*N*=1,273) supported the construct validity of the MGPQ.

Norms: Not cited. Psychometric data were reported for 986 children, ages 9-16 years old, and for 1,273 children drawn from schools and clubs in England.

**Availability: Contact Jean Whitehead, Chelsea School Research Centre, University of Brighton, Gaudick Road, Eastbourne, East Sussex, England BN20 7SP. (Phone # 01273-600900; FAX # 01273-643704; E-mail: jw73@bton.ac.uk)

Reference
Ewing, M. (1988) Psychometric properties of the Achievement Orientation Questionnaire and associated methodological issues [Abstract]. *Psychology of motor behavior and sport* (p. 91). Proceedings of the North American Society for the Psychology of Sport and Physical Activity annual convention. Scottsdale, AZ.

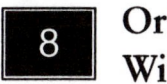

Orientations Toward Winning Scale (OTW)
Thomas R. Kidd and William F. Woodman

Source: Kidd, T. R., & Woodman, W. F. (1975). Sex and orientations toward winning in sport. *Research Quarterly, 46,* 476-483.

Purpose: To assess individual differences in the motive toward winning in sport.

Description: The OTW contains four items. Participants respond to each item using a 5-point Likert scale.

Construction: The scale was derived from the factor analyses of the responses of 451 male and female college students to a larger questionnaire.

Reliability: An alpha internal consistency coefficient of .76 was reported (*n*=451).

Validity: The OTW discriminated between men and women. As hypothesized, the men scored higher than the women on the OTW.

Norms: Not cited. Psychometric data were reported for 451 male and female college students representing one institution.

Availability: Last known address: Thomas R. Kidd, School of HPER, University of Nebraska, Omaha, NE 68182-0216.

References
Graham, R. H., & Carron, A. V. (1982). The impact of the national coaching certification program for hockey on coaching attitudes. In L. M. Wankel & R. B. Wilberg (Eds.), *Psychology of sport and motor behavior: Research and practice* (pp. 203-216). Proceedings of the Canadian Society for Psychomotor Learning and Sport Psychology, Edmonton, Alberta.

*Snyder, E. E., & Spretzer, E. (1979). Orientations toward sport: Intrinsic, normative, and extrinsic. *Journal of Sport Psychology, 1,* 170-175.

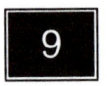 **9**

Parent-Initiated Motivational Climate Questionnaire-2 (PIMCQ-2)
Sally. A. White and Joan L. Duda

Source: White. S. A., & Duda, J. L. (1996). *The Parent-Initiated Motivational Climate Questionnaire-2: Construct, criterion, and predictive validity.* Manuscript in preparation.

Purpose: To assess the individual's perceptions of the motivational climate initiated by mothers and fathers in the learning and performance of physical skills.

---

*Note: This test summary was submitted by the first test author (S. A. White, personal communication, April 13, 1996).

Description: The PIMCQ-2 is a 36-item questionnaire containing three subscales: Learning/Enjoyment Climate, Worry Conducive Climate, and Success Without Effort Climate. For 18 items, participants respond to the stem, "I feel that my mother. . .", and for the other 18 items participants respond to the stem "I feel that my father. . ." A 5 point Likert scale with the anchorings 1 *(strongly disagree)* to 5 *(strongly agree)* is used to record responses.

Construction: The original 28-item version of the PIMCQ (White, Duda, & Hart, 1992) was adapted from an inventory developed by Papaioannous (1994) that examined the perceived motivational climate created by physical education teachers. The second version (PIMCQ-2) generated eight more items that focused on the enjoyment aspect of learning and performing physical skills. To determine the factor structure of the PIMCQ-2, two principal components factor analyses (PFA) were performed on participants' (N=301) responses. The first PFA for the mother items produced three factors accounting for 59.3% of the variance. The second PFA for the father items identified three factors and accounted for 65.5% of the variance.

Reliability: Both total sample and age group Cronbach alpha reliability coefficients were calculated. For the total sample (N=301), the coefficients were Learning/Enjoyment (.92), Worry Conducive Climate (.90), and Success Without Effort Climate (.84). The age group internal consistency coefficients were children Learning/Enjoyment (.91), children Worry Conducive Climate (.89), children Success Without Effort Climate (.81); young adolescents Learning/Enjoyment (.94), young adolescents Worry Conducive Climate (.89), young adolescents Success Without Effort Climate (.82); and older adolescents Learning/Enjoyment (.92), older adolescents Worry Conducive Climate (.90), older adolescents Success Without Effort Climate (.86).

Validity: The criterion-related validity of the PIMCQ-2 was assessed via a canonical correlation analysis. Specifically, two functions emerged with an eigenvalue greater than one (Wilks's lambda=.754; canonical correlation= .41, and .30 respectively). Function 1 reflected a task-involving perception of the motivational climate, with task orientation linked to a learning/enjoyment climate initiated by parents. The second function revealed that ego orientation was associated with the perception that parents valued a climate where success was coupled with low levels of effort, or ego-involving climate.

In addition, the discriminant validity of the PIMCQ-2 was determined. A 2 x 3 MANOVA analysis revealed gender and age group differences on the PIMCQ-2 subscales. For gender, differences were identified on the Success Without Effort Climate Subscale and Worry Conducive Climate Subscale. However, age-group differences were determined for the Worry Conducive Climate subscale only.

Norms: Not cited. Psychometric data were reported for 301 participants (n=152 males; n=149 females) involved in the following sports: soccer, basketball, ice hockey, and swimming. The sample included 96 children (M age= 11.7 years; SD=.46); 97 young adolescents (M age= 14.6 years; SD= .50); and 108 older adolescents (M age= 16.7 years; SD=.80). Specifically, there were 51 females and 45 males in the children's group, 50 females and 47 males in the young adolescent group, and 48 females and 60 males in the older adolescent group.

**Availability: Contact Sally A. White, 5120 Department of HPER, Illinois State University, P. O. Box 5120, Normal, IL 61790-5120. (Phone # 309-438-7501; FAX # 309-438-5559; E-mail: swhite@ilstu.edu).

References

Papaioannou, A. (1994). Development of a questionnaire to measure achievement orientation in physical education. *Research Quarterly for Exercise and Sport, 65*, 11-20.

*White, S. A. (1996). Goal orientation and perceptions of the motivational climate initiated by parents. *Pediatric Exercise Science, 6*, 45-54.

*White, S. A. (1996). *Perceptions of the parent-initiated motivational climate and competitive trait anxiety among sport participants high in task and ego orientation.* Manuscript submitted for publication.

*White, S. A., Duda, J. L., & Hart, S. (1992). An exploratory examination of the Parent-Initiated Motivational Climate Questionnaire. *Perceptual and Motor Skills, 75*, 875-880.

*White, S. A., & Guest, S. M. (1996). *Goal orientation, gender, and perceptions of the motivational climate created by significant others.* Manuscript submitted for publication.

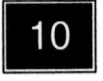

*[Perceived Effort Questionnaire] [PEQ]
Lavon Williams and Diane L. Gill

Source: Williams, L., & Gill, D. L. (1995). The role of perceived competence in the motivation of physical activity. *Journal of Sport & Exercise Psychology, 17*, 363-378.

Purpose: To assess children's perception of effort when participating in sport and related physical activity.

Description: The PEQ contains two subscales, (a) Behavioral Intensity ("How hard children try") and (b) Persistence ("How long they persist in physical activity"), each containing three items. Items are presented in a structured alternative format in which children respond to bipolar statements (e.g., really true for me) using a 4-point ordinal scale.

Construction: Principal components factor analysis (with varimax rotation) supported the existence of one factor (labeled Perceived Effort) that accounted for 45.5% of the variance. All six items loaded on this one factor.

Reliability: Pilot research resulted in Cronbach alpha internal consistency coefficients of .70 (Behavioral Intensity) and .64 (Persistence), and an overall alpha coefficient of .82 for the six items. In the current research, a Cronbach alpha coefficient (N=174) of .75 was reported for participants' responses to the six-item questionnaire (i.e., for Perceived Effort).

Validity: Moderate to high correlation coefficients (N=174) were obtained between participants' responses to the PEQ and their responses to measures of intrinsic interest, perceived competence, and task orientation. Perceived competence, interest, and task orientation (but not ego orientation) were predictors of effort, particularly among female participants.

Norms: Not cited. Psychometric data were reported for 103 female and 71 male physical education students, ages 11 to 15 (M= 12.7, SD= 1.07), from two middle schools in two school districts in the southeast region of the country. The students were enrolled in grades 6 thru 8.

**Availability: Contact Lavon Williams, Physical Education Department, Western Illinois University, Brophy Hall, Macomb, IL 61455. (Phone # 309-298-1702; FAX # 309-298-2981; E-mail: l-williams19@wiu.edu)

11   *Perceived Motivational Climate In Sport Questionnaire [PMCSQ]

Jeffrey J. Seifriz, Joan L. Duda, & Likang Chi

Source: Seifriz, J. J., Duda, J. L., & Chi, L. (1992). The relationship of perceived motivational climate to intrinsic motivation and beliefs about success in basketball. *Journal of Sport & Exercise Psychology*, 14, 375-391.

Purpose: "To assess players' perceptions of the degree to which their teams' motivational climates were characterized by an emphasis on mastery and performance goals" (p. 378).

Description: The PMCSQ contains two subscales: Performance Climate (12 items) and Mastery Climate (9 items). Players are asked to think what it was like playing on their teams during the season. For example, players respond to items such as "The coach favors some players" (Performance Climate subscale) or "All players have an important role" (Mastery Climate subscale). Responses to each item are made using a 5-point Likert scale with the anchorings of 1 (*strongly disagree*) to 5 (*strongly agree*).

Construction: An initial pool of 106 items was derived from the Classroom Achievement Goals Questionnaire (Ames & Archer, 1988) or developed by the investigators. The content validity of the PMCSQ was evaluated by eight experts, leading to the retention of 40 items. Exploratory and confirmatory principal components factor analysis ($N = 105$), using oblique and varimax rotations, led to a two-factor solution. These two factors were labeled Performance and Mastery, and accounted for 39.70% of the variance.

Reliability: Cronbach alpha internal consistency coefficients ($N = 105$) of .84 and .80 were reported for the Performance and Mastery subscales, respectively.

Validity: Discriminant validity was supported in that basketball athletes who perceived their basketball team environments to be strongly master-oriented reported (a) higher levels of enjoyment, (b) higher intrinsic motivation, and (c) stronger beliefs that high effort leads to success than did basketball athletes who perceived their basketball team environments to be low in mastery orientation. Conversely, perceptions of a performance-oriented climate were related to the view that superior ability leads to success.

Norms: Not cited. Psychometric data were reported for 105 male high school basketball players from nine teams in the Midwest.

**Availability: Contact Joan L. Duda, Department of Health, Kinesiology, and Leisure Studies, Purdue University, Lambert 113, West Lafayette, IN 47907. (Phone # 317-494-3172; FAX # 317-496-1239; E-mail: lynne@vm.cc.purdue.edu)

References

Ames, C., & Archer, J. (1988). Achievement goals in the classroom: Students' learning strategies and motivation processes. *Journal of Educational Psychology, 80,* 260-267.

*Andree, K. V., & Whitehead, J. (1995, June). *The interactive effect of perceived ability and dispositional or situational achievement goals on intrinsic motivation in young athletes.* Paper presented at the annual meeting of the North American Society for the Psychology of Sport and Physical Activity, Pacific Grove, CA .

*Boyd, M., Yin, Z, Ellis, D., & French, K. (1995). Perceived motivational climate, socialization influences, and affective responses in Little League baseball [Abstract]. *Journal of Sport & Exercise Psychology, 17* (Suppl.), S30.

*Chi, L., & Lu, S-E. (1995). The relationships between motivational climates and group cohesiveness in basketball [Abstract]. *Journal of Sport & Exercise Psychology, 17* (Suppl.), S 41.

*Duda, J. L., & Walling, M. D. (1995). Views about the motivational climate and their self-perceptions/affective correlates: The case of young elite female gymnasts [Abstract]. *Journal of Applied Sport Psychology, 7* (Suppl.), S58.

*Ebbeck, V., & Becker, S. L. (1994). Psychosocial predictors of goal orientations in youth soccer. *Research Quarterly for Exercise and Sport, 65,* 355-362.

*Hall, H. K., & Earles, M. (1995). Motivational determinants of interest, and perceptions of success in school physical education [Abstract]. *Journal of Sport & Exercise Psychology, 17* (Suppl.), S57.

*Newton, M. (1994). The perceived motivational climate: Affective and cognitive correlates in female team sports [Abstract]. *Journal of Sport & Exercise Psychology,16* (Suppl.), S23.

*Newton, M., & Duda, J. L. (1993). The Perceived Motivational Climate in Sport Questionnaire: Construct and predictive utility [Abstract]. *Journal of Sport & Exercise Psychology, 15* (Suppl.), S59.

*Rethorst, S., & Duda, J. L. (1993). Goal orientations, cognitions, and emotions in gymnastics. *Proceedings of the Eighth World Congress of Sport Psychology* (pp. 379 382). Lisbon, Portugal.

*Walling, M.D., & Duda, J. L. (1992). The psychometric properties of the Perceived

18

Motivational Climate in Sport Questionnaire: Further investigation [Abstract]. *Proceedings of the North American Society for the Psychology of Sport and Physical Activity annual convention* (p. 188). Pittsburgh, PA.

*Walling, M. D., Duda, J. L., & Chi , L. (1993). The Perceived Motivational Climate in Sport Questionnaire: Construct and predictive validity. *Journal of Sport & Exercise Psychology, 15,* 172-183.

*White, S. A., Duda, J. L., & Hart, S. (1992). An exploratory examination of the parent-initiated Motivational Climate Questionnaire. *Perceptual and Motor Skills, 75,* 875-880.

12 Perception Of Success Questionnaire* [PSQ]
Glyn C. Roberts and Gloria Balague

Source: Roberts, G. C., & Balague, G. (1989, August). *The development of a Social Cognitive Scale of Motivation.* Paper presented at the 7th World Congress in Sport Psychology, Singapore.

Purpose: To assess two major achievement goals that affect motivation in sport: Competitive goals and Mastery goals. Mastery goals enable individuals to focus upon improving ability and increasing mastery and skill in sport. Competitive goals lead people to focus on the adequacy of their abilities when compared to others.

Description: The PSQ contains 26 items and two subscales: Competitive goals and Mastery goals. Participants are asked to indicate the extent to which they feel most successful when playing sport when, for example, they beat other people (Competitive goal) or when they reach a goal (Mastery goal). Participants respond to each item using a 5-point Likert scale.

Construction: An initial pool of 48 items was developed, based on the work of major investigators in motivation and after a review of existing research questionnaires. A panel of experts evaluated the extent to which each item was pertinent to mastery or competitive goals, leading to the retention of 29 items.

The 29-item questionnaire was administered to 137 undergraduate students (n=66 females; n=71 males) who participated in an introductory psychology course and who had been involved in sports. Principal components factor analysis followed by varimax rotation led to the retention of two factors (labeled Mastery motivation and Competitive motivation) that accounted for 48% of the variance.

*Note: This test was titled the Social Cognitive Scale of Motivation in the first edition of this book.

Reliability: Cronbach alpha internal consistency coefficients (n=137) were .92 (Mastery subscale) and .90 (Competitive subscale). Split-half reliability coefficients were .91 (Mastery) and .88 (Competitive).

Validity: Convergent validity was supported in that participants' (n=137) responses to the SCSM were moderately correlated (r=.39) with their responses to Duda's (1989) Task and Ego Orientation in Sport Questionnaire. However, these participants' responses to the SCSM were not correlated with Vealey's (1986) Competitive Orientation Inventory.

Norms: Not presented. Psychometric data were based on the responses of 137 male and female undergraduate students.

Availability: Contact Glyn Roberts, Department of Kinesiology, 205 Louise Freer Hall, University of Illinois, 906 South Goodwin Ave., Urbana, IL 61801. (Phone # 217-333-6563; FAX # 217-244-7322; E–mail: glync@staff.uiuc.edu)

References

Famose,J.-P., Sarrazin, P., Cury, F., & Durand, M. (1993). Study of the effects of perceived ability, motivational goal and competitive context upon the selection of task difficulty in a free choice situation. *Proceedings of the Eighth World Congress of Sport Psychology* (pp. 656-659). Lisbon, Portugal.

*Hanrahan, S. (1993). Attributional style, intrinsic motivation, and achievement goal orientations. *Proceedings of the Eighth World Congress of Sport Psychology* (pp. 846-850). Lisbon, Portugal.

*Marsh, H. W. (1994). Sport motivation orientations: Beware of jingle-jangle fallacies. *Journal of Sport & Exercise Psychology, 16,* 365-380.

*Roberts, G. C., & Balague, C. (1989, August). *The development of a Social Cognitive Scale of Motivation.* Paper presented at the 7th World Congress of Sport Psychology, Singapore.

*Roberts, G. C., Jackson, S. A., Hall, H. K., Kimiecik, J. C., & Tonymon, P. (1990).Goal orientations and perceptions of the sport experience [Abstract]. *Proceedings of the Association for the Advancement of Applied Sport Psychology annual convention.* (p. 98). San Antonio, TX.

*Roberts, G. C., & Treasure, D. C. (1995). Achievement goals, motivational climate and achievement strategies and behaviors in sport. *International Journal of Sport Psychology, 26,* 64-80.

Tammen, V. V., Treasure, D. C. , & Power, K. T. D. (1992). The relationship between competitive and mastery achievement goals and dimensions of intrinsic motivation [Abstract]. *Journal of Sports Sciences, 10,* 630.

*Treasure, D. C., Lox, C., Rudolph, D., Bodey, K., & Roberts, G. C. (1993). The relationship between children's achievement goal orientations and affective responses in competitive sport [Abstract]. *Research Quarterly for Exercise and Sport, 64* (Suppl.), A-105.

*Treasure, D. C., & Roberts, G. C. (1994). Cognitive and affective concomitants of task and ego goal orientations during the middle school years. *Journal of Sport & Exercise Psychology, 16,* 15-28.

*Treasure, D. C., & Roberts, G. C. (1994). Perception of Success Questionnaire: Preliminary validation in an adolescent population. *Perceptual and Motor Skills, 79,* 607-610.

Treasure, D. C., Roberts, G. C., & Hall, H. K. (1992). The relationship between children's achievement goal orientations and their beliefs about the competitive sport experience [Abstract]. *Journal of Sports Sciences, 10,* 629-630.

13   Sport Orientation Questionnaire (SOQ)
Diane L. Gill and Thomas E. Deeter

Source: Gill, D. L., & Deeter, T. E. (1988). Development of the Sport Orientation Questionnaire. *Research Quarterly for Exercise and Sport, 59,* 191-202.

Purpose: To assess the disposition to strive for success in competitive and noncompetitive sport activities.

Description: The SOQ contains 25 items incorporating three subscales: (a) *competitiveness,* (b) the desire to *win* in interpersonal competition in sport, and (c) the desire to reach personal *goals* in sport. Participants respond to each item using a 5-point Likert format.

Construction: Items representing achievement orientation across sport and exercise activities were developed based on a literature review of achievement and sport competition, by consulting other sport psychologists and by collecting open-ended responses from independent samples of sport participants during several exploratory projects. A total of 58 items were evaluated by five graduate students in sport psychology for content validity and item clarity. The reduced pool of 32 items was placed into inventory format, further evaluated for item clarity and lack of ambiguity among 10 subjects, and then all 32 items were administered to two independent samples of undergraduate students ($n=237$; $n=218$) and 266 high school students. Exploratory and confirmatory factor analyses supported a three-factor structure (see subscales labeled above) and led to the retention of 25 items.

Reliability: Across the three samples, alpha reliability coefficients averaged .94 (competitiveness), .86 (win), and .81 (goal). Test-retest reliability coefficients obtained among the second sample of university students (n=218) across a 4-week interval were .89 (competitiveness), .82 (win), and .73 (goal). Intraclass correlation coefficients were .94 (competitiveness), .90 (win), and .84 (goal).

Validity: Concurrent validity was demonstrated by showing that participants' scores on the SOQ correlated with their scores on the Work and Family Orientation Questionnaire subscales. Construct validity was supported in that the competitiveness subscale differentiated students enrolled in competitive sport classes from students enrolled in noncompetitive classes. Competitive sport participants were also differentiated from nonparticipants. Win and goal orientation subscales appeared to be less discriminating variables.

Norms. Not reported. Psychometric data were cited for 455 undergraduate students and 266 high school students randomly selected from grades 9 through 12.

Availability: Contact Diane L. Gill, Exercise and Sport Science Department, University of North Carolina at Greensboro, Greensboro, NC 27412-5001. (Phone # 910-334-5744; FAX # 910-334-3238; E-mail: gilldl@iris.uncg.edu)

References

Acevedo, E. O., Dzewaltowski, D. A., Gill, D. L., & Noble, J. M. (1992). Cognitive orientations of ultramarathoners. *The Sport Psychologist, 6*, 242-252.

*Deeter, T. E. (1989). Development of a model of achievement behavior for physical activity. *Journal of Sport & Exercise Psychology, 11*, 13-25.

Deeter, T. E. (1990). Re-modeling expectancy and value in physical activity. *Journal of Sport & Exercise Psychology, 12*, 86-91.

*Gill, D. L. (1986). Competitiveness among females and males in physical activity classes. *Sex Roles, 15*, 233-247.

*Gill, D. L. (1988). Gender differences in competitive orientation and sport participation. *International Journal of Sport Psychology, 19*, 145-159.

*Gill, D. L. (1993). Competitiveness and competitive orientation in sport. InR. N. Singer, M. Murphey, & L. K. Tennant (Eds.), *Handbook of research on sport psychology* (pp. 314-327). New York: MacMillan Publishing Company.

Gill, D. L., & Dzewaltowski, D. A. (1988). Competitive orientations among intercollegiate athletes: Is winning the only thing? *The Sport Psychologist, 2*, 212-221.

*Gill, D. L., Dzewaltowski, D. A., & Deeter, T. E. (1988). The relationship of competitiveness and achievement orientation to participation in sport and nonsport activities.

Journal of Sport & Exercise Psychology, 10, 139-150.

*Gill, D. L., Kelley, B. C., Martin, J. J., & Caruso, C. M. (1991). A comparison of competitive-orientation measures. *Journal of Sport & Exercise Psychology, 13,* 266-280.

*Hayashi, C. T., & Weiss, M. R. (1991). A cross-cultural analysis of achievement motivation in Anglo-American and Japanese marathon runners. *International Journal of Sport Psychology, 25,* 187-202.

*Huddleston, S., & Garvin, G. W. (1995). Self-evaluation compared to coaches' evaluation of athletes' competitive orientation. *Journal of Sport Behavior, 18,* 209-214.

*Jones, G., & Swain, A. (1992). Intensity and direction as dimensions of competitive state anxiety and relationships with competitiveness. *Perceptual and Motor Skills, 74,* 467-472.

*Kang, L., Gill, D. L. Acevedo, E. O, & Deeter, T. E. (1990). Competitive orientations among athletes and nonathletes in Taiwan. *International Journal of Sport Psychology, 21,* 146-157.

*Lerner, B. S., & Locke, E. A. (1995). The effects of goal setting, self-efficacy, competition, and personal traits on the performance of an endurance task. *Journal of Sport & Exercise Psychology, 17,* 138-152.

*Marsh, H. W. (1993). Sport motivation orientations: Beware of jingle-jangle fallacies. *Journal of Sport & Exercise Psychology, 16,* 365-380.

*Martin, J. J., Eklund, R. C., & Smith, A. L. (1994). The relationships among competitiveness, age and ability in distance runners. *Journal of Sport Behavior, 17,* 258-268.

*Martin J. L., & Gill, D. L. (1995). The relationships of competitive orientations and self-efficacy to goal importance, thoughts, and performance in high school distance runners. *Journal of Applied Sport Psychology, 7,* 50-62.

Masters, K. S., Ogles, B. M., & Jolton, J. A. (1993). The development of an instrument to measure motivation for marathon runners: The Motivations of Marathoners Scales (MOMS). *Research Quarterly for Exercise and Sport, 64,* 134-143.

*Prapavessis. H., & Grove, J. R. (1994). Personality variables as antecedents of precompetitive mood states. *International Journal of Sport Psychology, 25,* 81-99.

Reeve, T. G., Kobayashi, M., & Eklund, R. C. (1994). Gender-role and competitiveness of female athletes [Abstract]. *Journal of Sports Sciences, 12,* 207.

*Swain, A., & Jones, G. (1991). Relationship between sport achievement orientation and competitive state anxiety. *The Sport Psychologist, 6,* 42-54.

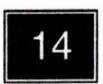

Sports Achievement Motivation Test [SAMT]

M. L. Kamlesh

Source: Kamlesh, M. L. (1990). Construction and standardization of Sports Achievement Motivation Test. *NIS Scientific Journal, 13*(3), 28-39.

Purpose: To differentiate high from low achievers in sport and to identify factors and conditions of high achievement motivation.

*This test summary was prepared by the test author (M. L. Kamlesh, personal communication, April 13, 1996).

Description: The SAMT contains 20 items. For example, participants respond to the item "I feel that winning in sports is (a) something to be proud of, or (b) everything for me" using a 2-point dichotomous scale. All items focus on the individual's desire to achieve higher in sport.

Construction: The theoretical framework for the SAMT items was derived from Murray et al. (1938), McClelland et al. (1953), Singer (1984), and Lazarevic and Bacanac (1985). Initially, 25 items with bipolar endings were developed that centered on such factors as "sports for health, perfecting skills, participation in sports seriously, individual effort, intention for high achievement" (p. 30). These items were evaluated by numerous experts in psychology and sport education before the final version of the SAMT was prepared.

Reliability: A test-retest reliability coefficient of .70 ($N = 79$) was reported.

Validity: Convergent validity was supported in that there was a positive relationship (.55) between actual sports achievement and responses to the SAMT.

Norms: Descriptive data were reported for 73 male and 48 female athletes, ages 19 27 years, from the Punjab Government College of Physical Education, Patiala. Additional data were collected among 53 male and 33 female athletes attending Yadevindra Public School, Patiala, India.

**Availability: Contact M. L. Kamlesh, Lakshmibai National College of Physical Education, Kariavattom P. O., P. O. Box 3, Trivandrum (Kerala) 695581, India. [Phone # (09) 0471-418712, 418722, FAX # 418769]

References

Lazarevic, L. J., & Bacanac, L. J. (1985). Relationship between achievement motive and personality traits [Abstract]. *Proceedings of the VI World Congress in Sport Psychology, 55.*

McClelland, D. C., et al. (1953). *The achievement motive.* New York: Appleton Century Crofts.

Murray,, H. A., et al. (1938). *Explorations in personality.* New York: Oxford University Press.

Singer, R. N. (1984). *Sustaining motivation in sport.* Tallahassee, FL: Sport Consultants International, Inc.

15 Sports Attitudes Inventory [SAI]
Joe D. Willis

Source: Willis, J. D. (1982). Three scales to measure competition-related motives in sport. *Journal of Sport Psychology, 4,* 338-353.

Purpose: To assess constructs related to sport competitiveness including the motives to approach success or avoid failure and the power motive.

Description: The SAI contains 40 items and three scales: Power motive (Pow), motive to achieve success (MAS), and motive to avoid failure (MAF). Participants respond to each item using a 5-point Likert scale.

Construction: Based on a review of the theoretical and empirical literature on achievement motivation and power, an initial pool of 140 items was developed. A factor analysis of the responses of 256 high school athletes (in three sports), plus the evaluation of the content validity by three experts (one professor and two graduate students in educational psychology), led to the retention of 40 items.

Reliability: Alpha reliability coefficients (n=764 male and 253 female athletes) reported were .76 (Pow), .78 (MAS), and .76 (MAF). Test-retest reliability coefficients across 8 weeks, using an independent sample of 46 participants, were .75 (Pow), .69 (MAS), and .71 (MAF).

Validity: Convergent validity was supported in that athletes' (n=158) scores on MAF correlated .65 with their responses to the Sport Competition Anxiety Test. Furthermore, participants' (n=191) scores on MAS correlated .23 with their scores on the Mehrabian Need for Achievement Scale, and their scores on the Pow scale correlated .22 with the Dominance scale of the California Psychological Inventory.

Discriminant function analysis indicated that the SAI could discriminate between athletes (n=463) rated as either good or poor competitors by coaches with a 71% correct classification. Furthermore, the correlation coefficients of participants' (n=132 high school students) scores on the three scales with their scores on the Crowne-Marlowe Social Desirability Scale were not statistically significant.

Norms: Normative data were presented for 764 male and 253 female athletes representing 17 sports at 22 high schools or colleges. Data were presented by gender and sport group.

Availability: Contact Joe D. Willis, Professor Emeritus, Department of Health, Physical Education, Recreation, and Dance, Georgia State University, Atlanta, GA 30303. (Phone # 404-651-2536).

References

*Bourgeois, A. E., Friend, J., & LeUnes, A. (1988). The identification of moderator variables that enhance the predictive utility of personality measures in sport research [Abstract]. *Proceedings of the Association for the Advancement of Applied Sport Psychology annual convention,* Nashua, NH.

Burkett, S., LeUnes, A., Bourgeois, T., Driggars-Bourgeois, T. (1995). Psychological predictors of intramural sports participation [Abstract]. *Journal of Applied Sport Psychology, 7* (Suppl.), S46.

Grove, J. R., Hanrahan, S. J., & Stewart, R. M. L. (1990). Attributions for rapid or slow recovery from sports injuries. *Canadian Journal of Sport Sciences, 15,* 107-114.

*Judice, T. N., Bourgeois, A., LeUnes, A., Friend, J., & Elledge, J. (1990). The relationship of the Willis Sports Attitudes Inventory and response style assessment to selected sport psychology measures [Abstract]. *Proceedings of the Association for the Advancement of Applied Sport Psychology annual convention* (p. 61). San Antonio, TX.

*Prapavessis, H., & Grove, J. R. (1994). Personality variables as antecedents of precompetitive mood states. *International Journal of Sport Psychology, 25,* 81-99.

*Willis, J. D., & Layne, B. H. (1988). A validation study of sport-related motives scales. *Journal of Applied Research in Coaching and Athletics, 3,* 299-307.

16 Sports Competition Trait Inventory (SCTI)
Lou Fabian and Marilyn Ross

Source: Fabian, L., & Ross, M. (1984). The development of the Sport Competition Trait Inventory. *Journal of Sport Behavior, 7,* 13-27.

Purpose: To assess the trait of competitiveness as expressed in sport.

Description: The SCTI contains 17 items. Examples of items include "I strive for supremacy in sports," and "I have a strong desire to be a success in sports." Participants respond to each item using a 7-point Likert scale, with the anchorings *hardly ever* to *almost always.*

Construction: Based on a literature review of competitiveness, 86 items were developed. These items were reviewed by three colleagues, which led to the retention of 76 items. These items were evaluated by six experts in the field of competition for content validity, resulting in the retention of 36 items. An item analysis of the responses of 104 high school students and 141 college students resulted in the final pool of 17 items.

Reliability: An alpha reliability coefficient of .96 was reported ($n=389$ high school and college students).

Validity: A discriminant function analysis resulted in a correct classification of 70.73% in differentiating varsity athletes from nonvarsity athletes ($n=389$). Also, the SCTI was successful in discriminating among swimmers of varying abilities. However, the correlation coefficient between the SCTI and the Sport Competition Anxiety Test was not statistically significant.

Norms: Not cited. Psychometric data were presented for 389 high school and college students.

**Availability: Contact Lou Fabian, Department of Health, Physical Education, and Recreation, 149 Trees Hall, University of Pittsburgh, Pittsburgh, PA 15261. (Phone # 412-648-8276; FAX # 412-648-7092; E-mail: fabian@fs1.sched.pitt.edu)

Reference
Fabian, L., Ross, M., & Hardwick, B. (1980). The human competitive process in intramurals and recreation. *National Intramural-Recreational Sports Association Journal, 4*(3), 46-50.

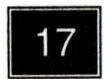 **17** # Task and Ego Orientation in Sport Questionnaire (TEOSQ)
Joan L. Duda and John G. Nicholls

Source: Duda, J. L. (1989). Relationship between task and ego orientation and the perceived purpose of sport among high school athletes. *Journal of Sport & Exercise Psychology, 11,* 318-335.

Purpose: To assess task versus ego orientation within a sport context.

Task orientation refers to individuals whose perceived ability is self-referenced and based on personal improvement task mastery. Individuals high on ego orientation perceive their ability in reference to others; subjective success means being better relative to other individuals competing in that sport.

Description: Participants are asked to think when they felt most successful in their sport and to respond to 13 items indicative of task or ego orientation. For example, responding to the item "I feel most successful in sport when I work really hard" is indicative of Task orientation, whereas responding to the item "I feel most successful in sport when I'm the best" is indicative of Ego orientation. Responses are evaluated based on a 5-point Likert scale with the anchorings *strongly agree* to *strongly disagree*.

Construction: The TEOSQ is a modified, sport-specific version of an inventory developed by Nicholls (1989) and his colleagues to assess task and ego orientation in an academic classroom environment.

Reliability: Alpha internal consistency coefficients were .82 (Task orientation) and .89 (Ego orientation) among 123 female and male high school varsity basketball athletes. Among 198 high school varsity athletes participating in other sports, alpha coefficients of .62 and .85 were reported for the Task and Ego orientation subscales, respectively.

Validity: Principal component factor analyses ($n=321$) followed by both orthogonal and oblique rotations indicated that task and ego orientations emerged as stable factors, supporting the construct validity of the TEOSQ. The concurrent validity of the TEOSQ was supported in that participants' ($n=321$) responses to the Task orientation subscale were correlated with their responses to a Purpose of Sport Questionnaire in terms of mastery/cooperation, active physical lifestyle, good citizen, and enhanced self-esteem. In contrast, their responses to the Ego orientation subscale were positively correlated with the competitiveness, high status career, enhance self-esteem, and social status/getting ahead subscales of the Purpose of Sport Questionnaire.

Norms: Not cited. Psychometric data were cited for 128 male and 193 female varsity interscholastic athlete participants representing six high schools in a midwestern community.

**Availability: Contact Joan L. Duda, Department of Health, Kinesiology, and Leisure Studies, Purdue University, Lambert 113, W. Lafayette, IN 47907. (Phone # 317-494-3172; FAX 317-496-1239; E-mail: lynne@vm.cc.purdue.edu)

References

*Andree, K. V., & Whitehead. J. (1995, June). *The interactive effect of perceived ability and dispositional or situational achievement goals on intrinsic motivation in young athletes*. Paper presented at the annual meeting of the North American Society for the Psychology of Sport and Physical Activity, Pacific Grove, CA.

Berger, B. G., Butki, B. D., & Berwind, J. S. (1995). Goal orientation and participation motivation for exercisers and for competitive sport participants [Abstract]. *Journal of Applied Sport Psychology, 7* (Suppl.), S40.

*Berlant, A. R., & Weiss, M. R. (1995). Modeling and motivational orientation: An integrated approach to motor skill learning [Abstract]. *Journal of Sport & Exercise Psychology, 17* (Suppl.), S27.

*Biddle, S., Aklande, A., Vlachopoulos, S., & Fox, K. (1995). Achievement goal orientations and beliefs about sport success: Cross-cultural validation of findings [Abstract]. *Journal of Sports Sciences, 13,* 48-49.

*Boone, K., Kuhlman, J., & Beitel, P. (1995). Goal orientation and its influence on cohesion [Abstract]. *Journal of Sport & Exercise Psychology, 17* (Suppl.), S29.

*Boyd, M., & Callaghan, J. (1994). Task and ego goal perspectives in organized youth sport. *International Journal of Sport Psychology, 25,* 411-424.

*Boyd, M., & Yin, Z. (1991). Ego-involvement and low competence in sport as a source of competitive trait anxiety [Abstract]. *Proceedings of the North American Society for the Psychology of Sport and Physical Activity annual convention* (p. 138). Pacific Grove, CA.

Boyd, M., Yin, Z., & Callaghan, J. (1992). Cognitive-affective predictors of sport enjoyment in adolescents [Abstract]. *Proceedings of the North American Society for the Psychology of Sport and Physical Activity annual convention* (p. 136). Pittsburgh, PA.

*Chi, L. & Duda, J. L. (1992). Confirmatory factor analysis of the Task and Ego Orientation in Sport Questionnaire [Abstract]. *Proceedings of the North American Society for the Psychology of Sport and Physical Activity annual convention* (p. 144). Pittsburgh, PA.

*Chi, L., & Duda, J. L. (1994). The effect of goal orientations on achievement-related behaviors in the physical domain [Abstract]. *Journal of Sport & Exercise Psychology, 16* (Suppl.), S23.

*Chi, L., & Duda, J. L. (1995). Multi-sample confirmatory factor analysis of the Task and Ego Orientation in Sport Questionnaire. *Research Quarterly for Exercise and Sport, 66*(2), 91-98.

*Chi, L., & Lin, H-H. (1995). The predictions of physical self-concept among youth dancers [Abstract]. *Journal of Sport & Exercise Psychology, 17* (Suppl.), S40.

*Damm, S. G., & Ashford, B. (1994). Physical self-perceptions and goal orientations in British schoolchildren aged 13-14 years: Gender and ability differences [Abstract]. *Journal of Sports Sciences, 12,* 188.

*Dempsey, J. M., Kimiecik, J. C., & Horn, T. S. (1993). Parental influence on children's moderate to vigorous physical activity participation: An expectancy-value approach. *Pediatric Exercise Science, 5,* 151-167.

*Duda, J. L. (1992). Motivation in sport settings: A goal perspective analysis. In G. Roberts (Ed.), *Motivation in sport and exercise* (pp. 57-91). Champaign, IL: Human Kinetics Publishers.

*Duda, J. L., Chi, L., Newton, M. L., Walling, M. D., & Catley, D. (1995). Task and ego orientation and intrinsic motivation in sport. *International Journal of Sport Psychology, 26,* 40-63.

Duda, J. L., Fox, K. R., Biddle, S. J. H., & Armstrong, N. (1992). Children's achievement goals and beliefs about success in sport. *British Journal of Educational Psychology, 62,* 313-323.

*Duda, J. L., & Hom, H. L. (1991). The interrelationships between children's and parent's goal orientations sport. *Pediatric Exercise Science, 5,* 234-241.

*Duda, J. L., & Huston, L. (1995). The relationship of goal orientation and degree of competitive sport participation to the endorsement of aggressive acts in American football. *In Integrating laboratory and field studies in sport psychology: Proceedings of the IXth European Congress on Sport Psychology.* Brussels, Belgium.

*Duda, J. L., & Nicholls, J. G. (1992). Dimensions of achievement motivation in schoolwork and sport. *Journal of Educational Psychology, 84,* 290-299.

*Duda, J. L., & Nicholls, J. G. (1993). The relationship of goal orientations to beliefs about success, perceived ability, and satisfaction in sport. In J. R. Nitsch and R. Seiler (Eds.), *Motivation, Emotion, Stress* (pp. 43-47). Proceedings of the VIII European Congress of Sport Psychology (Volume 1). Sankt Augustin, Germany: Academia Verlag.

*Duda, J. L., Olson, L. K., & Templin, T. J. (1991). The relationship of task and ego orientation to sportsmanship attitudes and the perceived legitimacy of injurious acts. *Research Quarterly for Exercise and Sport, 62,* 79-87.

*Duda, J. L., & White, S. A. (1992). Goal orientations and beliefs about the causes of sport success among elite skiers. *The Sport Psychologist, 6,* 334-343.

Ebbeck, V. (1994). Self-perception and motivational characteristics of tennis participants: The influence of age and skill. *Journal of Applied Sport Psychology, 6,* 71-86.

*Ebbeck, V., & Becker, S. L. (1994). Psychosocial predictors of goal orientations in youth soccer. *Research Quarterly for Exercise and Sport, 65,* 355-362.

*Goudas, M., & Biddle, S. (1993). Intrinsic motivation after fitness testing is affected by achievement goal orientations. *Proceedings of the Eighth World Congress of Sport Psychology* (pp. 788-791). Lisbon, Portugal.

*Goudas, M., Biddle, S., & Fox, K. (1994). Achievement goal orientations and intrinsic motivation in physical fitness testing with children. *Pediatric Exercise Science, 6,* 159-167.

*Goudas, M., Biddle, S., & Fox, K. (1994). Perceived locus of causality, goal orientations, and perceived competence in school physical education classes. *British Journal of Educational Psychology, 64,* 453-463.

*Goudas, M., Biddle, S., Fox, K., & Underwood, M. (1995). It ain't what you do, it's the way you do it! Teaching style affects children's motivation in track and field lessons. *The Sport Psychologist, 9,* 254-264.

*Goudas, M., Biddle, S., & Underwood, M. (1995). A prospective study of the relationships between motivational orientations and perceived competence with intrinsic motivation and achievement in a teacher education course. *Educational Psychology, 15,* 89-96.

*Grieve, F. G., Whelan, J. P., Kottke, R., & Meyers, A. W. (1994). Manipulating adults' achievement goals in a sport task: Effects on cognitive, affective and behavioral variables. *Journal of Sport Behavior, 17,* 227-245.

*Guest, S. M., & White, S. A. (1995). The role of goal orientations and beliefs about the causes of success in predicting gender and level of sport involvement in sport participants [Abstract]. *Journal of Applied Sport Psychology, 7* (Suppl.), S67.

*Guivernau, M., & Duda, J. L. (1995). The generality of goals, beliefs, interest and perceived ability across sport and school: The case of Spanish student athletes [Abstract]. *Journal of Sport & Exercise Psychology, 17* (Suppl.), S6.

*Guivernau, M., & Duda, J. L. (1995). Psychometric properties of a Spanish version of the Task and Ego Orientation in Sport Questionnaire (TEOSQ) and Beliefs about the Causes of Success Inventory. *Revista de Psicologia del Deporte, 5,* 31-51.

*Hall, H. K., & Earles, M. (1995). Motivational determinants of interest, and perceptions of success in school physical education [Abstract]. *Journal of Sport & Exercise Psychology, 17* (Suppl.), S57.

*Hall, H. K., & Finnie, S. (1995). Goals and perfectionism as antecedents of exercise addiction [Abstract]. *Journal of Sport & Exercise Psychology, 17* (Suppl.), S7.

*Harwood, C. G., & Swain, A. B. J. (1995). Antecedents of state goals in age group swimmers: An interactionist perspective [Abstract]. *Journal of Sports Sciences, 13,* 58-59.

*Hayashi, C. T., & Weiss, M. R. (1991). A cross-cultural analysis of achievement motivation in Anglo-American and Japanese marathon runners. *International Journal of Sport Psychology, 25,* 187-202.

*Hom, H., Duda, J. L., & Miller, A. (1993). Correlates of goal orientations among young athletes. *Pediatric Exercise Science, 5,* 168-176.

*James, D. W. G., & Fox, K. R. (1995). Goal profiles, beliefs and competitive cognitions among an elite bowls squad [Abstract]. *Journal of Sports Sciences, 13,* 60-61.

Kelly, S., & Duda, J. L. (1995). The motivation-related correlates of goal orientations in sport: An idiographic analysis [Abstract]. *Journal of Sport & Exercise Psychology, 17* (Suppl.), S6.

*Kim, B. J. (1995). Psychometric evaluation of the TEOSQ and the IMI in a Korean sport setting [Abstract]. *Journal of Sport & Exercise Psychology, 17* (Suppl.), S66.

*Kim, B. J., & Gill, D. L. (1995). Psychological correlates of achievement goal orientation in Korean youth sport [Abstract]. *Journal of Applied Sport Psychology, 7* (Suppl.), S80.

*Li, F., Chi, L., Harmer, P., & Vongjaturapat, N. (1994). The Task and Ego Orientation in Sport Questionnaire: Factorial validity across United States, Thailand, and Taiwan samples [Abstract]. *Journal of Sport & Exercise Psychology, 16* (Suppl.), S79.

*Li, F., & Harmer, P. (1993). Individual goal orientation in sport: Testing the assumption of equivalent structure across gender [Abstract]. *Research Quarterly for Exercise and Sport 64* (Suppl.), A-70-71.

*Li, F., Vongjaturapat, N., & Harmer, P. (1994). Confirmatory factor analysis of the TEOSQ: Thai version for males and female intercollegiate athletes [Abstract]. *Research Quarterly for Exercise and Sport, 65* (Suppl.), A-58.

*Li, F., Vongjaturapat, N., & Harmer, P. (1995). Confirmatory factor analysis models of factorial invariance: An examination of the Task and Ego Orientation in Sport Questionnaire in a cross-cultural setting [Abstract]. *Journal of Sport & Exercise Psychology, 17* (Suppl.), S72.

*Lloyd, J., & Fox, K. R. (1992). Achievement goals and motivation to exercise in adolescent girls: A preliminary study. *British Journal of Physical Education Research Supplement, 11,* 12-16.

*McCullagh, P., & Noble, J. (1994). Observational learning: Motivational and gender considerations [Abstract]. *Journal of Sport & Exercise Psychology, 16* (Suppl.), S87.

*Mills, B. D. (1995). Examining the relationship between trait sport confidence, goal orientation and competitive experience in female collegiate volleyball players [Abstract]. *Journal of Sport & Exercise Psychology, 17* (Suppl.), S81.

*Mitchell, S. A., & Chandler, T. J. L. (1993). Relationships between achievement orientation, perceived ability, perceptions of learning environment and intrinsic motivation in middle school physical education [Abstract]. *Research Quarterly for Exercise and Sport, 64* (Suppl.), A-91.

*Newton, M., & Duda, J. L. (1993). Elite adolescent athletes' achievement goals and beliefs concerning tennis. *Journal of Sport & Exercise Psychology, 15,* 437-448.

*Newton, M. L., & Walling, M. D. (1995). Goal orientations and beliefs about the causes of success among Senior Olympic Games participants [Abstract]. *Journal of Sport & Exercise Psychology, 17* (Suppl.), S81.

Nicholls, J. G. (1989). *The competitive ethos and democratic education.* Cambridge, MA: Harvard University Press.

*Papaioannou, A., & Macdonald, A. I. (1993). Goal perspectives and purposes of physical education as perceived by Greek adolescents. *Physical Education Review, 16,* 41-48.

*Pease, D. G., & Kozub, S. A. (1994). Role of goal orientations in athlete leadership behavior [Abstract]. *Research Quarterly for Exercise and Sport, 65* (Suppl.), A-90.

*Rethorst, S., & Duda, J. L. (1993). Goal orientations, cognitions, and emotions in gymnastics. *Proceedings of the Eighth World Congress of Sport Psychology* (pp. 379-382), Lisbon, Portugal.

Seifriz, J. J., Duda, J. L. , & Chi, L. (1992). The relationship of perceived motivational climate to intrinsic motivation and beliefs about success in basketball. *Journal of Sport & Exercise Psychology, 14,* 375-391.

*Swain, A. B. J., & Rankin, P. (1994). Achievement goal orientations and their impact on the social loafing phenomenon [Abstract]. *Journal of Sports Sciences, 12,* 211-212.

*Thorne, K., & White, S. (1993). The relationship of goal orientations to task choice among college-aged students [Abstract]. *Journal of Sport & Exercise Psychology, 15* (Suppl.), S83.

Vlachopoulos, S., & Biddle, S. (1995). Attributions and goal orientations as predictors of feelings, expectancy and intrinsic motivation after fitness testing with children [Abstract]. *Journal of Sports Science, 13,* 79.

*Vongjaturapt, N., Li, F., & Harmer, P. A. (1995). A confirmatory investigation of the dimensionality of the Task and Ego Orientation in Sport Questionnaire in a Thai college student sample with cross-validation [Abstract]. *Research Quarterly for Exercise and Sport, 66* (Suppl.), A-50.

*Walling, M. D., Catley, D., & Taylor, A. (1991). The interrelationships between goal perspectives, perceived competence, and indices of intrinsic motivation [Abstract]. *Proceedings of the North American Society for the Psychology of Sport and Physical Activity annual convention* (p. 201). Pacific Grove, CA.

*Walling, M. D., & Duda, J. L. (1995). Goals and their associations with beliefs about success in and perceptions of the purposes of physical education. *Journal of Teaching in Physical Education, 14,* 140-156.

Walling, M., Duda, J. L., Newton, M., & White, S. (1993). Task and Ego Orientation in Sport Questionnaire: Further analysis with youth sport participants [Abstract]. *Proceedings of the Association for the Advancement of Applied Sport Psychology annual convention* (p. 153). Montreal, Canada.

*White, S. A., & Duda, J. L. (1993). Dimensions of goals-beliefs about success among disabled athletes. *Adapted Physical Activity Quarterly, 10,* 125-136.

*White, S. A., & Duda, J. L. (1994). The relationship of gender, level of sport involvement, and participation motivation to Task and Ego Orientation. *International Journal of Sport Psychology, 25,* 4-18.

*White, S. A., Johnson, L. A., & Morgan, J. Q. (1995). Dimensions of goals and sport commitment among female volleyball players [Abstract]. *Journal of Applied Sport Psychology, 7* (Suppl.), S124.

*Williams, L. (1994). Goal orientations and athletes' preferences for competence information sources. *Journal of Sport & Exercise Psychology, 16,* 416-430.

*Williams, L., & Gill, D. L. (1995). The role of perceived competence in the motivation of physical activity. *Journal of Sport & Exercise Psychology, 17,* 363-378.

*Williams, L., Kim, B. J., & Gill, D. L. (1995). A cross-cultural study of achievement orientation and intrinsic motivation in young American and Korean athletes [Abstract]. *Journal of Sport & Exercise Psychology, 17* (Suppl.), S108.

Xiang, P., & Lee, A. (1995). Interaction of feedback and achievement goal during motor skill learning [Abstract]. *Research Quarterly for Exercise and Sport, 66* (Supplement), A72-73.

*Yin, Z. (1993). Influence of socializing agents, achievement goal orientation, and perceived competence as sources of sport enjoyment [Abstract]. *Research Quarterly for Exercise and Sport, 64* (Suppl.), A-105-106.

Yin, Z., Boyd, M., & Callaghan, J. (1991). Patterns between task/ego goal orientations and their cognitive/affective correlates in high school athletes [Abstract]. *Proceedings of the Association for the Advancement of Applied Sport Psychology annual convention* (p. 169). Savannah, GA.

*Yin, Z., Boyd, M., & Callaghan, J. (1992). Canonical analysis of goal orientation and its related variables [Abstract]. *Proceedings of the North American Society for the Psychology of Sport and Physical Activity annual convention* (p. 195). Pittsburgh, PA.

18 Will to Win Questionnaire [WW]
Vera Pezer and Marvin Brown

Source: Pezer, V., & Brown, M. (1980). Will to win and athletic performance. *International Journal of Sport Psychology, 11,* 121-131.

Purpose: To measure the desire to defeat an opponent or to exceed some performance standard in sport.

Description: The questionnaire contains 14 items to which participants respond in a true-false format.

Construction: A total of 34 items were selected from five personality tests. Items selected were reflective of the importance of winning, winning in relation to other reasons for competing, and personal feelings stemming from winning or losing. Fourteen additional items were created by the authors. Respondents ($n=254$ undergraduate students) answered these 48 items using a true-false format. Based on item and factor analyses, and an evaluation of the social desirability of each item using an independent sample of 62 physical education students, 25 items were retained. Additional item and factor analyses on data collected among another sample of 39 physical education undergraduate students and two samples of female curlers ($n=61$; $n=68$) led to a final 14-item version.

Reliability: A Kuder-Richardson-20 internal consistency coefficient of .66 was reported among 216 female curlers. A test-retest reliability coefficient of .87 was reported among a subsample of 47 female curlers across a 4-month interval.

Validity: A correlation coefficient of .78 was reported between female basketball players' ($n=10$) WW scores and their coaches' assessment of their will to win. Using an additional sample of 10 female basketball players, a correlation coefficient of .72 was reported between their WW scores and their teammates' and their own evaluations of their will to win. Similarly, a correlation coefficient of .72 was reported between female curlers' ($n=24$) WW scores and their teammates' ratings of their will to win. Thus, there was evidence supporting the concurrent validity of the WW scale.

Norms: Not cited. Psychometric data were reported for 248 Canadian female curlers and 20 female basketball players.

**Availability: Contact Vera Pezer, Student Affairs and Services, 60 Place Riel Campus Centre, University of Saskatchewan, 1 Campus Drive, Saskatoon, Saskatchewan, Canada S7N 5A3. (Phone # 306-966-4747; FAX # 306-966-5081; E-mail: pezer@admin.usask.ca)

References

Daino, A. (1985). Personality traits of adolescent tennis players. *International Journal of Sport Psychology, 16,* 120-125.

*Dorsey, B., Lawson, P., & Pezer, V. (1980). The relationship between women's basketball performance and will to win. *Canadian Journal of Applied Sport Sciences, 5,* 91-93.

*Hoffman, A. J. (1986). Competitive sport and the American athlete: How much is too much? *International Journal of Sport Psychology, 17,* 390-397.

*Woloschuk, W. (1986). Further evidence of a relationship between will to win and basketball performance. *Perceptual and Motor Skills, 62,* 253-254.

Chapter 2

Aggression

Tests in this chapter measure the aggressive tendencies of sport participants in terms of instrumental and reactive aggression, physical and nonphysical aggression, and perceptions among players and spectators of the legitimacy of aggressive behavior.

19 Aggressive Tendencies in Basketball Questionnaire [ATBQ]

Joan L. Duda, Linda K. Olson, and Thomas J. Templin

Source: Duda, J. L., Olson, L. K., & Templin, T. J. (1991). The relationship of task and ego orientation to sportsmanship attitudes and the perceived legitimacy of injurious acts. *Research Quarterly for Exercise and Sport, 62*, 79-87.

Purpose: To assess an individual's agreement with and reasoning about aggressive behaviors in basketball.

Description: The ATBQ contains six written scenarios depicting aggressive acts in basketball with intended consequences that become increasingly more serious. These consequences (in order of severity) include nonphysical intimidation, physical intimidation, miss a few minutes, miss the rest of the game, miss the rest of the season, and permanently disable an opponent. The scenarios are presented in random order with the participant being asked to indicate for each scenario whether this is legitimate to do and whether this is legitimate to do in order to win. Participants respond using a 5-point Likert scale with the anchorings *strongly disapprove* to *strongly approve*.

Construction: The ATBQ is a basketball-specific version of Bredemeier's (1985) Continuum of Injurious Sport Acts. Four experts developed the scenarios as typical examples of each type of injurious act within the context of interscholastic basketball.

Reliability: Not reported.

Validity: Discriminant validity was supported in that male high school basketball players (*n*=56) perceived the depicted intentionally injurious acts to be more legitimate than did female high school basketball players. This was true for each scenario except when the injured player would be permanently disabled.

Norms: Not cited. Psychometric data were reported for 56 male and 67 female interscholastic basketball players representing five high schools in a midwestern community.

Availability: Contact Joan L. Duda, Department of Physical Education, Health, and Recreation Studies, 113 Lambert Hall, Purdue University, West Lafayette, IN 47907. (Phone # 317-494-3172; FAX # 317-496-1239; E-mail: lynne@vm.cc.purdue.edu)

Reference

Bredemeier, B. (1985). Moral reasoning and the perceived legitimacy of intentionally injurious sport acts. *Journal of Sport Psychology, 7,* 110-124.

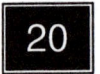 **20**

Bredemeier Athletic Aggression Inventory (BAAGI)

Brenda Bredemeier

Source: Bredemeier, B. (1975). The assessment of reactive and instrumental athletic aggression. In D. M. Landers (Ed.), *Psychology of sport and motor behavior-II* (pp. 71-83). State College, PA: Penn State HPER series.

Purpose: To assess reactive and instrumental athletic aggression.

Description: The BAAGI contains two 50-item scales measuring reactive and instrumental aggression, respectively. A reactive aggression response has as its primary goal the infliction of injury, whereas in instrumental aggression, the primary goal is the attainment of a particular reward. Participants respond to each item using a 4-point Likert scale.

Construction: Item development was guided by the need for clarity, an emphasis on athletic rather than pathological aggression, adaptability to different sport areas, the need for an item to tap different intensities of the same act or emotion, and minimization of social desirability contamination. A pilot instrument of 149 items was administered to 104 male and female high school and college students; in addition, six judges evaluated content validity. Subsequent item refinement plus the addition of items from existing scales such as the Buss Durkee Hostility Scale led to construction of a questionnaire containing 200 items. These items were administered to 166 female athletes in conjunction with the Buss Durkee Hostility Scale and the Crowne-Marlowe Social Desirability Scale. Further item analyses led to the retention of 50 reactive and 50 instrumental items.

Reliability: Alpha reliability coefficients of .90 (reactive aggression) and .86 (instrumental aggression) were reported (n=166).

Validity: Convergent validity was supported in that participants' (n=166) scores on the BAAGI were correlated with their responses to the Buss Durkee Hostility scale. However, there was also evidence of social desirability contamination in that these participants' scores on the BAAGI correlated with their responses to the Crowne Marlowe Social Desirability Scale. Concurrent validity was also enhanced in that these participants' responses on the BAAGI were correlated with their coaches' ratings of their aggressive behavior.

Norms: Not presented. Psychometric data were cited for 166 female athletes representing six sports at 11 state colleges, universities, or private schools.

Availability: Contact Brenda Jo Light Bredemeier, Department of Human Biodynamics, 206 Hearst Gymnasium, University of California, Berkeley, CA 94720-4482. (Phone # 510-642 1704; FAX # 510-642-7241; E-mail: brenda@uclink2.berkeley.edu)

References

*Rice, T. S., Ostrow, A. C., Ramsburg, I. D., & Brooks, D. D. (1989). A reactive aggression measure for baseball: A pilot investigation [Abstract]. In *Psychology of motor behavior and sport*. Kent, OH:Proceedings of the North American Society for the Psychology of Sport and Physical Activity annual convention.

*Wall, B. R., & Gruber, J. (1986). Relevancy of athletic aggression inventory for use in women's intercollegiate basketball: A pilot test. *International Journal of Sport Psychology*, 17, 23-33. (Developed 28-item short form of the BAAGI)

Worrell, G. L., & Harris, D. J. (1986). The relationship of perceived and observed aggression of ice hockey players. *International Journal of Sport Psychology, 17*, 34-40.

21 Collis Scale of Athletic Aggression [CSAG]
Martin L. Collis

Source: Collis, M. L. (October, 1972). The Collis Scale of Athletic Aggression. *Proceedings of the Fourth Canadian Symposium on Psycho-Motor Learning and Sport Psychology* (pp. 366-370). University of Waterloo, Waterloo, Ontario, Canada.

Purpose: To assess aggression as it relates to athletic success.

Description: The CSAG contains 50 items and measures two categories of aggression: legal aggression (25 items) and extra-legal aggression (25 items). Four response alternatives are presented for each item. Each alternative is weighted on a 4-point scale, with a score of 4 on an item designating high aggression.

Construction: "The Scale has been constantly refined on the basis of item analysis of individual questions for their discriminatory characteristics..." (p. 368).

Reliability: Not presented.

Validity: Ice hockey players' (n=20) scores on extra-legal aggression correlated positively with the number of minutes of penalties they had been assessed during the previous season.

Norms: Not cited. Descriptive data were presented for 240 male athletes (ages 10 and under, 11-14, and 15-18 years) representing soccer, swimming, hockey, and gymnastics.

Availability: Contact Martin L. Collis, Faculty of Education, University of Victoria, Victoria, British Columbia, Canada V8W 3N4. (Phone # 604-721-8385; FAX # 604-721-6601; E-mail: mcollis@uvic.ca)

Reference

Reid, R. M., & Hay, D. (1979). Some behavioral characteristics of rugby and association footballers. *International Journal of Sport Psychology, 10,* 239-251.

 22

Rice Reactive Aggression Measure for Baseball (RRAMB)
Timothy S. Rice, Andrew C. Ostrow, I. Dale Ramsburg, and Dana D. Brooks

Source: Rice, T. S., Ostrow, A. C., Ramsburg, I. D., & Brooks, D. D. (1989). A reactive aggression measure for baseball: A pilot investigation [Abstract]. *Proceedings of the North American Society for the*

Psychology of Sport and Physical Activity Annual Convention. Kent, OH.

Purpose: To assess the reactive aggression tendencies of baseball players.

Description: The RRAMB contains descriptions of four potentially reactive aggression evoking situations in baseball (e. g., a close play at second base). Each of the situations contains eight statements that require a 7-point Likert format response.

Construction: A panel of three experts evaluated the content validity of the four situations and 32 response alternatives of the RRAMB. These experts concurred that 3 of the 4 situations appeared to be measuring reactive aggression, but did not agree that the situation describing the conflict between a pitcher and batter was indicative of reactive aggression. Nevertheless, this situation was still included in this initial version of the RRAMB.*

Reliability: Alpha reliability coefficients for 58 high school baseball players ranged from .51 to .94 for each situation, with a value of .83 reported for the overall RRAMB score. Among 41 college varsity baseball players, alpha reliability coefficients ranged from .98 to .99 for each situation, with an overall RRAMB alpha reliability coefficient of .98.*

Validity: Concurrent validity was established by demonstrating that among these high school and college baseball players, the RRAMB correlated more highly with the reactive aggression subscale of the Bredemeier Athletic Aggression Inventory than the instrumental aggression subscale of this inventory. Furthermore, there was evidence that players' responses to the RRAMB were correlated with their assessments of other teams' members in terms of reactive aggression, as well as with their own self-assessments on reactive aggression.

Norms: Not reported. Psychometric data are cited for 58 high school and 41 college varsity baseball players.

**Availability: Contact Timothy S. Rice, Fairmont State College, Pence Hall, Fairmont, WV 26554. (Phone # 304-367-4289; 304-366-4870)

---

*Construction procedures and reliability coefficients cited are from a master's degree thesis by the first author, available at the Evansdale library, West Virginia University, Morgantown, WV 26506.

23 Scale of Children's Action Tendencies (SCATS)

Brenda Jo Bredemeier

Source: Bredemeier, B. J. (1994). Children's moral reasoning and their assertive, aggressive, and submissive tendencies in sport and daily life. *Journal of Sport & Exercise Psychology, 16,* 1-14.

Purpose: "...to assess children's behavioral responses to conflict situations within the realm of sport" (p. 5).

Description: The SCATS contains 10 stories within a sport context. Each of the ten stories is followed by three response alternatives--one aggressive, one assertive, and one submissive--which are presented in a paired-comparison format. Thus, the SCATS contains three pairs of choices per story. Scoring the SCATS involves summing the number of times assertive, aggressive, and submissive alternatives are selected. Aggression responses are subdivided into physical and nonphysical subscales.

Construction: Pilot research was conducted in which 15 children in grades 4 through 7 were asked to identify conflict situations they had experienced while participating in sport, and they were asked to identify their behavioral responses to these conflict situations.

Reliability: Kuder-Richardson 20 formula internal consistency coefficients of .68 (Assertion), .85 (Aggression), and .66 (Submission) were reported.

Validity: Concurrent validity was supported in that there were moderate-to-high, positive correlation coefficients reported between participants' responses to the subscales of the SCATS and their corresponding responses to the Children's Action Tendency Scale (CATS). Also low, but statistically significant correlation coefficients were reported between their scores on the SCATS and teachers' behavioral ratings.

Norms: Not cited.

Availability: Contact Brenda Jo Light Bredemeier, Department of

Human Biodynamics, 206 Hearst Gymnasium, University of California, Berkeley, CA 94720-4482. (Phone # 510-642-1704; FAX # 510-642-7241; E-mail: brenda@uclink2.berkeley.edu)

Reference

*Bredemeier, B. J., Weiss, M. R., Shields, D. L., & Cooper, B. A. B. (1987). The relationship between children's legitimacy judgments and their moral reasoning, aggression tendencies, and sport involvement. *Sociology of Sport Journal, 4,* 48-60. (This is source in which SCATS was originally reported.)

 24 ## Spectator Misbehavior Attitudinal Inquiry (SMAI)

Brian Cavanaugh and John Silva III

Source: Cavanaugh, B., & Silva, J. (1980). Spectator perceptions of fan misbehavior: An attitudinal inquiry. In C. H. Nadeau, W. R. Halliwell, K. M. Newell, & G. C. Roberts (Eds.), *Psychology of motor behavior and sport-1979* (pp. 189-198). Champaign, IL.: Human Kinetics Publishers.

Purpose: To assess spectator perceptions of factors that facilitate fan misbehavior.

Description: The SMAI is a 14-factor, 28-item attitudinal questionnaire. Spectators respond to each item using a 4-point Likert scale.

Construction: The factors derived for the questionnaire evolved from various theories of collective behavior. A total of 20 items were developed and then ranked by collegiate coaches, sport psychologists, sport sociologists, and former collegiate athletes in terms of each item's importance in facilitating spectator misbehavior. A total of 14 items were retained based on their consistently high rankings.

Reliability: An intraclass correlation coefficient (n=27 undergraduate physical education students) of .79 was reported across a 5-day test-retest interval.

Validity: Construct validity was examined through factor analysis. Principal components and alpha factoring were applied to the responses to the SMAI by 241 spectators randomly selected from a total sample of 1,747 participants. Items that loaded properly on factors across both methods were retained for the final questionnaire (J. Silva, personal communication, March 19, 1990).

Norms: Normative data are provided for 1,747 spectators attending one of three hockey games in either Buffalo, Rochester, or Brockport. A total of 1,006 males and 593 females participated in the study. The gender of 147 spectators was not identified.

Availability: Contact John Silva, Department of Physical Education, CB #8700, Fetzer Gym, University of North Carolina, Chapel Hill, NC 27599-8700. (Phone # 919-962-5176; FAX # 919-962-0489; E-mail: usilva@uncmvs.oit.unc.edu)

25 Sport Aggression Questionnaire (SAQ)
Mark Thompson

Source: Thompson, M. (1989). The development of a Sport Aggression Questionnaire for the study of justification of acts of aggression [Abstract]. *Proceedings of the Association for the Advancement of Applied Sport Psychology* (p. 104). Seattle, WA.

Purpose: To assess an individual's justification of acts of aggression occurring in specified sport situations.

Description: The SAQ focuses on five primary motivators of aggression in sport: injustice to self, injustice to teammate, frustration, aiding the team, and unprovoked aggression. An additional item on "no intent to harm" is included. Each sport situation identified is considered in relation to three possible outcomes signifying the severity of an injury due to the action.

Construction: Not discussed.

Reliability: A test-retest reliability coefficient ($n=32$ college males) of .84 was reported across a one-week interval.

Validity: Construct validity was supported in that male high school varsity basketball players (*n*=24) rated as high or low in aggression by their coaches were correspondingly high or low on aggression as measured by the SAQ. Players high on aggression as assessed by their coaches were more likely to justify actions of aggression in sport than were players rated as low on aggression.

Norms: Not presented. Psychometric data were based on the responses of 32 male college students and 24 male high school varsity basketball players.

Availability: Contact Mark A. Thompson, ESHS Dept., P. O. Box 19259, University of Texas, Arlington, TX 76019-0259. (Phone 817-273-3128; E-mail: mthompsn@utarlg.uta.edu)

References

*Thompson, M. A. (1991). Situation: An integral factor in the justification of sport aggression by NCAA Division I-A varsity basketball players [Abstract]. *Proceedings of the Association for the Advancement of Applied Sport Psychology annual convention* (p. 149). Savannah, GA.

Thompson, M. A. (1993). Gender and aggression in sport: A stereotype is challenged [Abstract]. *Proceedings of the Association for the Advancement of Applied Sport Psychology annual convention* (p. 147). Montreal, Canada.

Thompson, M. A., & Cook, D. L. (1992). Injury severity as a factor in the justification of sport aggression by NCAA Division I-A varsity basketball players [Abstract]. *Proceedings of the Association for the Advancement of Applied Sport Psychology annual convention* (p. 111). Colorado Springs, CO.

Chapter 3

Anxiety

Tests in this chapter measure anxiousness among sport participants in terms of cognitive and somatic trait and state anxiety, worry cognitions, and concerns regarding concentration disruption, social evaluation, and fear of injury. Coping strategies for dealing with anxiety are examined. Athlete burnout and sources of stress experienced by youth sport participants, officials, coaches, and cheerleaders are also assessed.

26 *Anxiety Rating Scale (ARS)
Richard H. Cox, William D. Russell, and Marshall Robb

Source: Cox, R. H., Russell, W. D., & Robb, M. (1996). Validity of the MRF and ARS competitive state anxiety rating scales for volleyball and basketball [Abstract]. *Research Quarterly for Exercise and Sport, 67* (Suppl.), A-98.

Purpose: To provide a quick and nonintrusive assessment of competitive state anxiety.

Description: The ARS is a three-item version of the CSAI-2. It is composed of the following three statements:

1. I feel concerned about performing poorly and that others will be disappointed with my performance (cognitive state anxiety);

2. I feel nervous, my body feels tight and/or my stomach tense (somatic state anxiety);

3. I feel secure, mentally relaxed, and confident of coming through under pressure (self-confidence).

Individuals respond to each statement using a 7-point ordinal scale with the anchorings 1 (*not at all*) to 7 (*intensely so*).

Construction: Utilizing 492 college-age intramural volleyball and basketball participants, multiple stepwise regression was used to determine the best three- variable model for predicting CSAI-2 subscales. Selected item aggregates formed the basis for the three statements in the ARS.

Reliability: Not indicated.

Validity: Participants' (N=418) responses to the ARS were positively correlated with their responses to the three subscales of the CSAI-2- .60, .72, and .59 with the cognitive, somatic, and confidence subscales, respectively. Using multiple regression analyses, it was observed that their scores on the ARS were a better predictor of cognitive and somatic competitive state anxiety, as measured by the CSAI-2, than were their scores on the Mental Readiness Form.

Norms: Not cited. Psychometric data were presented for 492 male and female participants of intramural volleyball and basketball at a large midwest university. The sample means and standard deviations for the 492 participants were 2.54 (SD=1.42), 2.11 (SD=1.23), 4.79 (SD=1.58), for cognitive state anxiety, somatic state anxiety, and self-confidence, respectively.

**Availability: Contact Richard H. Cox, Deparment of Educational & Counseling Psychology, 16 Hill Hall, University of Missouri, Columbia, MO 65211. (Phone # 573-882-7602; FAX # 573-884-4855; E-mail: rhcox@showme.missouri.edu).

References
*Cox, R. H., Russell, W. D., & Robb, M. (1994, October). Field testing an instrument designed to assess competitive state anxiety during or prior to competition. *Proceedings of the annual conference of the Association for the Advancement of Applied Sport Psychology*. Lake Tahoe, NV.

*Cox, R. H., Russell, W. D., & Robb, M. (1994, October). Phase one in the development of an instrument for assessing competitive state anxiety during and prior to competition. *Proceedings of the annual conference of the Association for the Advancement of Applied Sport Psychology*. Lake Tahoe, NV.

*Cox, R. H., Russell, W. D., & Robb, M. (1995). Comparative validity of the MRF and ARS competitive state anxiety rating scales [Abstract]. *Journal of Applied Sport Psychology, 7* (Suppl.), S52.

*Cox, R. H., Russell, W. D., & Robb, M. (1995). Development of an instrument for assessing competitive state anxiety during and prior to competition. *Research Quarterly for Exercise and Sport, 66* (1) (Suppl.), Abstract A-75.

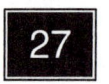

*Basketball Official's Sources of Stress Inventory (BOSSI)
Mark H. Anshel and Robert S. Weinberg

Source: Anshel, M. H., & Weinberg, R. S. (1995). Sources of acute stress in American and Australian basketball referees. *Journal of Applied Sport Psychology, 7*, 11-22.

Purpose: To assess the extent to which various sources of stress are experienced by basketball referees.

Description: The BOSSI contains 15 items (stressors). Officials are asked to rate each item from 1 (*not at all*) to 10 (*extremely*) indicating the extent to which they had experienced the stressor. Examples of stressors listed on the BOSSI include "Verbal abuse by coaches" and "Arguing with players." Respondents are also asked to provide a specific example from their officiating history to illustrate their experience with the stressor.

Construction: Items from the BOSSI were derived from (a) open-ended interviews with current ($n=8$) and former ($n=3$) American and Australian basketball officials; (b) a review of the anecdotal and research literature reporting on sources of stress among sport officials. Five former and 12 current American and Australian basketball officials helped establish the content validity of the 15 items.

Reliability: Not reported.

Validity: Discriminant function analysis indicated that American basketball officials ($N=70$) and Australian basketball officials ($N=62$) were differentiated in their responses to the BOSSI, particularly in terms of perceived stress sources such as verbal abuse by players and spectators and arguing with coaches and players.

Norms: Not cited. Psychometric data were reported for 70 American male basketball officials (M age= 32.6 years) and 62 Australian male basketball officials (M age= 29.8 years). All participants had at least 3 years of officiating experience in organized, competitive basketball

**Availabilty: Contact Mark H. Anshel, Department of Psychology, University of Wollongong, P. O. Box 1144, Wollongong, New South Wales, Australia 2522. (Phone # 61-42-213732; FAX # 61-42-214163; E-mail: m.anshel@uow.edu.au)

 [Basketball] S-R Inventory of Anxiousness(S-RSIA)
A. Craig Fisher, J. S. Horsfall, and H. H. Morris

Source: Fisher, A. C., Horsfall, J. S., & Morris, H. H. (1977). Sport personality assessment: A methodological re-examination. *International Journal of Sport Psychology, 8,* 92-102.

Purpose: To examine the relative contributions of the person and situation in accounting for anxiety responses in basketball.

Description: The S-RSIA contains 13 anxiety-eliciting situations in basketball. These situations focus on pregame, game, and postgame conditions. Participants respond to 13 response modes for each situation (such as "mouth gets dry") using a 5-point ordinal scale.

Construction: The 13 situations were reduced from a pool of 38 situations that had been developed by the investigators and a graduate sport psychology class. These basketball situations were felt to range from innocuous to potentially threatening. The modes of response were selected from Endler, Hunt, and Rosenstein's (1962) S-R Inventory of Anxiousness.

Reliability: The Cronbach alpha internal consistency coefficient ($n=106$ male college basketball players) for the total inventory was .81. The alpha coefficients for the situational scales ranged from .61 to .76, and for the modes of response from .56 to .83.

Validity: Not discussed.

Norms: Not cited. Psychometric data were based on the responses of 106 college male junior varsity and varsity basketball athletes representing nine teams in upstate New York.

**Availability: Contact A. Craig Fisher, Exercise and Sport Sciences Department, Ithaca College, Ithaca, NY 14850. (Phone # 607-274-3112; FAX # 607-274-1943; E-mail: cfisher@ithaca.edu)

References

*Dunn, J. G. H., & Nielsen, A. B. (1993). A between-sport comparison of situational threat perceptions in ice hockey and soccer. *Journal of Sport & Exercise Psychology, 15,* 449-465.

Endler, N. S., Hunt, J. M., & Rosenstein, A. J. (1962). An S-R Inventory of Anxiousness. *Psychological Monographs, 76* (17, Whole No. 536).

Fisher, A. C., & Dixon, L. R. (1985). Psychological analysis of athletes' anxiety responses: An attempt at explanation [Abstract]. *Proceedings of the annual conference of the Canadian Society of Psychomotor Learning and Sport Psychology* (pp. 52-53). Montreal, Canada.

Fisher, A. C., & Zwart, E. F. (1982). Psychological analysis of athletes' anxiety responses. *Journal of Sport Psychology, 4,* 139-158.

*Martin, J. W. (1995). A psychological analysis of levels 4.0, 4.5, and 5.0 competitive tennis players [Abstract]. *Journal of Applied Sport Psychology, 7* (Suppl.), S87.

*Burnout Inventory for Athletes (BIA)
Nico W. Van Yperen

Source: Van Yperen, N. W. (1993). *Team cohesion, parental support, burnout, and the performance level of talented young soccer players.* Paper presented at the Eighth World Congress of Sport Psychology, Lisbon, Portugal.

Purpose: To assess the extent to which soccer athletes feel burnout (i.e., feelings of energy depletion) from their sport.

Description: The BIA consists of seven items including "You do not feel like attending training" and "You considered leaving the club." Athletes respond on a 5-point ordinal scale with the anchorings 1 (*never*) to 5 (*always*).

Construction: The items of the BIA were developed based on a review of the burnout literature, particularly the work of Maslach and her colleagues (Maslach & Jackson, 1981).

Reliability: A test-retest reliability coefficient across a 7-month interval was reported to be .56. Cronbach alpha internal consistency coefficients computed at each of these two time intervals were .91. In a second study (Van Yperen, in press), a test-retest reliability coefficient of .58 was reported, and Cronbach alpha coefficients of .80 (Time 1) and .77 (Time 2) were also reported.

Validity: Concurrent validity was demonstrated by showing that scores on the BIA correlated positively with measures of psychosocial stress, including problems with coach and team manager (.39) and interpersonal stress with the team (.30), and correlated negatively (-.51) with perceptions of parental support. Construct validity was supported in that this burnout measure differentiated athletes who were rated below average by their coach (assuming that this was stressful for the athlete), particularly those who did not receive support from their parents.

The author also reported (N. W. Van Yperen, personal communication, April 6, 1996) that scores on the BIA were positively correlated (.59 Time 1; .32 Time 2) with intent to quit. Furthermore, athletes who felt underbenefitted in comparison to their peers playing for the same club reported the highest levels of energy depletion.

Norms: Not reported. Psychometric data were reported for 65 male soccer players (M age= 16.6 years) attending a prestigious soccer school in Ajax, Amsterdam.

**Availability: Contact Nico W. Van Yperen, Social and Organizational Psychology, University of Groningen, Grote Kruisstraat 2/I, 9712 TS Groningen, The Netherlands. (Phone # +31 50 363 63 32; FAX # +31 50 363 63 04; E-mail: n.van.yperen@ppsw.rug.nl)

References
Maslach, C., & Jackson, S. E. (1981). The measurement of experienced burnout. *Journal of Occupational Behavior, 2*, 99-113.

*Van Yperen, N. W. (in press). Inequity and dropping out: An exploratory causal analysis among highly skilled young soccer players. *The Sport Psychologist.*

 ## *[Cheerleading Anxiety Scale] (CHEER)
Justine J. Reel and Diane L. Gill

Source: Reel, J. J., & Gill, D. L. (1995). Psychosocial factors related to eating disorders among high school and college female cheerleaders [Abstract]. *Journal of Applied Sport Psychology, 7* (Suppl.), S103.

Purpose: To examine pressures experienced by cheerleaders.

Description: Not indicated.

Construction: Not indicated.

Reliability: A Cronbach alpha internal consistency coefficient (N=157) of .71 was reported.

Validity: Not indicated.

Norms: Not cited. Psychometric data were based on the responses of 73 college female cheerleaders and 84 high school female cheerleaders.

Availability: Contact Diane L. Gill, Exercise and Sport Science Department, University of North Carolina, Greensboro, NC 27412-5001. (Phone # 910-334-5744; FAX # 910-334-3238; E-mail: gilldl@iris.uncg.edu)

| 31 | *Children's Arousal Scale (CAS) Mark H. Anshel |

Source: Anshel, M. H. (1985). The effect of arousal on warm-up decrement. *Research Quarterly for Exercise and Sport, 56,* 1-9.

Purpose: To assess "...positive and negative levels of state arousal..." (p. 2).

Description: The CAS contains nine items: Four items indicate positive arousal (e.g., "excited"), and five items describe a negative arousal state (e.g., "nervous"). Items are listed as bipolar adjective pairs, and children respond to each pair using a 7-point semantic differential scale.

Construction: A pilot test established childrens' (N=42) understanding of 15 terms that had been derived from a list of emotions reported by people after experiencing success or failure.

Reliability: A Cronbach alpha internal consistency coefficient of (N=42) was reported.

Validity: Childrens' (N=15) responses to the CAS were correlated positively (.76 and .88) with different measurements obtained of heart rate. Also, these childrens' CAS scores were related to gymnastic vaulting performance. There was a statistically significant but low positive relationship with their CAS scores and their scores on the Sport Competition Anxiety Test.

Norms: Not cited. Psychometric data were reported for 15 female gymnasts (*M* age=11.3 years) and an additional sample of 42 children of similar age and educational background.

Availability: Contact Mark H. Anshel, Department of Psychology, University of Wollongong, P. O. Box 1144, Wollongong, New South Wales, Australia 2522. (Phone # 61-42-213732; FAX # 61-42-214163; E-mail: m.anshel@uow.edu.au)

32 | *Coaching Issues Survey (CIS)
Betty C. Kelley and Diane L. Gill

Source: Kelley, B. C., & Gill, D. L. (1993). An examination of personal/situational variables, stress appraisal, and burnout in collegiate teacher-coaches. *Research Quarterly for Exercise and Sport, 64,* 94-102.

Purpose: To measure "... the stress associated with various coaching issues" (p. 97).

Description: The CIS contains 32 items in which coaches rate on a 6-point ordinal scale the degree of stress they attribute to various coaching issues. Examples of these issues (items) include "placing pressure on myself to win" and "understanding my athletes' emotional responses and motivations." The scale anchorings are 0 (*no stress*) to 5 (*extreme stress*).

Construction: Initial content validity was established among 14 dual-role teacher-coaches who completed a 60-item survey and participated in an in-depth interview. The reduced 32-item questionnaire was then pilot tested among 52 Division III coaches.

Reliability: A Cronbach alpha internal consistency coefficient of .89 was reported ($N=52$). The current study reports an alpha reliability coefficient of .92 ($N=214$).

Validity: Multiple regression analysis indicated that subjects' ($N=214$) responses to the CIS were related to their scores on the burnout dimensions of emotional exhaustion, depersonalization, and personal accomplishments

Norms: Not cited. Psychometric data were reported for 52 NCAA Division III coaches, and an additional sample of 214 NCAA Division III and NAIA basketball coaches.

Availability: Contact Betty C. Kelley, Department of Physical Education, Central Missouri State University, Warrensburg, MO 64093. (Phone # 816-543-4732)

Reference

*Kelley, B. C. (1994). A model of stress and burnout in collegiate coaches: Effects of gender and time of season. *Research Quarterly for Exercise and Sport, 65,* 48-58.

33 *Cognitive Competitive Trait Anxiety Inventory (CCTAI)
Ye Ping

Source: Ping, Y. (1993). Competitive motives as predictors of cognitive trait anxiety in university athletes. *International Journal of Sport Psychology, 24,* 259-269.

Purpose: To assess individual differences in cognitive competitive trait anxiety.

Description: The CCTAI contains 50 items and six subscales: Game Preparation Anxiety, Failure Anxiety, Opponent's Ability Anxiety, Social Evaluation Anxiety, Injury Anxiety, and External Condition Anxiety. Participants respond to each item using a 4-point Likert scale with the anchorings 1 (*strongly disagree*) to 4 (*strongly agree*).

Construction: Items were generated from a review of the cognitive anxiety literature and from the open-ended responses of individuals in an exploratory investigation.

Reliability: Cronbach alpha internal consistency coefficients (N=406) ranged from .61 (External Condition Anxiety) to .89 (Game Preparation Anxiety).

Validity: Exploratory principal components factor analysis (N=406) with varimax rotation led to the retention of six factors noted above accounting for 53.3% of the total variance.

Norms: Not cited. Psychometric data were reported for 406 (254 males, 152 females) athletes attending a university in Japan.

Availability: Last known address: Jinnaka-cho 1-18-12, Toyota City, Aichi-ken 471 Japan.

34 Competitive Golf Stress Inventory (CGSI)
Peggy A. Richardson and Debra J. Norton

Source: Richardson, P. A., & Norton, D. J. (1983, February). *A competitive golf stress inventory*. Paper presented at the Texas Association for Health, Physical Education, Recreation, and Dance annual convention, Corpus Christi TX.

Purpose: To assess factors that contribute specifically to athletes' heightened anxiety levels in intercollegiate golf competition.

Description: The CGSI contains 40 items that focus on situation, spectator, expectation, opponent, and attitudinal influences. Participants are asked to respond on a 7-point Likert scale to items such as "I get tense when I am playing an important competitive round," or "I feel nervous when a crowd is watching my round."

Construction: Items for the CGSI were selected by analyzing and recording stress statements that appeared in newspapers and tournament reviews in *Golf Magazine*. A total of 75 items were evaluated by four LPGA Teaching Pros/ NCAA Division I coaches and one NCAA Division I golf coach for content validity, leading to the retention of 40 items.

Reliability: An uncorrected serial halves correlation coefficient of .93 was reported among 95 female college golfers.

Validity: Concurrent validity was supported in that participants' (n=95) responses to the CGSI correlated -.52 with their corresponding responses to the Sport Competition Anxiety Test. Furthermore, the CGSI discriminated between proficient and less proficient female intercollegiate golfers, where performance was defined as the average score over three 18-hole rounds.

Norms: Not cited. Descriptive and psychometric data were presented for 95 female intercollegiate golfers representing 15 golf teams from nine states.

**Availability: Contact Peggy A. Richardson, Department of Kinesiology, Health Promotion, and Recreation, P. O. Box 13857, University of North Texas, Denton, TX 76203-3857. (Phone # 817-565-3427; FAX # 817-565-4904; E-mail: rchrdsn@coefs.coe.unt.edu)

References
*Adler, W., & Thode, R. (1989). Beyond the SCAT: A specific sport-specific measure of competitive stress in golf [Abstract]. *Proceedings of the Association for the Advancement of Applied Sport Psychology annual convention* (p. 23). Seattle, WA.

*Lopes, P. (1991). *Human performance lab--Test file.* Unpublished manuscript, University of Ulster, Belfast, Ireland.

*Richardson, P. A., & Norton, D. J. (1984). A stress inventory for women's golf. *Scholastic Coach, 54,* 60-61, 72.

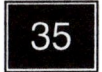

Competitive State Anxiety Inventory-2 (CSAI-2)
Rainer Martens, Damon Burton, Robin S. Vealey, Linda A. Bump, and Daniel E. Smith

Source: Martens, R., Vealey, R. S., & Burton, D. (1990). *Competitive anxiety in sport* (pp. 117-213). Champaign, IL: Human Kinetics Publishers.

Purpose: To assess cognitive and somatic components of competitive state anxiety and self-confidence in relation to competitive sport performance.

Description: The CSAI-2 is a 27-item self-report test designed to measure three relatively independent competitive states: cognitive state anxiety, somatic state anxiety, and confidence. Each of these three states is assessed by participants' responses to nine items using a 4-point Likert scale. An example of a cognitive A-state item is "I am concerned about losing." An example of a somatic A-state item is "I feel jittery." An example of a state self-confidence item is "I feel secure." Participants' total score on each subscale can range from a low of 9 to a high of 36.

The CSAI-2 was developed mainly as a research tool; its usefulness as a diagnostic instrument for clinical purposes has not been established.

Construction: Initially, the CSAI-2 was constructed to include fear of physical harm and generalized anxiety subscales, as well as cognitive and somatic A-state subscales. An initial pool of 102 items was developed from the first version of the CSAI-2 (called the CSAI) and by modifying items from existing general scales of somatic and cognitive A-state. An evaluation of these items for syntax, clarity, and face validity by three judges led to the retention of 79 items (Form A).

Form A was administered to 106 university football players prior to competition. It was also administered to 56 undergraduate physical education students who were asked to complete Form A based on a hypothetical competitive situation. On the bases of item analyses, item-to-subscale correlations, factor analyses, and discriminant analyses, 36 items (Form B) were retained comprising a 12-item somatic A-state subscale, a 12-item cognitive A-state subscale, a 10-item state self-confidence scale, and a 2-item fear-of-physical-harm subscale (which was subsequently eliminated based on further discrminant analysis).

Form C contained 6 additional self-confidence items, 6 new control items, and 12 internal-external locus of control items (hypothesized to be an important component of state self-confidence). Eight items were also deleted from Form B, resulting in a 52-item Form C containing four subscales. Form C was administered within one hour of competition to 80 male and female athletes who participated in collegiate swimming and track and field, high school wrestling, and road racing. Item analyses, item-to-subscale correlations, factor analyses, and discriminant analyses led to the deletion of the internal-external control subscale and the retention of cognitive A-state, somatic A-state, and state self-confidence subscales, each containing nine items (Form D). (One item from the cognitive A-state subscale was changed.)

It was found that both the cognitive and somatic A-state subscales were susceptible to social desirability contamination. The word *worry* was replaced by the word *concern* on all relevant items of the cognitive A-state subscale. This final version of the CSAI-2 was labeled Form E and also included a set of antisocial desirabilty instructions.

Reliability: Cronbach alpha reliability coefficients (across three samples of athletes) ranged from .79 to .83 for the cognitive A-state scale, from .82 to .83 for the somatic A-state scale, and from .87 to .90 for the state self-confidence scale.

Validity: Concurrent validity was demonstrated by showing that the responses of these three independent samples of athletes to the CSAI-2 correlated in the hypothesized directions with their responses to the Sport Competition Anxiety Test, general state and trait anxiety scales, Rotter's Internal-External Locus of Control Scale, the Zuckerman Affect Adjective Checklist, and Alpert and Haber's Achievement Anxiety Test.

Research by Gould, Petlichkoff, Simmons, and Vevera (1987) supported the predictive validity of the somatic A-state and state self-confidence subscales (but not the cognitive A-state scale) in relation to pistol shooting performance. Furthermore, Burton (1988a) found support for the inverted U relationship between somatic A-state and swimming performance among 33 collegiate swimmers and 70 swimmers chosen to compete at the 1982 National Sports Festival. However, there was a negative linear relationship between cognitive A-state and swimming performance and a positive linear relationship between state self-confidence and swimming performance.

Generally, the results are equivocal regarding the state anxiety-performance relationship. A most critical factor affecting this relationship seems to be the method by which performance is assessed.

Norms: Normative data are cited in the *Source* for 593 male and female high school athletes, 378 male and female college athletes, and 263 male and female elite athletes. In addition, normative data are presented for the sports of basketball, cycling, golf, swimming, track and field, and wrestling.

Availability: Permission is granted by the publisher of the *Source,* without written approval, for anyone to reproduce (but not publish) the CSAI-2 for research purposes. A copy of the CSAI-2 (Form E) is presented in the *Source.* The authors would like to receive reports of research findings resulting from the use of the CSAI-2.

References
*Bakker, F. C., & Kayser, C. S. (1994). Effect of a self-help mental training programme. *International Journal of Sport Psychology, 25,* 158-175.

*Barnes, M. W., Sime, W., Diensthbier, R., & Plake, B. (1986). A test of the construct validity of the CSAI-2 questionnaire on male elite collegiate swimmers. *International Journal of Sport Psychology, 17,* 364-374.

Bud, A. M., & Horn, M. A. (1990). Cognitive anxiety and mental errors in sport. *Journal of Sport & Exercise Psychology, 12,* 217-222.

*Burton, D. (1988a). Competitive state anxiety: Use and interpretation of the

Competitive State Anxiety Inventory-2 (abstract). In *Psychology of Motor Behavior and Sport* (p. 33). Proceedings of the North American Society for the Psychology of Sport and Physical Activity annual convention, University of Tennessee, Knoxville.

*Burton, D. (1988b). Do anxious swimmers swim slower? Reexamining the elusive anxiety-performance relationship. *Journal of Sport & Exercise Psychology, 10,* 45-61.

*Caruso, C. M., Dzewaltowski, D. A., Gill, D. L., & McElroy, M. A. (1990). Psychological and physiological changes in competitive state anxiety during noncompetition and competitive success and failure. *Journal of Sport & Exercise Psychology, 12,* 6-20.

*Coakley, L., & Terry, P. (1994). A comparison of the effectiveness of four intervention strategies in reducing pre-competition state anxiety among elite junior tennis players [Abstract]. *Journal of Sports Sciences, 12,* 186.

*Cogan, K. D., & Petrie, T. A. (1995). Sport consultation: An evaluation of a season-long intervention with female collegiate gymnasts. *The Sport Psychologist, 9,* 282-296.

*Copeland, B. W., Bonnell, R. J., & Reider, L. R. (1995). Introducing team cohesion and relaxation skills with junior U.S. national luge trainees [Abstract]. *Journal of Applied Sport Psychology, 7* (Suppl.), S50.

Couture, R. T., Bocksnick, J., & Kennedy, V. (1993). Effects of acute exercise programs on older adults [Abstract]. *Journal of Sport & Exercise Psychology, 15* (Suppl.), S19.

*Cox, R. H., Russell, W. D., & Robb, M. (1995). Development of an instrument for assessing competitive state anxiety during and prior to competition [Abstract]. *Research Quarterly for Exercise and Sport, 66* (Suppl.), A-75.

*Edwards, T. C., & Hardy, L. (1995). The interactive effects of intensity and direction of cognitive and somatic anxiety, self-confidence and performance [Abstract]. *Journal of Sports Sciences, 13,* 51-52.

*Eubank, M. R., & Smith, N. C. (1994). Intensity and direction of multidimensional competitive state anxiety: Relationships to performance [Abstract]. *Journal of Sports Sciences, 12,* 189-190.

*Eubank, M. R., Smith, N. C., & Smethurst, C. J. (1995). Intensity and direction of multidimensional competitive state anxiety: Relationships to performance in racket sports [Abstract]. *Journal of Sports Sciences, 13,* 52-53.

Finkenberg, M. E., DiNucci, J. N., McCune, E. D., & McCune, S. L. (1992). Cognitive and somatic state anxiety and self-confidence in cheerleading competition. *Perceptual and Motor Skills, 75,* 835-839.

Freigang, D. (1995). Psychological skills effects on training and competition in university swimmers [Abstract]. *Research Quarterly for Exercise and Sport, 66* (Suppl.), A75-76.

*George, T. R. (1994). Self-confidence and baseball performance: A causal examination of self-efficacy theory. *Journal of Sport & Exercise Psychology, 16,* 381-389.

*Gould, D., Petlichkoff, L., Simmons, J., & Vevera (1987). Relationship between Competitive State Anxiety Inventory-2 subscale scores and pistol shooting performance. *Journal of Sport & Exercise Psychology, 9,* 33-42.

*Gould, D., Petlichkoff, L., & Weinberg, R. S. (1984) Antecedents of temporal changes in, and relationships between CSAI-2 subcomponents. *Journal of Sport Psychology, 6,* 289-304.

Hall, H. K., & Kerr, A. (1994). The temporal patterning of pre competitive anxiety: A social-cognitive perspective [Abstract]. *Journal of Sport & Exercise Psychology, 16* (Suppl.), S63.

*Hammermeister, J., & Burton, D. (1993). Does anxiety reduce the limits of human endurance?: Perceived threat, control, and coping resources as antecedents of competitive anxiety [Abstract]. *Journal of Sport & Exercise Psychology, 15* (Suppl.), S39.

*Hammermeister, J., & Burton, D. (1995). Anxiety and the ironman: Investigating the antecedents and consequences of endurance athletes' state anxiety. *The Sport Psychologist, 9,* 29-40.

*Hanton, S., & Jones, G. (1994). Antecedents and levels of intensity and direction dimensions of state anxiety in elite and non-elite swimmers [Abstract]. *Journal of Sports Sciences, 12,* 193-194.

*Hanton, S., & Jones, G. (1995). Interpretation of anxiety symptoms and goal attainment expectations [Abstract]. *Journal of Sports Sciences, 13,* 57-58.

*Hardy, L., & Macgregor, G. (1994). Disruption of automatic processing as an explanation of the anxiety-performance effects [Abstract]. *Journal of Sports Sciences, 12,* 194-195.

*Hunt, R. L., Pemberton, C. L., & McSwegin, P. J. (1994). Coaches' ability to estimate athletes' levels of trait and state anxiety [Abstract]. *Research Quarterly for Exercise and Sport, 65* (Suppl.), A-87.

*Jambor, E. A., Rudisill, M. E., Weekes, E. M., & Michaud, T. J. (1994). Association among fitness components, anxiety, and confidence following aerobic exercise and aqua running. *Perceptual and Motor Skills, 78,* 595-602.

*Johnson, J., & Camburn, C. (1991). Cultural differences in the psychological characteristics of ultraendurance triathletes [Abstract]. *Proceedings of the Association for the Advancement of Applied Sport Psychology annual convention* (p. 75). Savannah, GA.

*Johnson, J., Wong, V., & Wainwright, T. (1993). Psychological characteristics of American, German and Japanese Ironman Triathletes. *Proceedings of the Eighth World Congress of Sport Psychology* (pp. 928-932). Lisbon, Portugal.

*Jones, G, & Swain, A. (1992). Intensity and direction as dimensions of competitive state anxiety and relationships with competitiveness. *Perceptual and Motor Skills, 74,* 467-472.

*Jones, G. & Swain, A. (1995). Predispositions to experience debilitative and facilitative anxiety in elite and nonelite performers. *The Sport Psychologist, 9,* 201-211.

*Jones, G, Swain, A., & Cale, A. (1991). Gender differences in precompetition temporal patterning and antecedents of anxiety and self-confidence. *Journal of Sport & Exercise Psychology, 13,* 1-15.

*Jones, G., Swain, A., & Hardy. L. (1993). Intensity and direction dimensions of competitive state anxiety and relationships with performance. *Journal of Sports Sciences, 11,* 525-532.

Kenow, L. J., & Williams, J. M. (1992). Relationship between anxiety, self-confidence, and evaluation of coaching behaviors. *The Sport Psychologist, 6,* 344-357.

Kingston, L., & Hardy, L. (1994). When are some goals more beneficial than others? [Abstract]. *Journal of Sports Sciences, 12,* 198-199.

*Kolt, G. S., & Kirby, R. J. (1994). Injury, anxiety, and mood in competitive gymnasts. *Perceptual and Motor Skills, 78,* 955-962.

*Krane, V., & Williams, J. M. (1994). Cognitive anxiety, somatic anxiety, and confidence in track and field athletes: The impact of gender, competitive level and task characteristics. *International Journal of Sport Psychology, 25,* 203-217.

*Krane, V., Williams, J., & Feltz, D. (1992). Path analyses examining relationships among cognitive anxiety, somatic anxiety, state confidence, performance expectations, and golf performance. *Journal of Sport Behavior, 15,* 279-294.

Lox, C. L. (1992). Perceived threat as a cognitive component of state anxiety and confidence. *Perceptual and Motor Skills, 75,* 1092-1094.

*Man, F., Stuchlikova, I., & Kindlmann, P. (1995). Trait-state anxiety, worry, emotionality, and self-confidence in top-level soccer players. *The Sport Psychologist, 9,* 212-224.

*Marchant, D. B., Andersen, M. B., & Morris, T. (1995). A test of the Martens, Vealey, and Burton (1990) Competitive Anxiety Model [Abstract]. *Journal of Applied Sport Psychology 7* (Suppl.), S86.

*Martin, J. J., & Gill, D. L. (1991). The relationships between competitive orientation, sport-confidency, self-efficacy, anxiety, and performance. *Journal of Sport & Exercise Psychology, 13,* 149-159.

*Matheson, H., & Mathes, S. (1991). Influence of performance setting experience and difficulty of routine on precompetitive anxiety and self-confidence of high school female gymnasts. *Perceptual and Motor Skills, 71,* 1099-1105.

*Maynard, I. W., & Cotton, P. C. J. (1993). An investigation of two stress-management techniques in a field setting. *Journal of Sport & Exercise Psychology, 15,* 375-387.

*Maynard, I. W., Hemmings, B., & Warwick-Evans, L. (1995). The effects of a somatic intervention strategy on competitive state anxiety and performance in semiprofessional soccer players. *The Sport Psychologist, 9,* 51-64.

*Maynard, I. W., Smith, M. J., & Warwick-Evans, L. (1995). The effects of a cognitive intervention strategy on competitive state anxiety and performance in semiprofessional soccer players. *Journal of Sport & Exercise Psychology, 17,* 428-446.

Murphy, S. M., Fleck, S. J., Dudley, G., & Callister, R. (1990). Psychological and performance concomitants of increased volume training in elite athletes. *Journal of Applied Sport Psychology, 2,* 34-50.

*Parfitt, G., & Hardy. L. (1993). The effects of competitive anxiety on memory span and rebound shooting tasks in basketball players. *Journal of Sports Sciences, 11,* 517-524.

*Parfitt, G., Hardy, L., & Pates, J. (1995). Somatic anxiety and physiological arousal: Their effects upon a high anaerobic, low memory demand task. *International Journal of Sport Psychology, 26,* 196-213.

*Perkins, T. G., & Williams, A. M. (1994). Self-report and psychophysiological measures of anxiety in novice and experienced abseilers [Abstract]. *Journal of Sports Sciences, 12,* 206-207.

*Perna, F. M. (1995). Competitive anxiety and sleep quality: An investigation of performance anxiety models in a health domain [Abstract]. *Journal of Applied Sport Psychology, 7* (Suppl.), S98.

Powell, F. M., & Verner, J. P. (1995). Pre-jump anxiety and sensation seeking characteristics of BASE jumpers [Abstract]. *Journal of Applied Sport Psychology, 7* (Suppl.), S100.

*Rodrigo, G., Lusiardo, M., & Pereira, G. (1990) Relationship between anxiety and performance in soccer players. International *Journal of Sport Psychology, 21,* 112-120.

*Russell, W. D., Robb, M., & Cox, R. H. (1994). Gender, sport, and situational effects on competitive state anxiety [Abstract]. *Journal of Sport & Exercise Psychology, 16* (Suppl.), S101.

*Scallen, S. (1993). Collegiate swimmers and the zone of optimal functioning theory [Abstract]. *Journal of Sport & Exercise Psychology, 15* (Suppl.), S68.

Serrano, A., & Pargman, D. (1993). The effects of a self-directed stress inoculation training program on collegiate football players. *Proceedings of the Eighth World Congress of Sport Psychology* (pp. 955 958). Lisbon, Portugal.

Smethurst, C. (1995). Performance catastrophes: A cognitive approach to testing the hysteresis hypothesis [Abstract]. *Journal of Sport & Exercise Psychology, 17* (Suppl.), S97.

Stratton, R. K. (1995). A test of the cyclical influence of game outcome on performer affect [Abstract]. *Journal of Applied Sport Psychology, 7* (Suppl.), S112.

Swain, A., & Jones, G. (1991). Relationship between sport achievement orientation and competitive state anxiety. *The Sport Psychologist, 6,* 42-54.

*Swain, A., & Jones, G. (1993). Intensity and frequency dimensions of competitive state anxiety. *Journal of Sports Sciences, 11,* 533-542.

*Swain, A. B. J., & Jones, G. (1994). The anxiety-performance relationship: Evidence of the need to assess the direction dimension [Abstract]. *Journal of Sports Sciences, 12,* 210-211.

*Terry, P., & Bowman, T. (1995). A comparison of state anxiety measures between novice and experienced parachutists [Abstract]. *Journal of Sports Science, 13,* 78.

*Wann, D. L. (1995). Competitive state anxiety in sport spectators [Abstract]. *Journal of Applied Sport Psychology, 7* (Suppl.), S122.

*White, S. A., & Barelay, J. A. (1990). Competitive state anxiety levels in youth and collegiate soccer players [Abstract]. *Proceedings of the Association for the Advancement of Applied Sport Psychology annual convention* (p. 125). San Antonio, TX.

*Whitehouse, A., & Hale, B. D. (1995). The effects of imagery manipulated perceptions on intensity and direction of competitive anxiety [Abstract]. *Journal of Applied Sport Psychology, 7* (Suppl.), S124.

*Williams, J. M., & Krane, V. (1992). Coping styles and self-reported measures of state anxiety and self-confidence. *Journal of Applied Sport Psychology, 4,* 134-143.

*Yang, G., & Pargman, D. (1993). An invesigation of relationships among sport-confidence, self-efficacy, and competitive anxiety and their ability to predict performance of a karate skill test. *Proceedings of the Eighth World Congress of Sport Psychology* (pp. 968-972). Lisbon, Portugal.

*Yang, G., & Pargman, D. (1995). The investigation of relationships among self-confidence, self-efficacy, competitive anxiety, and sport performance [Abstract]. *Journal of Applied Sport Psychology, 7* (Suppl.), S126.

*Competitive State Anxiety Inventory for Children (CSAI-2C)

Robert E. Stadulis, Thomas A. Eidson, Mary Jo MacCracken, and Carol Severance

Source: Stadulis, R. E., Eidson, T. A., MacCracken, M. J., & Severance, C. (1995, June). *Validation of the Competitive State Anxiety Inventory for children (CSAI-2C)*. Paper presented at the annual conference of the North American Society for the Psychology of Sport and Physical Activity, Pacific Grove, CA.

Purpose: To assess cognitive (worry) and somatic competitive state anxiety and confidence among children.

Description: The CSAI-2C has three subscales, each containing five items: cognitive state anxiety (e.g., "I am concerned that I may not play as well as I can today"); somatic state anxiety (e.g. " My heart is racing"); and confidence (e.g., "I feel secure"). Children respond to each item using a 4 point ordinal scale with the anchorings 1 (*not at all*) to 4 (*very much so*).

Construction: Using evaluative input from children and from language arts teachers, items from the Competitive State Anxiety Inventory-2 (Martens, Vealey, & Burton, 1990) were modified to be appropriate in language for childen ages 10 to 12 years (Stadulis, Eidson, & MacCracken, 1994). Based on exploratory factor analysis ($N=625$), the number of items on the CSAI 2C was reduced from seven items per subscale to five items per subscale; factor analysis did not support the addition of a concentration disruption scale (Stadulis, Eidson, & MacCracken, 1994).

Reliability: A Carmine's Theta internal consistency coefficient of .96 ($N=632$) was reported across all items. Cronbach alpha internal consistency cofficents ($N=632$) of .75 (cognitive anxiety), .78 (somatic anxiety) and .73 (confidence) were reported.

Validity: Principal factor analysis (oblique rotation) for the entire sample ($N=632$) as well as for the 10- to 12-year-old children only ($n=391$) supported the retention of three factors (cognitive anxiety, somatic anxiety, and confidence) accounting for 81% (entire sample) and 90% (older children) of the variance. Principal components analysis yielded similar results, thereby supporting the construct validity of the CSAI-2C.

Norms: Not cited. Psychometric data are presented for 632 elementary school children, ages 8 through 12 years of age, from a rural school district in northeastern Ohio.

Availability: Contact Robert E. Stadulis, School of Exercise, Leisure and Sport, Kent State University, P. O. Box 5190, Kent, OH 44242-0001. (Phone #330-672-2857; FAX 330-672-4106; E-mail: rstaduli@kentvm.kent.edu)

Reference

*Stadulis, R. E., Eidson, T. A., & MacCracken, M. J. (1994). A children's form of the Competitive State Anxiety Inventory (CSAI-2C) [Abstract]. *Journal of Sport & Exercise Psychology, 16* (Suppl.), S109.

37 *Competitive Thoughts Scale (CTS)
Rebecca Lewthwaite

Source: Lewthwaite, R. (1990). Threat perception in competitive trait anxiety: The endangerment of important goals. *Journal of Sport & Exercise Psychology, 12,* 280-300.

Purpose: To examine the frequency with which the cognitive component of competitive trait anxiety is experienced by young athletes (i.e., worries or concerns about performance inadequacy and its social evaluative consequences).

Description: The CTS contains 14 items dealing with thoughts about failure (e.g., "I am concerned about making mistakes/losing/not playing well") and about social evaluation (e.g., "I am concerned about what my coach/parents/teammates will think or say"). Participants respond to "how often you usually think or worry about the following things when you compete in sports and games" using a 7-point Likert scale with the anchorings 1 (*never*) to 7 (*very often*).

Construction: The CTS was developed on the basis of previous competitive anxiety research advocating the multidimensional measurement of somatic and cognitive anxiety components.

Reliability: An alpha reliability coefficient (N=102) of .92 was reported.

Validity: An iterated principal axis factor analyses (n=102) indicated that all items on the CTS loaded .40 or greater on a single factor accounting for 84.4% of the variance.

Norms: Not cited. Psychometric data were reported for 102 male soccer players, ages 9 to 15, representing 11 teams in the Los Angeles, CA, area.

Availability: Contact Rebecca Lewthwaite, Clinical Biokinesiology Program, Harriman 223/7601 E. Imp, Downey, CA 90242. (Phone 310-940-7061).

38	*Competitive Worries Inventory (CWI)

*Competitive Worries Inventory (CWI)
Vassilis Kakkos

Source: Kakkos, V., & Zervas, Y. (1995, July). Predictors of precompetitive cognitive-emotional states. In R. Vanfraechem-Raway & Y. Vanden Auweele (Eds.), *Proceedings of the IXth European Congress on Sport Psychology* (pp. 473-480). Brussels, Belgium.

Purpose: To assess the frequency and intensity of worry that athletes experience prior to competition.

Description: The CWI contains five subscales and 29 items: (a) performance worries, (b) social evaluation worries, (c) worries due to the importance and uncertainty of the situation, (d) worries due to feelings of personal inadequacy, and (e) worries caused by attribution to external factors. Participants rate their responses to each subscale based on frequency and intensity of experienced worry. Frequency is assessed using a 4-point ordinal scale with the anchorings 1 (*almost never*) to 4 (*almost always*). Intensity is assessed using a 7-point ordinal scale with the anchorings 1 (*not at all*) to 7 (*very much*).

Construction: The author (V. Kakkos, personal communication, May 7, 1996) summarized how the CWI was constructed. A preliminary investigation included three phases of data collection and evaluation involving 348 athletes from various sports. Specifically, the first phase (preliminary instrument planning) included the initial item pool generated by the investigator based on a review of the literature and the evaluation of content validity by three judges. The second phase (exploratory working) included structured open-ended interviews with athletes (*N*=25) in order to include or exclude items. The third phase (instrument development) included two studies (*N*=212; *N*=111) to assess the validity and reliability of the test.

Reliability: Cronbach alpha internal consistency coefficients (*N*=270) ranged from .73 to .81. The author also reported (V. Kakkos, personal communication, May 7, 1996) that test-retest reliability coefficients (*N*=99) ranged from .61 to .75 across a 2-week interval.

Validity: The author (V. Kakkos, personal communication, May 7, 1996) summarized the procedures used to establish the validity of the CWI. A principal components factor analysis (with a varimax rotation) yielded five factors accounting for approximately 65% of the variance. The discriminant validity of the CWI was supported in that gender, the type of sport (i.e., team versus individual) and the status of sport participation (i.e., participants versus dropouts) mediated participants' responses to the CWI. Further, the predictive validity of the CWI was supported in that athletes' ($N=90$; $N=270$)) scores on the CWI were predictive of their precompetitive cognitive and emotional state scores (cognitive and somatic anxiety; confidence, vigor, etc.). Finally, the concurrent validity of the CWI was supported in that participants' scores on the various CWI subscales were correlated with their scores on related trait variables (e.g., their competitive trait anxiety scores as measured by the Sport Competition Anxiety Test).

Norms: Not cited. Psychometric data were cited for 270 athletes (172 males and 92 females) with a mean age of 20.3 years ($SD=4.4$) and a mean competitive experience of 5.8 years ($SD=3.4$). The participants represented the following sports: track and field runners ($n=66$) and jumpers ($n=72$), swimmers ($n=63$), and target shooters ($n=69$).

**Availability: Contact Vassilis Kakkos, Laboratory of Motor Behavior and Sport Psychology, Department of Physical Education and Sport Science, University of Athens, 41 Olgas Street, Athens, Greece 17237. (Phone # 01-9752576; FAX # 01-9752576; E-mail: jzervas@atlas.uoa.gr)

Reference
*Kakkos, V., & Zervas, Y. (1995). Competitive worries and self-confidence as predictors of the precompetive cognitive-emotional state. *Proceedings of the Eighth World Congress of Sport Psychology* (pp. 855-859). Lisbon, Portugal.

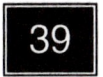

39 *Eades Athlete Burnout Inventory (EABI)
A. M. Eades

Source: Eades, A. M. (1991). An investigation of burnout in intercollegiate athletes: The development of the Eades Athlete Burnout Inventory [Abstract]. *Proceedings of the North American Society for the Psychology of Sport and Physical Actitivy annual convention* (p. 154). Pacific Grove, CA.

72

Purpose: To assess burnout in athletes.

Description: The EABI contains 41 items and six subscales: Negative Self Perception of Athletic Ability, Emotional and Physical Exhaustion, Psychological Withdrawal From and Devaluation by Coach and Teammates, Incongruent Coach-Athlete Performance Expectations and Evaluations, and Personal and Athletic Accomplishment.

Construction: The development of the EABI occurred through four pilot studies. Three pilot studies centered on (a) the item analyses of the responses of 56 current and former NCAA Division I athletes to items that were modified from the Maslach Burnout Inventory, (b) interviews with five of these athletes who had experienced burnout, (c) content analyses employing several sport psychology researchers and practitioners, and (d) administration of the revised EABI to 183 Division I athletes. A factor analysis of the responses of this latter sample led to the establishment of the six factors (subscales).

Reliability: Internal consistency coefficients for the six subscales ranged from .57 to .89.

Validity: Concurrent validity was supported in that subjects' scores on the EABI positively correlated with (a) years of sport participation and (b) number of experienced injuries.

Availability: Last known address: A. M. Eades, Department of Physical Education, University of California, Berkeley, CA 94720.

Reference
*Vealey, R. S., Comer, W., & Armstrong, L. (1995). Effects of coaching style and behavior on burnout and competitive anxiety in athletes [Abstract]. *Journal of Applied Sport Psychology, 7* (Suppl.), S119.

40 | [Fear of Social Consequences Scale] [FSCS]
Klaus Willimczik, S. Rethorst, and H. J. Riebel

Source: Willimczik, K., Rethorst, S., & Riebel, H. J. (1986). Cognitions and emotions in sports games--a cross-cultural comparative analysis. *International Journal of Physical Education, 23*(1), 10-16.

Purpose: To assess the fear that others might give a negative judgment of one's performance in a sport context.

Description: The FSCS contains 10 items. For example, "It depresses me when I am criticized by my teammates." Participants respond on a 7-point Likert scale.

Construction: Not discussed.

Reliability: Internal consistency coefficients of .73 ($n=137$ male and female German volleyball players) and .47 ($n=150$ male and female Indonesian volleyball players) were reported.

Validity: Not discussed.

Norms: Not cited. Psychometric data were based on the responses to the SCAQ of 68 German male volleyball players, 69 German female volleyball players, 90 Indonesian male volleyball players, and 60 Indonesian female volleyball players.

Availability: Contact Klaus Willimczik, Abteilung Sportwissenschaft, Universitat Bielefeld, Universitatsstr., Postfach 8640, D-4800 Bielefeld 1, Germany. (Phone # +521/106-5127)

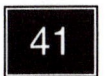 ## 41 *Gymnastics Anxiety Scale [GAS]
Kevin S. Spink

Source: Spink, K. S. (1990). Psychological characteristics of male gymnasts: Differences between competitive levels. *Journal of Sports Sciences, 8,* 149-157.

Purpose: To assess the anxiety levels of gymnasts at various points prior to competition.

Description: The GAS contains nine items.

Construction: Not discussed.

74

Reliability: A Cronbach alpha internal consistency coefficient of .80 was reported (*N*=38).

Validity: Discriminant validity was supported in that elite gymnasts (*n*=15) were more anxious than less elite gymnasts (*n*=23).

Norms: Not cited. Psychometric data were reported for 38 elite male gymnasts participating in an Australian gymnastic championship.

Availability: Contact Kevin S. Spink, College of Physical Education, 105 Gymnasium Place, University of Saskatchewan, Saskatoon, Saskatchewan, Canada S7N 0W0. (Phone # 306-966-6474; FAX # 306-966-6502; E-mail: spink@sask.usask.ca or spink@skyblu.usask.ca)

 ## Mental Readiness Form (MRF)
Shane M. Murphy, Michael Greenspan, Douglas Jowdy, and Vance Tammen

Source: Murphy, S. M., Greenspan, M., Jowdy, D., & Tammen, V. (1989). Development of a brief rating instrument of competitive anxiety: Comparisons with the Competitive State Anxiety Inventory-2 [Abstract]. *Proceedings of the Association for the Advancement of Applied Sport Psychology* (p. 82). Seattle, WA.

Purpose: To assess precompetitive state anxiety.

Description: The MRF is a three-item instrument employing a bipolar continuous scale assessment method. The MRF was developed so that the three ratings obtained would correspond to the cognitive anxiety, somatic anxiety, and self-confidence subscales of the Competitive State Anxiety Inventory-2 (CSAI-2). Participants respond to thoughts, bodily feelings, and self-confidence before competition using calm-worried, tense-relaxed, and scared-confident bipolar adjective pairs, respectively.

Construction: The test authors were seeking to develop a self-report assessment of anxiety that would take athletes only seconds to complete prior to competing and that would produce little distraction. They selected the three subscales of the CSAI-2 as a basis for the bipolar continuous scale assessment.

Reliability: Not discussed.

Validity: Concurrent validity correlation coefficients between participants' (*n*=105 elite cyclists; *n*=19 elite table tennis players; *n*=15 elite junior figure skaters) responses to the MRF and the appropriate subscales of the CSAI-2 were .63 (cognitive anxiety/thoughts), .59 (somatic anxiety/bodily feelings), and .63 (self-confidence/self-confidence).

Norms: Not cited. Psychometric data were cited for 105 male and female senior and junior cyclists, 19 senior and junior table tennis players, and 15 junior figure skaters.

Availability: Contact Shane M. Murphy, Gold Medal Psychological Consultants, 500 B Monroe Turnpike, Suite 106, Monroe, CT 06468 (Phone # 203-452-7409; FAX # 203-459-2744; E-mail: the zonedoc@aol.com)

References
*Cox, R. H., Russell, W. D., & Robb, M. (1995). Comparative validity of the MRF and ARS competitive state anxiety rating scales [Abstract]. *Journal of Applied Sport Psychology, 7* (Suppl.), S52.

Daw, J., & Burton, D. (1994). Evaluation of a comprehensive psychological skills training program for collegiate tennis players. *The Sport Psychologist, 8,* 37-57.

*Edwards, T. C., & Hardy, L. (1995). Further dimensions of anxiety: Validating a short self-report scale [Abstract]. *Journal of Applied Sport Psychology, 7* (Suppl.), S59.

*Krane, V. (1994). The Mental Readiness Form as a measure of competitive state anxiety. *The Sport Psychologist, 8,* 189-202.

*Krane, V., Joyce, D., & Rafeld, J. (1994). Competitive anxiety, situation criticality, and softball performance. *The Sport Psychologist, 8,* 58-72.

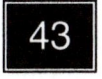 **43** **Precompetitive Stress Inventory (PSI)**
John M. Silva, Charles J. Hardy, R. K. Crace, and N. E. Slocum

Source: Silva, J. M., Hardy, C. J., Crace, R. K., & Slocum, N. E. (1987). Establishment of the psychometric properties of the Precompetitive Stress Inventory. *Research abstracts of the American Alliance for Health, Physical Education, Recreation, and Dance annual convention,* Las Vegas, NV.

Purpose: To assess individual differences in the proneness toward experiencing precompetitive stress.

Description: The PSI is a 10-item questionnaire designed to assess sources of precompetitive stress. Participants are asked to indicate the frequency with which certain stressors occur 24 hours pregame; they are also asked to rate the impact (positive, negative, or none) the stressors had on performance.

Construction: A panel of experts from sport psychology and clinical psychology were used to establish the content validity of the PSI.

Reliability: An alpha internal consistency coefficient of .98 was reported among 45 female and 78 male youth sport participants (ages 12-18).

Validity: A principal component factor analysis (n=123) led to the emergence of 14 factors accounting for 75.82% of the variance; comparative factor analyses across two studies led to the retention of seven factors. These seven factors (and the corresponding accountable variance) were Group Motivation (21.13%), Self-confidence (15.56%), Performance Achievement (13.87%), Guilt/Fear of Misfortune (13.30%), Playing Time (12.97%), Material Rewards (11.68%), and Family Involvement (11.45%). Concurrent validity was supported in that participants' (n=123) scores on the PSI correlated with their responses to the Sport Competition Anxiety Test (r=.56).

Norms: Not cited. Psychometric properties were reported for 123 youth sport participants, ages 12-18, with 1 to 13 years' experience in youth sport.

Availability: Contact John M. Silva, Department of Physical Education, CB #8700, 203 Fetzer Gym, University of North Carolina, Chapel Hill, NC 27599-8700. (Phone # 919-962-5176; FAX # 919-962-0489; E-mail: usilva@uncmvs.oit.unc.edu)

References

*Cornelius, A. E., & Silva, J. M. (1992). Sources of stress in athletes: A validation of the Precompetitive Stress Inventory [Abstract]. *Proceedings of the North American Society for the Psychology of Sport and Physical Activity annual convention* (p. 145). Pittsburgh, PA

*Finch, L., Silva, J., & Hardy, C. (1988). An assessment of the factor validity of the

Precompetitive Stress Inventory [Abstract]. *Proceedings of the Association for the Advancement of Applied Sport Psychology*. Nashua, NH.

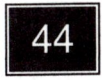 **44**

Pre-race Questionnaire (PRQ)
J. Graham Jones, Austin Swain, and Andrew Cale

Source: Jones, J. G., Swain, A., & Cale, A. (1990). Antecedents of multidimensional competitive state anxiety and self-confidence in elite intercollegiate middle-distance runners. *The Sport Psychologist, 4,* 107-118.

Purpose: To examine the antecedents of competitive state anxiety and self-confidence that exist prior to participating in a middle-distance running event.

Description: The PRQ contains 19 items that focus on situational variables perceived as contributing most to how runners feel during the period immediately preceding a race. (For example, "How important is it for you to do well in this race?") Participants respond to each item using a 9-point ordinal scale.

Construction: The PRQ was developed using a series of structured interviews with middle-distance runners. Potential items were formulated from these interviews and administered to a group of middle-distance runners who assessed the suitability of the questions for such athletes. The 19 items that emerged from this review were evaluated in a pilot study of six middle-distance athletes prior to competition. Based on these athletes' feedback, adjustments were made to some items of the PRQ.

Reliability: Cronbach's alpha coefficients for the five factors (see validity section) ranged from .63 to .78 among 125 male middle-distance runners.

Validity: Principal component factor analysis using both varimax and oblique rotations supported the existence of five factors that were labeled Perceived Readiness, Attitude Toward Previous Performance, Position Goal, External Environment, and Coach Influence. These factors accounted for 63.10% of the variance in participants' responses to the PRQ.

Stepwise multiple regression analyses indicated that individuals' (n=125) scores on the cognitive anxiety subscale of the Competitive State Anxiety Inventory-2 (administered one hour before a race) were predicted by the first three factors of the PRQ (identified above).

Norms: Not cited. Psychometric data were based on the responses of 125 male middle-distance runners (M age=22.18 years; SD=3.36). All participants were elite intercollegiate runners.

Availability: Contact J. Graham Jones, Department of Physical Education, Sports Science, and Recreation Management, Loughborough University, Loughborough, Leicestershire, LE11 3TU, United Kingdom. (Phone # +44 1509 263171; FAX # +44 1509 223971; E-mail: j.g.jones@lboro.ac.uk)

Reference

*Hanton, S., & Jones, G. (1994). Antecedents and levels of intensity and direction dimensions of state anxiety in elite and non-elite swimmers [Abstract]. *Journal of Sports Sciences, 12*, 193-194.

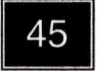 ## *Soccer Officials Stress Survey (SOSS)
Adrian H. Taylor

Source: Taylor, A. H., & Daniel, J. (1988). Sources of stress in soccer officiating: An empirical study. In T. Reilly, A. Lees, K. Davids, & W. J. Murphy (Eds.), *Science and football: Proceedings of the First Congress of Science and Football* (pp. 538-544). Liverpool, England: Spon.

Purpose: To identify different sources of stress perceived by soccer officials.

Description: The original SOSS contained 53 items reflecting potential sources of stress for the official. Participants responded to each item on an intensity basis (i.e, "How much did the item contribute to the amount of stress you felt during the past season?") using a 4-point ordinal scale with the anchorings 0 (*did not*) to 3 (*strongly*). They also responded to 39 of the items on a frequency basis (i.e., "How often did you experience the item?") using a 4-point ordinal scale with the anchorings 0 (*never*) to 3 (*often*). A subsequent version employed just the intensity subscale and included 30 items.

Construction: Extensive interviews with soccer officials from all levels of certification (Youth to FIFA) in Ontario, Canada, led to a 90-item pool of potential officiating stressors. A 12-member panel with expertise in psychometric construction, stress research, or soccer officiating reduced this number to 53 items by eliminating items that were ambiguous or overlapping. The items spanned a broad range of potential acute and chronic stressors. The SOSS was then mailed to 400 randomly selected Ontario male officials from all levels of certification. A total of 215 officials responded. The correlation coefficient describing the relationship between participants' responses to the frequency and intensity scales was 0.59. Using the intensity subscale items, a principal components factor analysis revealed six factors with a minimum of three items each, and accounted for 35.4% of the variance. These factors (representing 28 items) were labeled: interpersonal conflicts; fear of physical harm; time pressures; peer conflicts; role culture conflict; and fear of failure.

In subsequent research (Taylor, 1990; Taylor, Daniel, Leith, & Burke, 1990), all 1,269 registered officials in Ontario were mailed the Ontario Soccer Officals Survey 3 months into the soccer season and 4 months later at the end of the season. This included sections on sources of stress, burnout, satisfaction, intentions to quit, and background variables. The sources of stress section included 25 of 28 intensity subscale items from the SOSS, and 5 additional items to reflect fitness concerns and time pressures. Exploratory and confirmatory factor analyses were conducted on these participants' responses to the 30 items using both assessments ($n=733$ and $n=529$, respectively). Seven factors emerged accounting for 60% of the variance explained on both occasions.

Reliability: Hoyt's estimate of reliability for the six initial subscales ranged from .67 to .87. Cronbach alpha reliability coefficients ranged from .65 to .88 for the seven subscales at both data collection points (Taylor, 1990; Taylor et al., 1990).

Validity: Construct validity has been supported in that significant relationships between scores on the SOSS and the hypothesized outcomes of burnout, satisfaction, intentions to quit, and actual turnover have been revealed. Low to moderate correlations between the stressor scales also suggest independent constructs (Taylor, 1990; Taylor et al., 1990).

Norms: Not cited. Psychometric data were cited for male soccer officials residing in Ontario, Canada.

**Availability: Contact Adrian Taylor, Chelsea School Research Centre, University of Brighton, Gaudick Roìxbourne, East Sussex, BN20 7SP, England. (Phone # 01273-643743; FAX # 01273-643704; E-mail: aht@bton.ac.uk)

References
Hemmings, B., & Graydon, J. (1994). Sources of stress and the incidence of burnout in National List and Junior League status football referees in the 1992-93 season [Abstract]. *Journal of Sports Sciences, 12,* 195.

*Rainey, D. (1995). Sources of stress among baseball and softball umpires. *Journal of Applied Sport Psychology, 7,* 1-10.

*Rainey, D. W. (1995). Stress, burnout, and intention to terminate among umpires. *Journal of Sport Behavior, 18,* 312-323.

*Taylor, A. (1993). Satisfaction among soccer officials. In J. R. Nitsch and R. Seiler (Eds.), *Motivation, emotion, stress* (pp. 197-202). Proceedings of the VIII European Congress of Sport Psychology (Volume 1). Sankt Augustin: Academia Verlag.

Taylor, A. H. (1990). Psycho-social factors preceding actual dropout from soccer officiating [Abstract]. *Journal of Sport Sciences, 8(1),* 70-71.

*Taylor, A. H., Daniel, J. V., Leith, L., & Burke, R. (1990). Perceived stress, psychological burnout and paths to turnover intentions among sport officials. *Journal of Applied Sport Psychology, 2,* 84-97

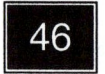

[Sources of Stress Scale] [SSS]
Daniel Gould, Thelma Horn, and Janie Spreeman

Source: Gould, D., Horn, T., & Spreeman, J. (1983). Sources of stress in junior elite wrestlers. *Journal of Sport Psychology, 5,* 159-171.

Purpose: To assess perceived sources of competitive stress in wrestlers.

Description: Wrestlers respond to 33 items on a 7-point Likert scale in terms of how often a potential source of stress makes them nervous or worried.

Construction: Items were developed based on a previous review of the research literature on stress and athletics. The content validity of the items was established by two sport psychologists.

Reliability: A pilot research study produced a test-retest reliability coefficient of .74 for all items combined.

Validity: Principal component factor analysis of the responses of 458 elite wrestlers led to the identification of three factors: fear of failure-feelings of inadequacy, external control-guilt, and social evaluation. These factors accounted for 75%, 14%, and 11%, respectively, of the variance in the factorial model. Using multiple regression analyses, it was determined that participants' scores on the Sport Competition Anxiety Test were predictive of the fear of failure-feelings of inadequacy factor.

Norms: None available. Psychometric data were cited for 458 elite wrestlers (ages 13-19) participating in the United State Wrestling Federation Junior National Championships.

**Availability: Contact Daniel Gould, Department of Exercise and Sport Science, University of North Carolina, 250 HHP Building, Greensboro, NC 27412-5001. (Phone # 910-334-3037; FAX # 910-334-3238; E-mail: gouldd@iris.uncg.edu)

References

*Gould, D., & Weinberg, R. S. (1983). Sources of worry in successful and unsuccessful intercollegiate wrestlers [Abstract]. In *Psychology of motorbehavior and sport--1983* (p. 80). Proceedings of the North American Society for the Psychology of Sport and Physical Activity annual convention, Michigan State University, East Lansing, MI.

*Silva, J. M., & Hardy, C. J. (1984). Detecting and predicting perceptions of stress factors in senior elite wrestlers. *Proceedings of the 1984 Olympic Congress* (p. 104). Eugene, OR: College of Human Development and Performance Microform Publications.

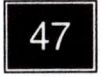 **47 Sport Anxiety Interpretation Measure (SAD)**
Dieter Hackfort

Source: Hackfort, D., & Schwenkmezger, P. (1989). Measuring anxiety in sports. Perspectives and problems. In D. Hackfort & C. D. Spielberger (Eds.), *Anxiety in sports: An international perspective* (pp. 55-74). New York: Hemisphere Publishing Corporation.

Purpose: To measure sport-specific trait anxiety among children across different sports.

Description: The SAD assesses fear of disgrace, fear of competition, fear of failure, fear of the unknown, and fear of injury using 22 items in the form of pictures. Response categories are also nonverbal (sketches of facial expressions portraying different degrees of anxiety).

Construction: Not discussed.

Reliability: Test-retest reliability coefficients ranged from .87 to .94.

Validity: Not discussed.

Norms: Not cited.

Availability: Contact Dieter Hackfort, ISWS der Uni BWM, Werner Heisenberg-Weg 39, 85577 Neubiberg, Germany (Phone # 49 89 6004 4180/81; FAX # 49 89 6004 4179; E-mail: p51bdhp5@rz.unibw-muenchen.de)

Reference

*Hackfort, D., & Schwenkmezger, P. (1993). Anxiety. In R. N. Singer, M. Murphey, & L. K. Tennant (Eds.). *Handbook of Research on Sport Psychology* (pp. 328-364). New York: MacMillan Publishing Company.

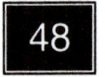 ## Sport Anxiety Scale (SAS)
48 Ronald E. Smith, Frank L. Smoll, and Robert W. Schutz

Source: Smith, R. E., Smoll, F. L., and Schutz, R. W. (1990). Measurement and correlates of sport-specific cognitive and somatic trait anxiety: The Sport Anxiety Scale. *Anxiety Research, 2,* 263-280.

Purpose: To assess cognitive and somatic dimensions of competitive trait anxiety.

Description: The SAS is a 21-item questionnaire containing three sub-scales: Somatic Anxiety (9 items), Worry (7 items), and Concentration Disruption (5 items). Examples of items: "My body feels tight" (Somatic Anxiety), "I am concerned about choking under pressure" (Worry), and "My mind wanders during sport competition" (Concentration Disruption). Participants respond to each item using a 4-point ordinal scale.

Construction: Some of the initial items of the SAS were developed from existing measures of cognitive and somatic anxiety. Pilot work led to the retention of 15 cognitive and 15 somatic items that were administered in questionnaire format to 250 male and 201 female high school athletes in basketball, wrestling, and gymnastics at 41 high schools; 123 college football players were also administered the questionnaire. Principal component factor analysis followed by varimax rotation led to the retention of three factors (somatic anxiety, worry, and concentration distruption) and 22 items that accounted for 48% of the variance in the high school samples, and 53% of the variance in the college football sample. Confirmatory factor analysis using the postseason data of 300 of these subjects supported a 22-item three-factor model. However, cross-validiation with an independent sample (n=490) led to the elimination of one Concentration Disruption item.

Reliability: Cronbach alpha coefficients (n=490) were .88 (somatic), .82 (Worry), and .74 (Concentration Disruption). Test-retest reliability coefficients (n=64) over 7 days exceeded .85 across all scales.

Validity: Convergent validity was supported in that high school athletes' (n=837) responses to the SAS correlated with their responses to the Sport Competition Anxiety Test (particularly the Somatic scale), and to a lesser extent with their responses to Spielberger's State-Trait Anxiety Inventory. Predictive validity was evident in that football players' (n=47) scores on the SAS were predictive 2 weeks later of their pregame Tension and Confusion subscale scores on a shortened version of the Profile of Mood States. In addition, football players (n=48) categorized as high or low on performance, based on coaches' gradings of game films over an entire season, differed on the Concentration Disruption scale.

Norms: Not presented. However, normative data were derived for 489 male and 348 female high school varsity athletes involved in one of six sports, and for 123 college football athletes competing at an NCAA Division I school.

**Availability: Contact Ronald E. Smith, Department of Psychology NI-25, Box 351525, University of Washington, Seattle, WA 98195-1525. (Phone # 206-543-8817; FAX # 206-685-3157; E-mail: resmith@u.washington.edu)

References

*Barnett, N. P., Smoll, F. L., & Smith, R. E. (1993). Reduction of competitive trait anxiety in youth sports: Effects of a coach training intervention [Abstract]. *Proceedings of the Association for the Advancement of Applied Sport Psychology annual convention* (p. 8). Montreal, Canada.

*Finch, L., Krane, V., Gould, D., Eklund, R., & Kelley, B. (1990). Factors influencing coaches' ability to predict anxiety levels in their athletes: Part II-Trait anxiety [Abstract]. *Proceedings of the Association for the Advancement of Applied Sport Psychology annual convention* (p. 42). San Antonio, TX.

*Krane, V., Joyce, D., & Rafeld, J. (1994). Competitive anxiety, situationcriticality, and softball performance. *The Sport Psychologist, 8, 58-72.*

*Krane, V., & Leibold, B. (1994). Psychological factors related to the incidence of injury in collegiate soccer players [Abstract]. *Journal of Sport & Exercise Psychology, 16* (Suppl.). S71.

*Leffingwell, T. R., & Williams, J. M. (1995). Cognitive interpretations of competitive trait anxiety as facilitative or debilitative [Abstract]. *Journal of Applied Sport Psychology, 7* (Suppl.), S85.

*Leffingwell, T. R., & Williams, J. M. (1995). Comparison of the Sport Anxiety Scale (SAS) and Sport Competition Anxiety Test (SCAT) at predicting multidimensional state anxiety [Abstract]. *Journal of Sport & Exercise Psychology, 17* (Suppl.), S74.

*Millhouse, J. I., Willis, J. D., & Layne, B. H. (1989). The clinical utility of three recent psychological instruments with advanced female gymnasts: A preliminary study [Abstract]. *Proceedings of the Association for the Advancement of Applied Sport Psychology annual convention,* Seattle, WA.

*Newton, M. L., & Duda, J. L. (1992). The relationship of goal perspectives to multidimensional trait anxiety in adolescent tennis players [Abstract]. *Proceedings of the North American Society for the Psychology of Sport and Physical Activity annual convention* (p. 167). Pittsburgh, PA.

Shewokis, P. A., Krane, V., Snow, J., & Greenleaf, C. (1995). A preliminary investigation of the influence of anxiety on learning in a contextual interference paradigm [Abstract]. *Journal of Sport & Exercise Psychology, 17* (Suppl.), S94.

*Smith, R. E. (1989). Conceptual and statistical issues in research involving multidimensional anxiety scales. *Journal of Sport & Exercise Psychology, 11,* 452-457.

*Smith, R. E., Schutz, R. W., Smoll, F. L., & Ptacek, J. T. (1995). Development and validation of a multidimensional measure of sport specific psychological skills: The Athletic Coping Skills Inventory-28. *Journal of Sport & Exercise Psychology, 17,* 379-398.

*Stadulis, R. E., MacCracken, M. J., LeVan, C., & Fender-Scarr, L. (1993). Using both quantitative and qualitative methodology in sport psychology research: A competitive golf example. *Proceedings of the Eighth World Congress of Sport Psychology* (pp. 493-497). Lisbon, Portugal.

*Tamen, V. V., & Murphy, S. M. (1991). Establishing validity for the Sport Anxiety Scale [Abstract]. *Proceedings of the North American Society for the Psychology of Sport and Physical Activity annual convention* (p. 196). Pacific Grove, CA.

*Trantow, C. B., Lewthwaite, R., & Snyder, A. C. (1991). Competitive trait anxiety, training demands, and children's sport-related avoidance preferences [Abstract]. *Proceedings of the North American Society for the Psychology of Sport and Physical Activity annual convention.* (p. 198).Pacific Grove, CA.

*Vealey, R. S., Comar, W., & Armstrong, L. (1995). Effects of coaching style and behavior on burnout and competitive anxiety in athletes [Abstract]. *Journal of Applied Sport Psychology, 7* (Suppl.), S119.

 ## Sport Competition Anxiety Test (SCAT)
Rainer Martens, Diane Gill, Tara Scanlan, and Julie Simon

Source: Martens, R., Vealey, R. S., & Burton, D. (1990). *Competitive anxiety in sport* (pp. 3-115). Champaign, IL: Human Kinetics Publishers, Inc.

Purpose: To assess individual differences in competitive trait anxiety, or the tendency to perceive competitive situations as threatening and/or to respond to these situations with elevated state anxiety.

Description: The SCAT contains 15 items. Participants are asked to indicate how they *generally* feel when they compete in sports and games and respond to each item using a 3-point ordinal scale (hardly ever, sometimes, or often). Ten of the items assess individual differences in competitive trait anxiety proneness (e.g., "Before I compete I worry about not performing well"); five spurious items are also included to reduce possible response bias. Total scores on the SCAT range from 10 (low competitive trait anxiety) to 30 (high competitive trait anxiety).

The SCAT was developed as a research instrument, and its usefulness as a diagnostic instrument for clinical evaluation has not been established. Both child (ages 10 thru 14) and adult versions of SCAT exist. Furthermore, SCAT has been translated into Spanish, French, German, Russian, Japanese, and Hungarian.

Construction: Psychometric development of the SCAT was guided by the theoretical conceptualization of competitive trait anxiety as a situation-specific form of anxiety proneness that mediates, in part, an individual's perceptions of and/or responses to threat within the competitive process. Several criteria guided the format of SCAT including the need for an objective rather than projective psychological test, the need to minimize response bias, the desirability of unambiguous administration procedures, a short completion time, and easy scoring procedures.

SCAT was initially constructed for use with children (ages 10 to 15).

An initial pool of 75 items was developed by modifying items from existing general trait anxiety scales and by adding additional sport-specific items. Based on item evaluations by six judges, a total of 21 items were retained (Version 1). The first version, consisting of 21 items retained from the original item pool plus 9 spurious items, was administered to 193 male junior high school students. Item analyses, correlation analyses between item responses and total SCAT scores, and discriminant analyses led to the retention of 14 items (Version 2). The second version, consisting of the 14 accepted items and 7 spurious items, was administered to two additional male junior high school samples ($N=175$). Item analyses, triserial correlations, and discriminant analyses led to the retention of 10 items, which when combined with 5 spurious items, formed Version 3. The third version was administered to two samples: 106 male and female fifth and sixth graders, and 98 male and female junior high school students. Item analyses, triserial correlations, and discriminant analyses led to the final 15-item (including 5 spurious items) child form of SCAT.

An adult version of SCAT was developed by simply modifying the instructions and by changing one word for one item. Item analyses, triserial correlations, and discriminant analyses, using a sample of 153 male and female university students, supported the item integrity of this adult version of SCAT.

Reliability: Test-retest reliability coefficients for the child form (SCAT-C) among four samples of boys and girls in grades 5, 6, 8, and 9 ranged from .57 to .93 (mean $r=.77$) across four time intervals: 1 hour, 1 day, 1 week, and 1 month. ANOVA reliability coefficients, computed on the basis of the first test administrations among these four samples, were slightly higher (mean $r=.81$) than the test-retest reliability coefficients reported. A higher ANOVA reliability coefficient ($r=.85$) was obtained for the adult version of SCAT (SCAT-A) ($n=153$).

Kuder-Richardson formula 20 (KR-20) internal consistency coefficients, computed for the four samples used to confirm the item integrity of Version 3 of SCAT-C and for two SCAT-A samples of 268 male and female undergraduate students, ranged from .95 to .97 for both forms of SCAT.

Validity: Content validity was evident during the initial item selection phase; six judges who were qualified researchers in sport psychology or motor learning, and who had either conducted or were knowledgeable about research on anxiety in sport, evaluated systematically the integrity of each item selected for Version 1 of SCAT-C. The convergent validity of SCAT was supported by showing that participant responses to SCAT were positively correlated to measures of sport-specific dispositions of fear of failure, ineffective attentional focus, and cognitive and somatic anxiety. Conversely, divergent validity was demonstrated by showing participant SCAT scores to be inversely related to sport-specific dispositions of need for power and self-confidence. Concurrent validity was also supported by the low, but statistically significant positive correlation coefficients with general measures of trait anxiety and external locus of control assessments, and negative correlation coefficients with internal locus of control and self-esteem measures. Generally, SCAT demonstrated stronger correlations with sport-specific measures than with general personality tests as hypothesized.

The predictive validity of SCAT was supported in that participant responses to SCAT related positively to future assessments of both general and competitive state anxiety. Participants' SCAT scores correlated more highly with their competitive than with their noncompetitive A-state responses. A meta-analysis using the validity generalization model indicated that the average correlation coefficient between SCAT responses and competitive A-state was .61. Also, SCAT was a better predictor of athletes' A-state responses than were the coaches' ratings of their players.

However, the predictive validity of SCAT in relation to self-confidence and motor performance is equivocal. Furthermore, SCAT responses do not appear to be predictive of pre- and postcompetition performance expectancies.

Norms: Updated normative data on SCAT-C were provided for male and female youth sport participants ($n=1094$), and on SCAT-A for male and female high school ($n=352$) and college ($n=565$) athletes. Also, normative data were provided on SCAT-A for baseball, basketball, football, soccer, swimming, tennis, volleyball, and wrestling participants.

Availability: Permission is granted by publishers of the *Source*, without written approval, for anyone to reproduce (but not publish) the SCAT for research purposes. SCAT can be found in the *Source*. The authors would like to receive reports of research findings resulting from use of the SCAT.

References

Allyson, B., & Murray. J. H. (1990). An investigation of competitive anxiety as positive affect [Abstract]. *Proceedings of the 3rd Southeast Sport and Exercise Psychology Symposium*. Greensboro, NC.

*Bakker, F. C., & Kayser, C. S. (1994). Effect of a self-help mental training programme. *International Journal of Sport Psychology*. 25, 158 175.

*Barnett, N. P., Smoll, F. L., & Smith, R. E. (1993). Reduction of competitive trait anxiety in youth sports: Effects of a coach training intervention [Abstract]. *Proceedings of the Association for the Advancement of Applied Sport Psychology annual convention* (p. 8). Montreal, Canada.

*Brand, H. J., Hanekom, J. D. M., & Scheepers, D. (1988). Internal consistency of the Sport Competition Anxiety Test. *Perceptual and Motor Skills, 67*, 441-442.

Burkett, S., LeUnes, A., Bourgeois, T., & Driggars-Bourgeois, T. (1995). Psychological predictors of intramural sports participation [Abstract]. *Journal of Applied Sport Psychology, 7*, S46.

Daw, J., & Burton, D. (1994). Evaluation of a comprehensive psychological skills training program on collegiate tennis players. *The Sport Psychologist, 8*, 37-57.

Ebbeck, V. (1994). Self-perception and motivational characteristics of tennis participants: The influence of age and skill. *Journal of Applied Sport Psychology, 6*, 71-86.

*Finkenberg, M. E., DiNucci, J. M., McCune, E. D., & McCune, S. L. (1992). Analysis of the effects of competitive trait anxiety on performance in Taekwondo competition. *Perceptual and Motor Skills, 75*, 239-243.

Frost, R. O., & Henderson, K. J. (1991). Perfectionism and reactions to athletic competition. *Journal of Sport & Exercise Psychology, 13*, 323-335.

Hanson, S. J., McCullagh, P., & Tonymon, P. (1992). The relationship of personality characteristics, life stress, and coping resources to athletic injury. *Journal of Sport & Exercise Psychology, 14*, 262-272.

*Hunt, R. L., Pemberton, C. L., & McSwegin, P. J. (1994). Coaches' ability to estimate athletes' levels of trait and state anxiety [Abstract]. *Research Quarterly for Exercise and Sport, 65* (Suppl.), A-87.

*Kang, L., Gill, D. L., Acevedo, E. O., & Deeter, T. E. (1990). Competitive orientations among athletes and nonathletes in Taiwan. International *Journal of Sport Psychology, 21*, 146-157.

Kenow, L. J., & Williams, J. M. (1992). Relationship between anxiety, self-confidence, and evaluation of coaching behaviors. *The Sport Psychologist, 6*, 344-357.

*Kerr, G., & Leith, L. (1993). Stress management and athletic performance. *The Sport Psychologist, 7*, 221-231.

*Krane, J., Williams, J., & Feltz, D. (1992). Path analysis examining relationship among cognitive anxiety, somatic anxiety, state confidence, performance expectations, and golf performance. *Journal of Sport Behavior, 15*, 279-295.

*Leffingwell, T. R., & Williams, J. M. (1995). Comparison of the Sport Anxiety Scale (SAS) and Sport Competition Anxiety Test (SCAT) at predicting multidimensional state anxiety [Abstract]. *Journal of Sport & Exercise Psychology, 17* (Suppl.). S74.

Mahoney, C. A., Kremer, J., & Scully, D. M. (1994). The evaluation of mental skills training in swimming [Abstract]. *Journal of Sports Sciences, 12*, 200.

*Ostrow, A. C., & Ziegler, S. G. (1977). Psychometric properties of the Sport Competition Anxiety Test. In B. Kerr (Ed.), *Human performance and behavior* (pp. 139-142). Banff, Alberta: Proceedings of the 9th Canadian Psycho-motor Learning and Sport

Psychology symposium.

*Petrie, T. A. (1993). Coping skills, competitive trait anxiety, and playing status: Moderating effects on the life stress-injury relationship. *Journal of Sport & Exercise Psychology, 15*, 261-274.

*Prapavessis, H., & Grove, J. R. (1994). Personality variables as antecedents of precompetitive mood states. *International Journal of Sport Psychology, 25*, 81-99.

*Randle, S. M., Weinberg, R. S., & Hodge, K. (1992). Competitive anxiety and sources of stress experienced by high school athletes [Abstract]. *Proceedings of the Association for the Advancement of Applied Sport Psychology annual convention* (p. 85). Colorado Springs, CO

*Rupnow, A., & Ludwig, D. A. (1981). Psychometric note on the reliability of the Sport Competition Anxiety Test. *Research Quarterly for Exercise and Sport, 52*, 35-37.

*Ryska, T. D. (1993). The relationship between trait and precompetitive state anxiety among high school athletes. *Perceptual and Motor Skills, 76*, 413-414.

*Scanlan, T. K. (1978). Perceptions and responses of high- and low-competitive trait-anxious males to competition. *Research Quarterly, 49*, 520-527.

*Stadulis, R. E., MacCracken, M. J., LeVan, C., & Fender-Scarr, L. (1993). Using both quantitative and qualitative methodology in sport psychology research: A competitive golf example. *Proceedings of the Eighth World Congress of Sport Psychology* (pp. 493-497). Lisbon, Portugal.

Takahashi, K. The effect of cognitive and coping processes on the exertion of skills in judo athletes. *Proceedings of the Eighth World Congress of Sport Psychology* (pp. 398-401). Lisbon, Portugal

Tremayne, P., & Barry, R. (1990). Repression of anxiety and its effects on psychophysiological responses to stimuli in competitive gymnastics. *Journal of Sport & Exercise Psychology, 12*, 333-352.

*Vealey, R. S. (1988). Competitive trait anxiety: Use and interpretation of the Sport Competition Anxiety Test [Abstract]. In *Psychology of motor behavior and sport* (p. 35). Proceedings of the North American Society for the Psychology of Sport and Physical Activity annual convention, Knoxville, TN.

*Williams, J. M., & Krane, V. (1992). Coping styles and self-reported measures of state anxiety and self-confidence. *Journal of Applied Sport Psychology, 4*, 134-143.

Yang, G., & Pargman, D. (1993). An investigation of relationships among sport-confidence, self-efficacy, and competitive anxiety and their ability to predict performance on a karate skill test. *Proceedings of the Eighth World Congress of Sport Psychology* (pp. 968-972). Lisbon, Portugal.

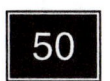

*SPORT GRID [SG]
Thomas D. Raedeke, Gloria L. Stein, and G. W. Schmidt

Source: Raedeke, T. D., Stein, G. L., & Schmidt, G. W. (1993). A new look at arousal: A two-dimensional conceptualization [Abstract]. *Journal of Sport & Exercise Psychology, 15* (Suppl.), S64.

Purpose: To assess one's current level of arousal and thoughts/feelings.

Description: Respondents complete a grid by marking an "X" in the box that best represents their current level of arousal and thoughts/feelings.

Construction: Not discussed.

Reliability: Not presented.

Validity: Convergent validity was supported in that participants' responses to the Sport Grid were correlated with their responses to the Competitive State Anxiety Inventory-2. Furthermore, the predictive validity of the Sport Grid was evidenced by demonstrating that high arousal--positive thoughts/feelings--were positively related to higher performance scores.

Norms: Not cited. Sample characteristics that psychometric data were based on were not presented.

Availability: Contact Thomas Raedeke, Department of Kinesiology, University of Colorado, Campus Box 354, Boulder, CO 80309-0354. (Phone # 303-492-5362; FAX # 303-492-4009)

51 Sport Pressure Checklist [SPC]
Brent S. Rushall and Cheyne A. Sherman

Source: Rushall, B. S., & Sherman, C. A. (1987). A definition and measurement of pressure in sport. *The Journal of Applied Research in Coaching and Athletics, 2,* 1-23.

Purpose: To assess elite athletes' perceptions of pressure prior to or during competition.

Description: The SPC contains 16 items and four subscales: Positive pressure, negative pressure, internal pressure, and external pressure. Items focus on areas such as coach expectations, audience effects, parental expectations, and the anticipated difficulty of the contest. Participants respond to each item on a 7-point ordinal scale.

Construction: Items were derived based on a review of the stress and pressure research literature, an examination of stress and anxiety assessment tools, and interviews with 13 coaches. Item analyses ($n=70$) and content analyses using 7 sport psychologists who had international coaching or competition experiences supported the retention of 16 items.

Reliability: Cronbach alpha internal consistency coefficients of .87 (internal subscale) and .82 (external subscale) were reported ($n=70$). Test-retest reliability coefficients among 9 female and 9 male swimmers across one hour, one day, and 2 weeks ranged from .98 (Negative subscale-one-day interval) to .46 (Negative subscale-2-week interval). Test-retest reliability coefficients among 14 members of the Canadian cross-country ski team across five different time intervals were all higher than .97. Similar encouraging results were reported among nine intercollegiate basketball players.

Validity: Content validity was established using seven experts (above).

Norms: Not cited. Psychometric data were based on the responses of 70 elite athletes.

Availability: Contact Brent S. Rushall, Department of Exercise and Nutritional Science, San Diego State University, San Diego, CA. 92182-0171. (Phone # 619-594-4094; FAX # 619-594-6553; E-mail: brushall@mail.sdsu.edu)

References

*Franseen, L. M., & McCann, S. (1995). A comparison of perceived pressures and the prevalence of eating disturbances in elite female athletes [Abstract]. *Journal of Applied Sport Psychology, 7* (Suppl.), S62.

Rushall, B. S. (1984). Pressure in Olympic athletes--measurement and four case studies [Abstract]. *Proceedings of the Canadian Society of Psychomotor Learning and Sport Psychology annual conference* (p. 5). Kingston, Ontario, Canada.

52 *Stressful Situations in Basketball Questionnaire (SSBQ)

Christopher C. Madden, Jeffrey J. Summers, and David F. Brown

Source: Madden, C. C., Summers, J. J., & Brown, D. F. (1990). The influence of perceived stress on coping with competitive basketball. *International Journal of Sport Psychology, 21,* 21-35.

Purpose: "...to determine the perceived relative degree of stress experienced across a range of sporting situations in competition basketball" (p. 23).

Description: The SSBQ contains 20 situations or game states. Items relate to a range of offensive, defensive, and neutral situations. For example, participants are asked to indicate how stressful are situations such as "Missing outside shots," "Having the ball stolen from me," and "Missing lay-ups." Participants respond on a 5-point Likert scale ranging from 0 (*not stressful*) to 4 (*very stressful*).

Construction: The twenty game situations were "...chosen from an initial list of items developed by analyses of the range of game states occurring in competitive basketball" (p. 25). These items were pilot tested among basketball players. Items were deleted, altered, or additional items were included based on their feedback.

Reliability: A Cronbach alpha internal consistency coefficient of .84 (*N*=133) was reported.

Validity: Not discussed.

Norms: Not cited. Psychometric data were reported for 133 basketball players (*n*=84 males; *n*=49 females; *M* age = 24 years) residing in Victoria, Australia.

Availability: Contact Christopher C. Madden, Department of Behavioural Health Sciences, Lincoln School of Health Sciences, La Trobe University, Carlton Campus, 625, Swanston Street, Carlton, Victoria 3053, Australia. (Phone # 03 9479 1741)

53 *Test of Archers' Competitive State Anxiety (TACSA)

Byung Hyun Kim, Kee Woong Kim, and Seon Jin Kim

Source: Kim, B. H., Kim, K. W., & Kim, S. J. (1993). The development of a Test of Archers' Competitive State Anxiety (TACSA). *Korean Journal of Sport Science, 5,* 111-122.

Purpose: To evaluate cognitive and somatic state anxiety and self confidence among competitive archers.

Description: The TACSA contains cognitive state anxiety (7 items), somatic state anxiety (7 items), and self-confidence (7 items) subscales. Archers respond to each item using a 5-point ordinal scale with the anchorings 1 (*not at all*) to 5 (*very much so*).

Construction: Items for the TACSA were developed based on Martens and his colleagues' conceptualization of competitive state anxiety and construction of the Competitive State Anxiety Inventory-2. Items were also derived based on an examination of the literature on state anxiety and self-confidence. "...Factors related to the context of archery as mode of competing, equipment, competing place, and activities of competition" (p. 114) were considered in order to ensure that the items were specific to archery competition.

Initially, two coaches asked 10 archers to describe every possible situation that affected their performances in practice and in competition. A total of 162 terms were selected and categorized into 12 areas. The research team selected 73 main terms, and with the assistance of coaches and archers and expert analyses, developed 45 items from these 73 terms. These items were grouped into cognitive and somatic state anxiety, and self-confidence subscales. Item analyses and exploratory factor analysis using varimax rotation ($N=94$) reduced the item pool to 21 items.

Reliability: Cronbach alpha internal consistency coefficients ($N=94$) of .71 (Cognitive state anxiety), .84 (Somatic state anxiety), and .75 (Self confidence) were reported.

Validity: Not reported.

Norms: Not cited. Psychometric data were reported for 94 male and female archers who were participating in the Korean National Archery Championship Contest.

Availability: The items are listed in the *Source.*

*The Officials' Stress Test (OST)
Patrick A. Goldsmith and Jean M. Williams

Source: Goldsmith, P. A., & Williams, J. M. (1992). Perceived stressors for football and volleyball officials from three rating levels. *Journal of Sport Behavior, 15,* 106-118.

Purpose: To evaluate perceived sources of stress among sport officials.

Description: Participants evaluate 31 items (e.g., "Spectators too close to the field") in terms of their contribution to personal stress experienced during the officiating season. Participants respond on a 4-point ordinal scale to each item using the anchorings 1 (*did not*) to 4 (*strongly*).

Construction: The OST was modified from the Soccer Officials' Stress Survey (Taylor & Daniel, 1988) so as to be applicable to other sports. Principal components factor analyses (varimax rotation) of the respones of 99 officials to the OST resulted in the retention of five factors accounting for 60% of the variance. These factors were labeled Fear of Physical Harm, Pressure Game, Verbal Abuse by Players or Coaches, Time Pressures, and Fear of Failure.

Reliability: Cronbach alpha internal consistency coefficients ($N=99$) of .83 (Fear of Physical Harm), .72 (Pressure Game), .71 (Verbal Abuse), .71 (Time Pressure), and .63 (Fear of Failure) were reported.

Validity: Not reported

Norms: Not cited. Psychometric data were reported for 99 officials ($n=24$ male volleyball officials; $n=14$ female volleyball officials; and *n*=61 male football officials) who were either University of Arizona intramural officials or noncertified or certified Arizona Interscholastic Association officials.

Availability: Contact Jean M. Williams, Department of Psychology, University of Arizona, 109 Ina Gittings Building, Tucson, AZ 85721. (Phone # 602-621-6984; FAX # 602-621-8170; E-mail: williams@u.arizona.edu)

Reference

Taylor, A. H., & Daniel, J. V. (1988). Sources of stress in soccer officiating: An empirical study. In T. Reilly, A. Lees, K. Davids, & W. J. Murphy (Eds.), *Science and football: Proceedings of the First World Congress of Science and Football* (pp. 538-544). Liverpool, England: Spon.

 **55** | ***Trait Anxiety Inventory for Sports (TAIS)**
Kimio Hashimoto, Mikio Tokunaga, Hideo Tatano, and Ryozo Kanezaki

Source: Hashimoto, K., Tokunaga, M., Tatano, H., & Kanezaki, R. (1993). Reliability and validity of the Trait Anxiety Inventory for Sports (TAIS). *Journal of Health Science, 15,* 39-49.

Purpose: To measure competitive trait anxiety in sport situations.

Description: The TAIS contains 25 items and five independent factors: Mental Agitation, Cognitive Worry Concerning Victory or Defeat, Tendency of Somatic Anxiety, Flight From Situation, and Loss of Confidence.

Construction: The TAIS was derived from Spielberger's conceptualization of trait-state anxiety, and Martens' theoretical framework for competitive anxiety.

Reliability: An internal consistency coefficient, using a split-half technique adjusted by the Spearman-Brown Prophesy formula, was .94 (*N*= 457). A test-retest reliability coefficient of .81 was reported.

Validity: Convergent validity was supported in that participants' (*N*= 457) responses to the TAIS were positively related to their responses to the trait anxiety scale of Spielberger's State-Trait Anxiety Scale (.56) and to their responses to the Sport Competition Anxiety Scale (.68).

Norms: Not cited. Psychometric data were reported for 167 junior high school, 188 high school, and 102 college athletes.

Availability: Contact Mikio Tokunaga or Kimio Hashimoto, Institute of Health Science, Kyushu University, 6-1 Kasuga kouen, Kasuga city, Fukuoka, 816 Japan. (Phone/fax #s 011-81-92-583-7846; E-mail: tokunaga@ihs.kyushu-u.ac.jp)

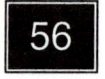 **56**

Worry Cognition Scale [WCS]
Maureen R. Weiss, Kimberley A. Klint, and Diane M. Wiese

Source: Weiss, M. R., Klint, K. A., & Wiese, D. M. (1989). Head over heels with success: The relationship between self-efficacy and performance in competitive youth gymnastics. *Journal of Sport & Exercise Psychology, 11*, 444-451.

Purpose: To assess worry cognitions about gymnastic performance and negative social evaluation among youth participants.

Description: The WCS contains two subscales: performance cognitions (9 items) and evaluation cognitions (8 items). However, given the correlation (.81) between subscales, a composite worry score is derived. Items specific to gymnastics include "I worry about poor judging" and "I worry about doing better than another competitor." Participants respond to each item on the WCS using a 5-point Likert scale.

Construction: The WCS was derived and adapted from previous sport-specific sources of stress and prematch cognition scales.

Reliability: Cronbach alpha reliability coefficients of .84 (performance cognition subscale) and .90 (evaluation cognition subscale) were reported.

Validity: Frequency of worry cognitions (in combination with self-efficacy, years of experience, and precompetitive anxiety) were predictive of the all-around gymnastic performance of 22 boys.

Norms: Not cited. Psychometric data were reported for 22 boys ranging in age from 7 to 18 years who were members of a competitive youth gymnastics club participating in the state gymnastics tournament.

Availability: Contact Maureen R. Weiss, Department of Exercise and Movement Science, 131 Esslinger Hall, University of Oregon, Eugene, OR 97403-1240. (Phone # 541-346-4108; FAX # 541-346-2841; E- mail: mrw@oregon.uoregon.edu)

Chapter 4

Attention

Four of the five tests in this chapter are sport-specific versions of Nideffer's (1976) Test of Attention and Interpersonal Style. This instrument is based on a two-dimensional conceptual framework of attention, containing broad/narrow and internal/external components. The test developed by Etzel examines attention among elite rifle shooters from a multidimensional perspective.

57 Baseball Test of Attentional and Interpersonal Style (B-TAIS)

Richard R. Albrecht and Deborah L. Feltz

Source: Albrecht, R. R., & Feltz, D. L. (1987). Generality and specificity of attention related to competitive anxiety and sport performance. *Journal of Sport Psychology, 9,* 231-248.

Purpose: To assess attentional style as it relates to baseball/softball batting.

Description: The B-TAIS is a 59-item sport-specific version of Nideffer's (1976) Test of Attention and Interpersonal Style (TAIS). Six attentional subscales and the cognitive-information processing subscale from the TAIS were restructured to be specific to baseball/softball batting. The attentional subscales include Broad External Attention, External Overload, Broad Internal Attention, Internal Overload, Narrow Attention, and Reduced Attention.

Construction: All 59 items of the TAIS were converted to a baseball/softball batting-specific reference. As much of the TAIS context, grammatical structure, and wording were retained as was possible. Five experts who had used the TAIS in their research evaluated the revised items of the B-TAIS for content validity. Each item was also evaluated by an intercollegiate varsity baseball and softball coach.

Reliability: Cronbach's alpha internal consistency coefficients ($n=29$) ranged from .50 (Reduced Attention) to .85 (External Overload). Test-retest reliability coefficients across a 2-week interval ranged from .72 (Internal Overload) to .95 (Broad Internal Attention). None of the reliability coefficients statistically exceeded those computed for the TAIS.

Validity: Convergent validity was supported in that participants' ($n=29$) scores on the B-TAIS correlated .50 with their scores on the TAIS. Construct validity was supported in that participants' scores on designated subscales of the B-TAIS correlated with their competitive trait anxiety scores. Also, participants' scores on the B-TAIS were predictive of their seasonal batting performance scores.

Norms: Not cited. Psychometric data were based on the responses of 15 male varsity intercollegiate baseball players and 14 female varsity intercollegiate softball players attending Michigan State University.

**Availability: Contact Richard R. Albrecht, Office of Medical Education Research and Development, A-209 East Fee Hall, Michigan State University, East Lansing, MI 48824 1316. (Phone # 517-353-9656; FAX # 517-353-3146; E-mail: albrech5@pilot.msu.edu)

Reference

Nideffer, R. M. (1976). Test of Attentional and Interpersonal Style. *Journal of Personality and Social Psychology, 34,* 397-404.

58 Riflery Attention Questionnaire (RAQ)
Edward F. Etzel, Jr.

Source: Etzel, E. F., Jr. (1979). Validation of a conceptual model characterizing attention among international rifle shooters. *Journal of Sport Psychology, 1,* 281-290.

Purpose: To assess the attentional style of elite international style rifle shooters.

Description: The RAQ is a 25-item self-report test containing five attention subscales: Capacity, Duration, Intensivity, Flexibility, and Selectivity. Participants respond to each item using a 4-point Likert scale.

Construction: An original pool of 60 items was derived by the author using an intuitive-rational strategy plus a general item-developmental approach. All items were derived based on a hypothesized multidimensional conceptual model of attention in elite shooters. Two judges with background experience in both psychology and riflery assigned each item to the appropriate hypothesized subscale. Based on their review, 30 items were retained of which 25 items were included in the RAQ.

Reliability: Alpha reliability coefficients (n=71 elite rifle shooters) ranged from .10 (Capacity) to .82 (Selectivity).

Validity: The construct validity of the RAQ was partially supported through principal component factor analysis in which four of the five hypothesized attention factors emerged accounting for 85% of the variance in participants' (*n*=71) responses to the RAQ. The predictive validity of the RAQ was partially supported. Elite shooters, classified as successful or unsuccessful based on 3-day smallbore shooting aggregate scores of the 1978 United States World Shooting Championship Team Tryouts, could not be distinguished based on their RAQ scores. However, multiple regression analysis supported the low but statistically significant relationship of these elite shooters' scores on Selectivity and Intensivity to their shooting performances.

Norms: Psychometric data were cited for 71 elite rifle shooters who represented 75% of the foremost male and female international rifle shooters in the United States.

**Availability: Contact Edward F. Etzel, School of Physical Education, P. O. Box 6116, West Virginia University, Morgantown, WV 26506-6116. (Phone # 304-293-3295, x589; FAX # 304-293-4641)

Reference
*Boutcher, S. H., & Crews, D. J. (1984). Multidimensional attentional measures of collegiate golfers [Abstract]. *Proceedings of the 1984 Olympic Scientific Congress.* Eugene, OR: College of Human Development and Performance Microform Publications.

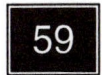 **Tennis Test of Attentional and Interpersonal Style (T-TAIS)**
Stephen R. Van Schoyck and Anthony F. Grasha

Source: Van Schoyck, S. R., & Grasha, A. F. (1981). Attentional style variations and athletic ability: The advantages of a sports-specific test. *Journal of Sport Psychology, 3,* 149-165.

Purpose: To assess the attentional style of tennis players

Description: The T-TAIS is a 59-item sport-specific version of Nideffer's (1976) Test of Attention and Interpersonal Style (TAIS). Six attentional scales and one control scale from the TAIS were restructured to be tennis-specific. These scales include Broad External Attention, External Overload, Broad Internal Attention, Internal Overload, Narrow Attention, Reduced Attention, and Information Processing.

Construction: A rational approach to test construction was employed. Two item writers, one male and one female, with extensive backgrounds in tennis and psychology, converted the items from the TAIS to describe analogous situations in tennis. The writers independently listed their first association to tennis for each TAIS item, resulting in the retention of 39 common items. The remaining 20 items were included after extensive discussion and final agreement among the writers.

Reliability: Alpha reliability coefficients (n=45 male tennis players; n=45 female tennis players) ranged from .16 (Reduced Attention) to .83 (Narrow Attention; Internal Overload). Test-retest reliability coefficients (n=83 tennis players) across a mean test-retest interval of 29.2 days (SD=17.1) ranged from .68 (Reduced Attention) to .91 (External Overload). All reliability coefficients were higher than those obtained for the TAIS among these participants (except for the Reduced Attention scale).

Validity: Principal component factor analysis (n=90) led to the retention of two primary factors accounting for 79.2% of the variance. Evaluation of these two factors led to the interpretation that bandwidth was multidimensional and not bipolar as suggested by Nideffer; the direction of attention dimension did not appear as a strong component of participants' responses.

The T-TAIS differentiated better among tennis skill levels (n=90) than did the TAIS. Furthermore, the T-TAIS better predicted match play tennis performance among advanced tennis players (n=14 male intercollegiate tennis players) than did the TAIS.

Norms: Psychometric data were presented for 45 male and 45 female tennis players solicited from two local tennis clubs, public tennis facilities in Cincinnati, and the University of Cincinnati men's and women's tennis teams. (M age=29 years; SD=9.8)

**Availability: Contact Stephen R. Van Schoyck, 148 West Marshall Avenue, Langhorne, PA 19047. (Phone #215-752-7111; FAX # 215-968-5263)

Reference

Nideffer, R. M. (1976). Test of Attentional and Interpersonal Style. *Journal of Personality and Social Psychology, 34,* 397-404.

60 Test of Soccer Attentional Style (TSAS)
A. Craig Fisher and Adrian H. Taylor

Source: Fisher, A. C., & Taylor, A. H. (1980). Attentional style of soccer players. Reston, VA: *Research abstracts-American Alliance for Health, Physical Education, Recreation, and Dance* (p. 71). Annual convention, Detroit, MI.

Purpose: To assess attentional style as it relates specifically to soccer performance.

Description: The 72-item TSAS contains the six scales of Nideffer's (1976) TAIS, but is operationally defined to soccer. These scales include broad external focus, broad internal focus, overload external focus, overload internal focus, narrow effective focus, and underinclusive focus. Participants respond to each item using a 5-point ordinal scale, with the anchorings *never* to *always*.

Construction: Not discussed.

Reliability: Alpha internal consistency coefficients ranged from .67 to .83 across the six subscales (*n*=104). Test-retest reliability coefficients ranged from .81 to .92.

Validity: The TSAS more effectively discriminated between high- and low-ability soccer players than did Nideffer's (1976) more general Test of Attentional and Interpersonal Style.

Norms: Not cited. Psychometric data were based on 104 college soccer athletes.

**Availability: Contact A. Craig Fisher, Exercise and Sport Sciences Department, Ithaca College, Ithaca, NY 14850. (Phone # 607-274-3112; FAX # 607-274-1943; E-mail: cfisher@ithaca.edu)

References

Fisher, A. C. (1984). Specificity of attention in sport: The data speak clearly [Abstract]. *Proceedings of the Canadian Society of Psychomotor Learning and Sport Psychology annual conference* (p. 3). Kingston, Ontario, Canada.

Nideffer, R. M. (1976). Test of Attentional and Interpersonal Style. *Journal of Personality and Social Psychology, 34,* 397-404.

Wilson, V. E., & Parolini, J. (1984). Assessment and training of soccer players [Abstract]. *Proceedings of the Canadian Society of Psychomotor Learning and Sport Psychology annual conference* (p. 5). Kingston, Ontario, Canada.

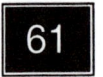

*The Basketball Concentration Survey (BCS)

Thomas A. Bergandi

Source: Bergandi, T. A., Shryock, M. G., & Titus, T. G. (1990). The Basketball Concentration Survey: Preliminary development and validation. *The Sport Psychologist, 4,* 119-129.

Purpose: To identify a basketball athlete's strengths and weaknesses in attention or concentration.

Description: The BCS is a 59-item sport-specific version of Nideffer's (1976) Test of Attention and Interpersonal Style (TAIS). The items of seven subscales of the TAIS (broad-external; broad-internal; narrow-attention; overload-external; overload internal; reduced-attention; and information processing) were converted so as to be appropriate for basketball.

Construction: Each of the 59 items constituting the BCS was revised with a "...strong effort to maintain as much of the original grammatical structure and syntax as possible" (p. 121) of the TAIS. Two coaches and two players then critiqued each item based on relevance to basketball.

Reliability: Cronbach alpha internal consistency coefficients ranged from .45 (reduced-attention) to .85 (narrow-attention) among 20 male and 23 female college basketball players. One-month test-retest reliability coefficients ranged from .75 (overload-external; reduced-attention) to .89 (narrow-attention) among these athletes.

Validity: Concurrent validity was demonstrated, in part, by the statistically significant correlation coefficients between these basketball athletes' scores on three subscales of the BCS and their corresponding scores on the Sport Competition Anxiety Test. Predictive validity was supported in that these athletes' scores on the "ineffective attention factor" (derived from three BCS subscale scores) correlated with seven basketball performance assessments.

Norms: Not cited. The psychometric data reported were based on the responses of 20 male members of two different intercollegiate basketball teams and 23 female members of two intercollegiate teams.

**Availability: Contact Thomas A. Bergandi, Department of Psychology, Spalding University, 851 South Fourth Street, Louisville, KY 40203. (Phone # 502-585-9911; FAX # 502-585-7156)

References

Nideffer, R. M. (1976). Test of Attention and Interpersonal Style. *Journal of Personality and Social Psychology, 34,* 397-404.

*Wendi, R., & Vealey, R. S. (1992). Attention in sport: Measurement issues, psychological concomitants, and the prediction of performance [Abstract]. *Proceedings of the Association for the Advancement of Applied Sport Psychology* (p. 89). Colorado Springs, CO.

Chapter 5

Attitudes Toward Exercise and Physical Activity

Tests in this chapter assess attitudes of children, college students, physical education teachers, and other groups toward the values of participating in exercise and related physical activities. Enjoyment of physical activity, attraction to being physically active, pathological attitudes toward exercise, and the attitudinal beliefs among nonexercisers are also evaluated.

62 *Attitude Strength Scale [ASS]
Yannis Theodorakis

Source: Theodorakis, Y. (1994). Planned behavior, attitude strength, role identity, and the prediction of exercise behavior. *The Sport Psychologist, 8,* 149-165.

Purpose: To examine attitudes towards exercise within a multicomponents structure.

Description: The Attitude Strength scale examines six strength-related attitude dimensions: importance, confidence, certainty, centrality, skill, and knowledge. For example, respondents are asked to rate "How certain are you about regular participation in the program of the gym during the next two months?" using a 5-point ordinal scale with the anchorings *very certain-very uncertain*. The Attitude Strength scale contains nine items.

Construction: Items for the Attitude Strength scale were derived from an extensive review of the literature (Y. Theodorakis, personal communication, March 29, 1996).

Reliability: A Cronbach alpha coefficient (N=395) of .90 was reported.

Validity: A factor analysis (varimax rotation) supported the unidimensionality of the Attitude Strength scale among 395 exercise participants. A single factor emerged from the analysis accounting for 55.1% of the total variance. In an earlier pilot research study, it was found that 230 high school students' responses to the Attitude Strength scale were correlated with intentions to participate in exercise (r=.75) and actual participation in physical activities (r=.35). In the current investigation, it was found that participants' (N=395) responses to the Attitude Strength scale were predictive of exercise intention and exercise behavior (i.e., the total number of hours exercised in each of 2 months).

Norms: Not cited. Psychometric data were reported for 395 female exercise participants (M age= 29.27 years; SD= 8.75) who were selected, using stratified random sampling techniques, from 50 exercise classes in four fitness clubs in Salonika, Greece.

112

Availability: Contact Yannis Theodorakis, Department of Physical Education and Sport Science, Democritus University of Thrace, 69100, Komotini, Greece. (Phone # +0531 27192; FAX # +0531 33582). Items can also be found in the second reference listed below.

References

*Theodorakis, Y., & Bagiatis, K. (1995, July). Predicting and understanding physical education student's career orientations: Application of planned behavior, role-identity and attitude strength theories. In R. Vanfraechem-Raway and Y. Vanden Auweele (Eds.), *Proceedings of the IXth European Congress on Sport Psychology* (pp. 493-500). Brussels, Belgium.

*Theodorakis, Y., Bagiatis, K., & Goudas, M. (1995). Attitudes toward teaching individuals with disabilities: Application of planned behavior theory. *Adapted Physical Activity Quarterly, 12,* 151-160.

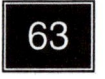

63 Attitude Toward Physical Activity Inventory(ATPA)

Gerald S. Kenyon

Source: Kenyon, G. S. (1968). Six scales for assessing attitude toward physical activity. *Research Quarterly, 39,* 566-574.

Purpose: To assess the perceived instrumental value held for physical activity.

Description: The ATPA assesses values held for physical activity participation in terms of physical activity as a social experience, as a catharsis, as a form of health and fitness, as the pursuit of vertigo, as an aesthetic experience, and as an ascetic experience. Both Likert and semantic differential versions of the ATPA are available.

Construction: The construct validities of two initial conceptual models characterizing the perceived instrumental (satisfaction) values held for physical activity were examined based on the factor analyses of the responses of independent samples (n=756 college students; n=100 college students; n=176 college students) to 73 Likert-type attitude statements. Partial support was found for the second conceptual model in terms of physical activity as a social experience, as a form of health and fitness, as the pursuit of vertigo, and as an aesthetic experience, but not as a recreational or competitive experience.

A third model, in which the subdomains of physical activity as an ascetic experience and as a catharsis were added, was examined based on the responses of 355 male and 215 female college students to 42 Likert-type items thought to be representative of each subdomain. Separate inventories for men and women were developed.

Reliability: Hoyt reliability (internal consistency) coefficients ranged from .70 (social experience) to .89 (pursuit of vertigo) among 215 female and 353 male college students.

Validity: The construct validity of the third model was support through factor analyses. Five of the six scales discriminated between appropriate high and low preference groups in terms of values held for physical activity.

Norms: Not presented. Psychometric data cited were based on the responses of independent samples of 200 to 360 male and female college students.

Availability: Contact Gerald Kenyon, Department of Sociology, University of Lethbridge, 4401 University Drive, Lethbridge, Alberta, Canada T1K3M4. (Phone 403-329-2551)

References

*Dotson, C. O., & Stanley, W. J. (1972). Values of physical activity perceived by male university students. *Research Quarterly, 43,* 148-156.

Farmer, R. J. (1992). Surfing: Motivations, values, and culture. *Journal of Sport Behavior, 15,* 241-257.

*Hallinan, C. J., Snyder, E. E., Drowatzky, J. N., & Ashby, A. A. (1990). Values held by prospective coaches towards women's sport participation. *Journal of Sport Behavior, 13,* 167-180.

*Martindale, E., Devlin, S., & Vyse, S. A. (1990). Participation in college sports: Motivational differences. *Perceptual and Motor Skills, 71,* 1139-1150.

*Milner, E. K., & Baker, J. A. W. (1985). Attitude changes among male and female high school athletes toward physical activity as a result of a one-week training programme in a summer sports camp setting. *Carnegie Research Reports, 1*(7), 12-17.

Nahas, M. V. (1992). Knowledge and attitudes changes of low-fit college students following a short-term fitness education program. *The Physical Educator, 49,* 152-159.

*Onifade, S. A. (1985). Relationship among attitude, physical activity behavior and physical activity belief of Nigerian students toward physical activity. *International Journal of Sport Psychology, 16,* 183-192, 1985.

*Singer, R., Eberspaecher, H., Rehs, H-J., & Boss Kl. (1978). Experience with a German version of the Kenyon-Scale (ATPA). In U. Simri (Ed.), *Proceedings of the*

International Symposium on Psychological Assessment in Sport (pp. 171-180). Netanya, Israel: Wingate Institute for Physical Education and Sport.

*Smoll, F. L., Schutz, R. W., Wood, T. M., & Cunningham, J. K. (1979). Parent-child relationships regarding physical activity attitudes and behaviors. In G. C. Roberts and K. M. Newell (Eds.), *Psychology of motor behavior and sport-1978* (pp. 131-143) Champaign, IL: Human Kinetics Publishers.

*Williams, L. R. T., & Coldicott, A. G. (1982). High school students: Their self-esteem, body esteem and attitudes toward physical activity. *New Zealand Journal of Health, Physical Education, and Recreation, 15,* 62-65.

*Yoo, J. (1993). Analyses of multidimensional factors influencing adherence to exercise. *Proceedings of the Eighth World Congress of Sport Psychology* (pp. 906-910). Lisbon, Portugal.

64 [Attitude Toward Warm-Ups Scale] [AWS]
Judith L. Smith and Margaret F. Bozymowski

Source: Smith, J. L., & Bozymowski, M. F. (1965). Effect of attitude toward warm-ups on motor performance. *Research Quarterly, 36,* 78-85.

Purpose: To evaluate attitudes of college women toward the value of the warm-up prior to motor performance.

Description: The scale contains 34 items. Participants respond using a 5-point Likert scale.

Construction: Responses to 42 statements pertaining to warm-ups in relation to performance, endurance, injury, fatigue, and efficiency while participating in sports were evaluated among 200 college women using the Flanagan Index of Discrimination. A total of 34 items were retained.

Reliability: A coefficient of equivalence of .94 was reported among 100 college women.

Validity: Discriminant validity was supported in that college women (n=86) with more favorable attitudes toward warm-up performed better in an obstacle race than did women with less favorable attitudes, when warm-ups were given prior to the race.

Norms: Not reported. Psychometric data reported were based on the responses of 186 college women.

Availability: The scale is presented in the original *Source*.

 **[Attitudes Toward Exercise and Physical Activity] [AEPA]**
Barry D. McPherson and M. S. Yuhasz

Source: McPherson, B. D., & Yuhasz, M. S. (1968). An inventory for assessing men's attitudes toward exercise and physical activity. *Research Quarterly, 39,* 218-220.

Purpose: To assess attitudes of individuals toward exercise and physical activity.

Description: The attitude inventory contains 50 items. Participants respond using a 5-point Likert scale.

Construction: The investigators compiled a series of statements depicting common opinions, beliefs, attitudes, and fallacies about exercise and physical activity. Statements that appeared irrelevant or ambiguous were discarded.

Reliability: A split-half odd-even corrected internal consistency coefficient of .95 was obtained among 25 male physical education teachers. A test-retest reliability coefficient ($n=25$) of .92 was reported across a 7-day interval.

Validity: A *t*-test indicated that the inventory successfully discriminated between male physical education teachers ($n=25$) and a group of male teachers ($n=20$) identified by the physical education teachers as having unfavorable attitudes toward exercise and physical activity.

Norms: Not cited.

Availability: See McPherson, B. D. (1965). *The psychological effects of exercise for normal and post-cardiac males.* Unpublished master's thesis, University of Western Ontario, London, Ontario, Canada. (Available through interlibrary loan)

Reference

*McPherson, B. D., Paivio, A., Yuhasz, M. S., Rechnitzer, P. A., Pickard, H. A., & Lefcoe, N. M. (1967). Psychological effects of an exercise program for post-infarct and normal adult men. *The Journal of Sports Medicine and Physical Fitness, 7,* 95-102.

*[Attitudes Toward Exercise Questionnaire] [ATEQ]
Mark H. Anshel

Source: Anshel, M. H. (1991). A psycho-behavioral analysis of addicted versus non-addicted male and female exercisers. *Journal of Sport Behavior, 14,* 145-154.

Purpose: To assess participants' attitudes and beliefs about their exercise-related habits and behavioral tendencies.

Description: The ATEQ contains four content areas: (a) pre-exercise affect (e.g., "I feel the urge to exercise on a day-to-day basis"), (b) post-exercise affect (e.g., "I feel fatigued after a typical exercise session"), (c) feelings about missing exercise bouts (e.g, "If I do not exercise on a given day, I feel depressed"), and (d) physical and psychological responses to injury and illness (e.g., "I tend to miss a day of exercise if I do not feel well"). Each content area contains four items. Participants respond to each item from 1 (*not at all*) to 7 (*very much so*).

Construction: Items were derived from interviews with exercise participants and staff, from an examination of related literature, and from an evaluation of the feelings and behavioral tendencies of individuals characterized as positively addicted to exercise.

Reliability: Cronbach alpha internal consistency coefficients ($N=60$) were .81 (pre-exercise affect), .77 (post-exercise affect), .68 (feelings about missing exercise bouts), and .83 (physical and psychological responses to injury and illness).

Validity: Discriminant validity was supported in that participants categorized as addicted to exercise ($n=30$), when contrasted with participants who were not addicted ($n=30$), were more restless and stressed prior to exercising, were more depressed, anxious, and angry after missing a workout, and tended to ignore feelings of illness or injury.

Norms: Not cited. Psychometric data were reported for 30 males and 30 females (*M* age=27.8 years) exercising at a private health and fitness center in New South Wales, Australia.

**Availability: Contact Mark H. Anshel, Psychology Department, University of Wollongong, P. O. Box 1144, Wollongong, New South Wales, Australia 2522. (Phone # 61-42-213732; FAX # 61-42-214163; E-mail: m.anshel@uow.edu.au)

 **[Attitudes Toward Jogging Questionnaire] [AJQ]**
Patricia K. Riddle

Source: Riddle, P. K. (1980). Attitudes, beliefs, behavioral intentions, and behaviors of women and men toward regular jogging. *Research Quarterly for Exercise and Sport, 51,* 663-674.

Purpose: To assess attitudes toward and beliefs about jogging.

Description: The questionnaire was based on Fishbein's Behavioral Intention Model. The questionnaire contained 68 items, of which 19 items measured the beliefs an individual had about the consequences (advantages/disadvantages) of jogging, and 19 items assessed the evaluation of the consequences corresponding to those beliefs. Seven items measured beliefs about the expectations of those referents who might approve or disapprove of jogging regularly. In addition, 14 attitudinal items were included in the questionnaire. Participants respond to each of the 68 items using 7-point bipolar adjective scales that employed the semantic differential technique.

Construction: The questionnaire was based on the responses of 40 participants to a pilot study concerning beliefs about participation in regular jogging. The subject pool consisted of an equal number of female and male joggers and nonexercisers.

Reliability: Test-retest reliability coefficients (n=63) ranged from .72 to .87 across the four derived summary scores.

Validity: Discriminant validity was demonstrated in that joggers (n=100 males and 49 females) were more likely than nonexercisers (n=98 males and 49 females) to believe that regular jogging would have positive effects, and they evaluated being in good physical and mental condition more positively than did nonexercisers. Nonexercisers thought jogging required too much discipline, took too much time, and made them too tired. Furthermore, there was a positive relationship (r=.82) between the intention to jog and jogging behavior.

Norms: Not cited. Psychometric data were reported for 296 males and females, 30 years or older, who were either joggers (n=149) or nonexercisers (n=147).

Availability: Unknown. Test items are not available in the *Source*.

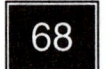 ## [Attitudinal Beliefs Regarding Exercise Questionnaire] [ABEQ]
Gaston Godin, Roy J. Shephard, and Angela Colantonio

Source: Godin, G., Shephard, R. J., & Colantonio, A. (1986). The cognitive profile of those who intend to exercise but do not. *Public Health Reports, 101*(5), 521-526.

Purpose: To examine among people who intend to but do not exercise their attitudinal beliefs about exercise, their evaluation of the associated consequences, and their normative beliefs and motivation to comply with these norms.

Description: The ABEQ contains 14 items focusing on one's exercise beliefs (B) and values (V) (e.g., "I think that participation in active sports or vigorous physical activities long enough to get sweaty at least twice a week in my leisure time during the next two months would help me look younger"). In addition, the ABEQ contains 5 items focusing on normative beliefs (NB) regarding exercise, and 5 items focusing on the motivation to comply (MC). Participants respond to all items on a 7-point scale (-3 to +3).

Construction: The theoretical frameworpp questionnaire was based on Fishbein-Ajzen's model of behavioral intentions.

Reliability: Internal consistency coefficients were reported as .71 (B), .74 (V), .67 (NB), and .72 (MC).

Validity: There were few differences on the ABEQ among individuals with positive intentions to exercise who eventually did exercise, versus individuals with positive intentions to exercise who did not then participate in exercise.

Norms: Not cited. Psychometric data were based on the responses of 163 male and female employees (*M* age = 39 years) obtained from a larger survey on corporate fitness.

**Availability: Contact Gaston Godin, School of Nursing, Laval University, Quebec, Canada G1K 7P4. (Phone # 418-656-7900; FAX # 418-656-7747; E-mail: gaston.godin@esi.ulaval.ca)

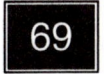

69 Children's Attitudes Toward Physical Activity Inventory (CATPA)
Robert W. Schutz, Frank L. Smoll, and Terry M. Wood

Source: Schutz, R. W., Smoll, F. L., Carre, F. A., & Mosher, R. E. (1985). Inventories and norms for children's attitudes toward physical activity. *Research Quarterly for Exercise and Sport, 56*, 256-265.

Purpose: To assess among children the perceived instrumental value held for physical activity.

Description: The CATPA utilizes a semantic differential format. Attitudes children hold regarding physical activity participation are assessed within seven subdomains or scales: physical activity as an aesthetic experience, as the pursuit of vertigo, as an ascetic experience, as a form of health and fitness, as a means of social growth, as a catharsis, and as a means of continuing social relations. Children are asked to respond to five bipolar adjectives on a 5-point scale for each of these seven domains. The health and fitness domain, although a unitary concept, is scored separately for Health & Fitness: Value and Health & Fitness: Enjoyment.

Construction: The original CAPTA (Simon & Smoll, 1974) was an adaption of Kenyon's (1968) semantic differential Attitudes toward Physical Activity (ATPA) inventory and was prepared for use with elementary school children. The current revised version is viewed as psychometrically superior and less time-consuming to administer, and is appropriate for individuals from ages 12 to adulthood (R. W. Schutz, personal communication, March 28, 1990).

Reliability: Alpha reliability coefficients (n=1,038 males and females-grade 7; n=857 males and females-grade 11) ranged from .76 (Health) to .91 (Aesthetic) for Grade 7 participants, and from .77 (Health) to .94 (aesthetic) for Grade 11 participants. Reliability coefficients did not statistically differ as a function of gender. Test stability coefficients (Schutz & Smoll, 1986) ranged from .80 to .87 across a 6-month test-retest interval among grades 10 and 11 students.

Validity: The construct validity of the seven hypothesized attitude domains was supported through principal component factor analyses among the Grade 7 (n=1,038) and Grade 11 (n=857) participants. However, among 127 boys and 137 girls in grades 4, 5, and 6, there was no evidence of a relationship between their attitudes toward physical activity and motor skill (running, jumping, and throwing). Furthermore, the correlation coefficients between attitudes and self-reported levels of actual participation in physical activity, although statistically significant, were low.

Norms: Psychometric data were reported for 1,038 males and females in Grade 7, and 857 males and females in Grade 11 from the Canadian province of British Columbia. Stratified random sampling techniques were used to select these subjects from 67 schools in the province.

**Availability: Contact Robert W. Schutz, School of Human Kinetics, University of British Columbia, 210 War Memorial Gym, 6081

University Blvd., Vancouver, British Columbia, CanadaV6T 1Z1. (Phone # 604-822-2457; FAX # 604-822-6842; E-mail: rschutz@unixg.ubc.ca)

References

*Birtwistle, G. E., & Brodie, D. A. (1991). Canonical relationships between two sets of variables representing the CATPA subdomains and health-related fitness. *International Journal of Physical Education, 28*(1), 25.

Bocket, T. J. (1995). Differences in physical activity attitudes and fitness knowledge between aerobic capacity standard, sex, and grade groups [Abstract]. *Research Quarterly for Exercise & Sport, 66* (Suppl.), A-73.

Brodie, D. A., & Birtwistle, M. A. (1990). Children's attitudes to physical activity, exercise, health and fitness before and after a health related fitness measurement. *International Journal of Physical Education, 27*(2), 10-14.

Kenyon, G. S. (1968). Six scales for assessing attitude toward physical activity. *Research Quarterly, 39,* 566-574.

*Martin, C. J., & Williams, L. R. T. (1985). A psychometric analysis of an instrument for assessing children's attitudes toward physical activity. *Journal of Human Movement Sciences, 11,* 89-104.

*Mott, D. S., Virgilio, S. J., Warren, B. L., & Berenson, G. S. (1991). Effectiveness of a personalized fitness module on knowledge, attitude, and cardiovascular endurance of fifth-grade students: "Heart Smart." *Perceptual and Motor Skills, 73,* 847-858.

*Patterson, P., & Faucette, N. (1990). Attitudes toward physical activity of fourth and fifth grade boys and girls. *Research Quarterly for Exercise and Sport, 61,* 415-418.

*Politino, V., & Smith, S. L. (1989). Attitude toward physical activity and self-concept of emotionally disturbed and normal children. *Adapted Physical Activity Quarterly, 6,* 371-378.

*Schutz, R. W., & Smoll, F. L. (1985). The (in)stability of attitudes toward physical activity during childhood and adolescence. In B. D. McPherson (Ed.), *Sport and aging* (pp. 187-197). Champaign, IL: Human Kinetics.

*Schutz, R. W., Smoll, F. L., & Wood, T. M. (1981). A psychometric analysis of an inventory for assessing children's attitudes toward physical activity. *Journal of Sport Psychology, 4,* 321-344.

*Simon, J. A., & Smoll, F. L. (1974). An instrument for assessing children's attitudes toward physical activity. *Research Quarterly, 45,* 407-415.

*Theodorakis, Y., Doganis, G., & Bagiatis, K. (1992). Attitudes toward physical activity in female physical fitness program participants. *International Journal of Sport Psychology, 23,* 262-273.

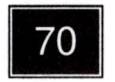

70 *Children's Attraction to Physical Activity Scale (CAPA)

Robert J. Brustad

Source: Brustad, R. J. (1993). Who will go out and play? Parental and psychological influences on children's attraction to physical activity. *Pediatric Exercise Science, 5,* 210-223.

Purpose: To measure children's attraction to physical activity or their desire to be physically active.

Description: The CAPA contains 22 items and five subscales: (a) liking of vigorous exercise, (b) liking of games and sports, (c) perceived importance of exercise to health, (d) peer acceptance in games and sports, and (e) fun of physical exertion. Items are presented in a structured-alternative format, and children respond to each item using a four-choice response format.

Construction: Open-ended group discussions with third- and fourth-grade children in their physical education classes served to identify various dimensions of physical activity that children viewed as attractive or unattractive. These dimensions included liking/disliking: (a) vigorous physical activity and exercise, (b) competitive games and sports, and (c) peer interactions in games and sports, as well as differences in the perceived importance of health benefits of physical activity.

Items were then developed based on these dimensions using a structured-alternative format. A total of 34 items were pilot tested with children enrolled in five physical education classes. Items exhibiting high mean scores and/or low variability were deleted leading to the retention of 22 items.

Exploratory principal component factor analysis (N=231), using both orthogonal and oblique rotations, supported a five-factor structure. These five factors accounted for 53% of the variance (varimax rotation) in children's responses to the items of the CAPA.

Reliability: Cronbach alpha internal consistency coefficients (N=231) ranged from .62 to .78 for the five subscales of the CAPA. The author reported (R. J. Brustad, personal communication, April 4, 1996) acceptable internal consistency coefficients (.70-.78) for four of the subscales among fourth- through seventh-grade children; the perceived importance of exercise to health subscale, however, has evidenced low (.44) internal consistency.

The author also reported that test-retest reliability coefficients exceeded .80 for third-grade children across a 2-week period (Brustad, 1991).

Validity: The author reported (R. J. Brustad, personal communication, April 4, 1996) that predictive validity of the CAPA has been supported by research that indicates that higher levels of attraction to physical activity are significantly related to more extensive sport involvement (Brustad, 1991) and to higher physical fitness levels (Brustad, 1994).

Norms: Not available. The author noted (R. J. Brustad, personal communication, April 4, 1996) that research indicates that separate norms will be necessary according to age, gender, and perhaps, ethnicity or socioeconomic status; further, the CAPA is intended for use among children in the third through seventh grades.

**Availability: Contact Robert J. Brustad, School of Kinesiology and Physical Education, University of Northern Colorado, Greeley, CO 80639. (Phone #970-351-1737; FAX # 970-351-1762; E-mail: bbrustad@goldng8.univnorthco.edu)

References

*Brustad, R. J. (1991, June). *Attitudinal and self-perception correlates of children's physical activity and sport involvement.* Paper presented at the annual conference of the North American Society for the Psychology of Sport and Physical Activity, Pacific Grove, CA.

*Brustad, R. J. (1994, April). *Psychological correlates of children's physical activity.* Paper presented at the annual conference of the American Alliance for Health, Physical Education, Recreation, and Dance, Denver, CO.

*Brustad, R. J. (in press). Attraction to physical activity in urban children: Parental socialization influences. *Research Quarterly for Exercise and Sport.*

*Walling, M. D., & Duda, J. L. (1992). The relationship between goal orientations and positive attitudes towards sport and exercise among young athletes [Abstract]. *Proceedings of the Association for the Advancement of Applied Sport Psychology annual convention* (p. 128). Colorado Springs, CO.

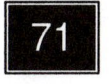

71 *Exercise Decisional Balance Measure [EDB]

Bess H. Marcus, William Rakowski, and Joseph S. Rossi

Source: Marcus, B. H., Rakowski, W., & Rossi, J. S. (1992). Assessing motivational readiness and decision making for exercise. *Health Psychology, 11,* 257-261.

Purpose: To evaluate an individual's perceptions regarding the benefits and detriments of exercising.

Description: The EDB contains 10 "pro" items (e.g., "I would feel more confident if I exercise regularly" and 6 "con" items (e.g., "Regular exercise would take too much of my time"). Participants respond to how important each item is with respect to their decision to exercise or not to exercise using a 5-point Likert-type scale with the anchorings 1 (*not at all important*) to 5 (*extremely important*).

Construction: A small group of male or female regular exercisers and nonexercisers was used to generate an initial pool of 75 items reflecting their perceptions of the positive (pros) and negative (cons) aspects of exercise. After reviewing the item pool for clarity and representativeness, and to eliminate redundancy among items, 40 items were retained. Seventeen items (3 pros, 14 cons) were eliminated due to excessive positive or negative responses (N=778).

Reliability: Cronbach alpha internal consistency coefficients of .95 (Pro) and .79 (Con) were reported.

Validity: Exploratory principal components factor analysis (N= 778) with varimax rotation led to the retention of 16 items. These 16 items loaded on either a pro or con factor accounting for 60.4% of the variance.

Norms: Not cited. Psychometric data were reported for 778 employees of four worksites. Fifty-four percent of the sample was female, and the average age of participants was 41.5 years (SD= 11.0 years).

Availability: Contact Bess H. Marcus, Division of Behavioral Medicine, The Miriam Hospital, Brown University School of Medicine, RISE Building, 164 Summit Avenue, Providence, RI 02906. (Phone # 401-331-8500, Ext. 3707; FAX # 401-331-2453). The items are also listed in the *Source*.

References

*Marcus, B. H., Eaton, C. A., Rossi, J. S., & Harlow, L. L. (1994). Self efficacy, decision-making, and stages of change: An integrative model of physical exercise. *Journal of Applied Social Psychology, 24,* 489-508.

*Marcus, B. H., & Owen, N. (1992). Motivational readiness, self efficacy and decision-making for exercise. *Journal of Applied Social Psychology, 22,* 3-16.

*Marcus, B. H., Pinto, B. M., & Simkin, L. R., Audrain, J. E., & Taylor, E. R. (1994). Application of theoretical models to exercise behavior among employed women. *American Journal of Health Promotion, 9*(1), 49-55.

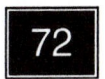 ## *Generalized Attitude to Physical Activity Scale (GAPAS)

Nigel Gleeson, Bill Tancred, and Michael Banks

Source: Gleeson, N., Tancred, B., & Banks, M. (1989). Psycho-biological factors influencing habitual activities in male and female adolescents. *Physical Education Review, 12,* 110-124.

Purpose: To assess attitudes toward physical activity.

Description: The GAPAS is a 24-item scale "...covering beliefs about physical activity, commitment to exercise, intentions to exercise and attitude to competition...." (p. 111). Participants respond to each item on a 5-point Likert scale with the anchorings 1 (*strongly disagree*) to 5 (*strongly agree*).

Construction: Not discussed.

Reliability: A Cronbach alpha reliability coefficient of .88 was reported.

Validity: A factor analysis generated five factors accounting for 46% of the variance; the first factor accounted for 23% of the variance. Further, stepwise multiple discriminant analysis indicated that the GAPAS was able to discriminate between physically inactive (n=83) and active young females (n=18).

Norms: Descriptive statistics were cited for 412 male or female students (M age=15.25 years) in Year 4 at four secondary schools in Sheffield, South Yorkshire, England.

**Availability: Contact Bill Tancred, Faculty of Leisure and Tourism, Buckinghamshire College of Higher Education, Wellesbourne Campus, Kingshill Road, High Wycombe, Buckinghamshire HP13 5BB, England.

(Phone # 01494 603042; FAX # 01494 465432; E-mail: wtancr01@buckscol.ac.uk)

73 [Perceptions of Movement Activities Questionnaire] [PMAQ]
Linda L. Bain

Source: Bain, L. L. (1979). Perceived characteristics of selected movement activities. *Research Quarterly, 50,* 565-573.

Purpose: To assess individual differences in perceptions of the meaning of various physical activities.

Description: Participants respond to one or more physical activities related to sport, dance or exercise using a semantic differential technique. The participant must differentiate between 21 bipolar adjectives using a 9-point ordinal scale.

Construction: In a pilot study, 67 college students rated 25 physical activities on 21 word pairs. These word pairs were derived from a literature review of conceptual models characterizing values or motives for participating in physical activity. A factor analysis of their responses led to the retention of four factors accounting for 38.7% of the variance. Only word pairs loading .40 or greater on one of these factors were retained.

Reliability: Not reported.

Validity: Alpha and incomplete principal components factor solutions led to the retention of seven factors accounting for 37.19% of the variance.

Norms: Psychometric data were presented for 1,435 students enrolled in the physical education basic instructional program at a large urban university in the southwestern United States.

**Availability: Contact Linda L. Bain, Provost and Vice President for Academic Affairs, San Jose State University, One Washington Square, San Jose, CA 95192-0020. (Phone # 408-924-2400; FAX # 408-924-2410; E mail: lbain@sjsuvm1.sjsu.edu)

74 | *Physical Activity Enjoyment Scale (PACES)
Deborah Kendzierski and Kenneth J. DeCarlo

Source: Kendzierski, D., & DeCarlo, K. J. (1991). Physical Activity Enjoyment Scale: Two validation studies. *Journal of Sport & Exercise Psychology, 13,* 50-64.

Purpose: To assess the "...extent to which an individual experiences a particular physical activity as enjoyable at a given point in time...." (p. 52)

Description: The PACES is an 18-item scale that employs bipolar adjectives in a 7-point semantic differential format. For example, participants are asked to respond to how they feel, at the moment, about the physical activity they are doing using bipolar adjectives such as "I enjoy it- I hate it"; "it's very invigorating- it's not at all invigorating"; and "it's very pleasant- it's very unpleasant."

Construction: A preliminary set of 39 seven-point items evolved from a review of the exercise adherence/enjoyment literature; an examination of dictionary and thesaurus entries; discussions between test authors about affective experiences regarding physical activity (including those informally reported by undergraduate student research subjects and acquaintances); and formal interviews of 16 individuals (*M* age=41.50 years; *SD*= 14.59) regarding their likes/dislikes about physical activity, in general, and about physical activities they did for exercise. Three experts on exercise adherence evaluated each item for construct relevance leading to the retention of 16 items. Three additional items were included based on the unanimous recommendations of these experts. Item analyses of students' (*n*=24 females; *n*=39 males) responses lead to the retention of 18 of 19 items.

Reliability: Cronbach alpha coefficients of .93 (*N*=30 students), .93 (*N*=33 students), and .96 (*N*=37 undergraduate students) were reported in separate investigations. Intraclass correlations (*N*=37) of .60 and .93 were reported for the physical activities of bicycling and jogging on a minitrampoline, respectively, supporting test-retest reliability.

Validity: Participants' (*N*=44 undergraduate students) PACES scores correlated negatively with their proneness toward boredom while riding

128

an exercise bicycle in a sterile laboratory environment. Furthermore, the construct validity of PACES was supported by demonstrating that individuals (N=44) who listened to music while exercising on a stationary bicycle reported enjoying their exercise session more than when exercising on the bicycle without music. In a further study, when participants (N=37 undergraduate students) were permitted to self-select either a bicycle or minitrampoline for exercise, their choice was compatible with the activity they rated as most enjoyable, based on their PACES scores for that activity.

Norms: Not cited. Psychometric data were reported for four studies employing male or female undergraduate students.

Availability: Contact Deborah Kendzierski, Department of Psychology, Villanova University, Villanova, PA 19805. (Phone # 610-519-4753)

References
*Crocker, P. R. E. (1992). Measuring affective states after youth physical activity: A comparison of PACES and PANAS measures [Abstract]. *Proceedings of the Association for the Advancement of Applied Sport Psychology annual convention.* (p. 181). Colorado Springs, CO.
*Crocker, P. R. E., Bouffard, M., & Gessaroli, M. E. (1995). Measuring enjoyment in youth sport settings: A confirmatory factor analysis of the Physical Activity Enjoyment Scale. *Journal of Sport & Exercise Psychology, 17,* 200-205.
Ekkekakis, P., & Zervas, Y. (1993). The effect of a single bout of aerobic exercise on mood: Co-examination of biological and psychological paramenters in a controlled field study. *Proceedings of the Eighth World Congress of Sport Psychology* (pp. 543-547). Lisbon, Portugal.
Zervas, Y., Ekkekakis, P., Emmanuel, C., Psychoudaki, M., & Kakkos, V. (1993). The acute effects of increasing levels of aerobic exercise intensity on mood states. *Proceedings of the Eighth World Congress of Sport Psychology* (pp. 620-624). Lisbon, Portugal.

75 | *[Physical Fitness Values Scale] [PFVS]
John E. Bezjak and Jerry W. Lee

Source: Bezjak, J. E., & Lee, J. W. (1990). Relationship of self-efficacy and locus of control constructs in predicting college students' physical fitness behaviors. *Perceptual and Motor Skills, 71,* 499-508.

Purpose: To assess participants' "...general values held toward health related physical fitness" (p. 502).

Description: The PFVS contains nine items. Individuals respond on a 6 point Likert scale, with the anchorings 1 (*strongly disagree*) to 6 (*strongly agree*), to items such as "Happiness is more important than physical fitness."

Construction: Adapted from a previous scale of terminal values.

Reliability: A Cronbach alpha internal consistency coefficient of .85 ($N=300$ approximate) was reported.

Validity: Not reported.

Norms: Not cited. Psychometric data were reported for approximately 300 undergraduate students ($n=161$ females; $n=139$ males), and descriptive statistics and psychometric data were reported for 211 undergraduate students ($n=114$ females; $n=97$ males). Participants were recruited from colleges and universities in the Riverside, California, area.

Availability: Contact John E. Bezjak, Department of Institutional Research, University of Phoenix, 4615 E. Elwood Street, Phoenix, AZ 85040.

Reference
*Bezjak, J. E., & Langga-Sharifi, E. (1991). Validation of the Physical Fitness Opinion Questionnaire against marathon performance. *Perceptual and Motor Skills, 73,* 993-994.

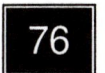 *Pictorial Risk-Taking Preference (PRTP)
Hezkiah Aharoni

Source: Aharoni, H. (1987, April). *The identification of risk-taking in children's movement patterns: Assessment and implications.* Paper presented at the American Alliance for Health, Physical Education, Recreation, and Dance annual convention, Las Vegas, NV.

Purpose: To assess the degree and willingness of children, ages 3-6 years, to take physical risks.

Description: The PRTP includes seven illustrated pictures of seven different gross motor activities that evidence varied levels of physical risk:

sliding down a wooden slide, jumping off a gymnastic box to the floor, playing with a ball, walking a balance beam, jumping off the top of three steps forward to the ground, climbing a horizontal ladder, and walking an inclined board (bleacher attached to the wall). These seven pictures formed 10 pairs of pictures. One task in each pair had been previously rated by children as riskier than the others. One point is assigned if the child selects the risky task; 0 points are assigned if the child selects the less risky task. The author noted (H. Aharoni, personal communication, April 15, 1996) that the PRTP has two versions, one illustrated with a boy and the other with a girl, for the same identical gross motor activities described above.

Construction: A total of 44 boys and girls, ages 3-5, helped establish the content validity of the PRTP by rating the extent to which physical activity tasks presented in paired illustrations varied in perceived physical risk.

Reliability: A test-retest reliability coefficient of .77 was reported across a 1-3 week interval among 104 children. The author reported (personal communication, April 15, 1996) that the reliability coefficents were .72 for age 3, .81 for age 4, .72 for age 5, and .85 for age 6.

Validity: Correlation coefficients were used to establish criterion-related validity using various dependent variables. Children's ($N=104$) movement confidence scores, in which their performances on the seven motor tasks were videotaped, analyzed, and scored, correlated .48 with their responses to the PRTP, and .54 with the Life Preference (LP), which is the selection and preference among pairs of the actual tasks that were set up in the gymnasium (H. Aharoni, personal communication, April 15, 1996).

Norms: Not cited. Psychometric data were reported for 104 boys and girls, ages 3 to 6 years old, who lived in central Ohio. Pilot data to establish content validity were obtained from 44 boys and girls, ages 3 to 5 years old, who were enrolled at The Ohio State University Day Care Center.

**Availability: Contact Hezi Aharoni, The Zinman College of Physical Education, Wingate Institute, Netanya, 42902 Israel (Phone # 972-9-639222; FAX # 972-9-650960)

Reference

*Aharoni, H. (1988, December). *Assessment of children's risk taking behavior as reflected in motor activity.* Paper presented at the International Early Childhood Conference, Washington, DC.

*Role Identity Scale [RIS]
Yannis Theodorakis

77

Source: Theodorakis, Y. (1994). Planned behavior, attitude strength, role identity, and the prediction of exercise behavior. *The Sport Psychologist, 8,* 149-165.

Purpose: To assess one's social role identification with respect to participation in an exercise program.

Description: The RIS contains seven items. For example, participants are asked to respond on a 5-point Likert scale to "I would feel a loss if I gave up exercising during the next 2 months" or "To participate in the program of this gym during the next 2 months is an important part of myself."

Construction: Some of the items were derived from previous literature (Y. Theodorakis, personal communication, March 29, 1996).

Reliability: A Cronbach alpha internal consistency coefficient ($N=395$) of .86 was reported.

Validity: An initial factor analysis (varimax rotation) supported the unidimensionality of the Role Identity scale. One factor emerged from the factor analysis accounting for 55.3% of the total variance. In addition, hierarchical regression analysis revealed that participants' responses to the Role Identity scale were predictive of their ($N=395$) intentions to exercise and exercise behavior (i.e., the number of hours exercised during each of two months).

Norms: Not presented. Psychometric data were based on the responses of 395 females (M age= 29.27 years; SD=8.75) who were selected using stratified random sampling procedures from 50 classes in four fitness clubs in Salonika, Greece.

132

Availability: Contact Yiannis Theodorakis, Department of Physical Education and Sport Science, Democritus University of Thrace, 69100, Komotini, Greece. (Phone # +0531 27192; FAX # +0531 33582). The items can also be found in the second reference source listed below.

References

*Theodorakis, Y., & Bagiatis, K. (1995, July). Predicting and understanding physical education student's career orientations: Applications of planned behavior, role-identity and attitude strength theories. In R. Vanfraechem-Raway and Y. Vanden Auweele (Eds.), *Proceedings of the IXth European Congress on Sport Psychology* (pp. 403-500). Brussels, Belgium.

*Theodorakis, Y., Bagiatis, K., & Goudas, M. (1995). Attitudes toward teaching individuals with disabilities: Application of planned behavior theory. *Adapted Physical Activity Quarterly, 12,* 151-160.

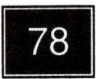

*The Exercise Salience Scale (TESS)
Julian Morrow and Philip Harvey

Source: Morrow, J., & Harvey, P. (1991). Analysis of data derived from the Exercise Salience Scale (TESS) [Abstract]. *Proceedings of the Association for the Advancement of Applied Sport Psychology annual convention* (p. 108). Savannah, GA.

Purpose: "To examine pathological attitudes towards and inappropriate use of exercise" (p. 108).

Description: TESS is a 40-item inventory focusing on inappropriate prioritization, compulsivity, mood states, and so forth. Participants respond to each item on a 4-point scale with the anchorings 0 (*not at all*) to 3 (*extremely*). Scores range from 0 to 120 with a higher score indicating greater dependence on exercise.

Construction: Not discussed

Reliability: A Cronbach alpha internal consistency coefficient of .93 was reported.

Validity: Not discussed.

Norms: Not cited. Descriptive data are reported for 50 females and 50 males who registered for the 1990 New York Marathon and for 720 individuals who completed the TESS when it was published in *American Health* magazine.

Availability: Contact Julian Morrow, John Jay College, City University of New York, 899 10th Ave., New York, NY 10019.

Chapter 6

Attitudes/Values Toward Sport

Tests in this chapter assess the attitudes of sport participants towards the values of sport participation, professional versus play orientations expressed during sport participation, sportsmanship attitudes, and the values youth sport coaches hold regarding the potential outcomes of competition for children. Tests assess children's beliefs about the purposes of sport, perceptions of coaching behaviors, attitudes toward sport officials, and the values of professional sport to the community as perceived by spectators.

Tests in this chapter also assess role expectancies for female versus male participation in sport. Attitudes toward female involvement in sport and perceived and experienced role conflict among female athletes are also evaluated.

79 [Athlete Sex Role Conflict Inventory] [ASRCI]
George H. Sage and Sheryl Loudermilk

Source: Sage, G. H., & Loudermilk, S. (1979). The female athlete and role conflict. *Research Quarterly, 50,* 88-96.

Purpose: To assess perceived and experienced role conflict among female athletes in enacting the roles of both female and female athlete.

Description: The 20-item inventory contains two parts, with the same 10 items used in both parts. The first part measures role conflict perception (RCP) and the second part measures role conflict experience (RCE). Content areas relate to attitudes of society toward females and athletic participation, physical appearance and motor skills that may be incompatible with femininity, and incompatibility of expectations of parents, friends, and others regarding sex roles and athlete roles. Participants respond to each item on the inventory using a 5-point ordinal scale.

Construction: Item content was partially derived from the literature on sex role stereotypes and the literature describing athletic role expectations. Other sources included interviews with female athletes and coaches. The content validity of the items was evaluated by professionals in sociology, psychology, and physical education.

Reliability: Test-retest reliability (*n*=24 female athletes) coefficients over a 2-to 3-week period were .72 for RCP and .76 for RCE.

Validity: Female athletes (*n*=30) differing on the Spence-Helmreich Attitudes Toward Women Scale also differed on RCP in that athletes with a traditional orientation toward women's role in society perceived greater role conflict in terms of involvement in athletics.

Norms: Psychometric data were presented for 268 collegiate female athletes from nine sports, representing 13 colleges.

**Availability: Contact George H. Sage, 1933-26th Avenue, Greeley, CO 80631 (Phone # 970-352-4611; FAX # 970-353-1908; E-mail: pdwd45a@prodigy.com)

[Attitudes of Athletes Toward Male Versus Female Coaches] [AAMFC]

Robert Weinberg and Margie Reveles

Source: Weinberg, R., Reveles, M., and Jackson, A. (1984). Attitudes of male and female athletes toward male and female coaches. *Journal of Sport Psychology, 6,* 448-453.

Purpose: To assess the attitudes and feelings of male and female athletes toward having a female coach versus a male coach.

Description: The athlete is presented a paragraph describing a male or female coach who (hypothetically) was to be the athlete's coach the following year. The athlete is asked to respond to 11 items using an 11-point Likert scale (with the anchorings *not at all* to *very much*). Examples of items include "I would like her as a coach" and "I could not take orders from him easily."

Construction: Not discussed.

Reliability: Test-retest reliability coefficients ($n=60$) were reported as .80 and .77 for the male and female questionnaires across a 2-week interval.

Validity: Construct validity was supported by demonstrating among 34 junior high, 27 high school, and 24 college basketball athletes that males displayed more negative attitudes toward female coaches than did females; however, male and female athletes did not differ in their view of male coaches.

Norms: Not cited. Test-retest reliability data were reported for an independent sample of 60 subjects.

Availability: Contact Robert Weinberg, Department of Physical Education, Health, and Sport Studies, Phillips Hall, Miami University, Oxford, OH 45056. (Phone # 513-529-2700; FAX # 513-529-5006; E-mail: rweinber@miamiu.muohio.edu)

81 [Attitudes to Male and Female Athletes Questionnaire] [AMFAQ]

Joan Vickers, Michael Lashuk, and Terry Taerum

Source: Vickers, J., Lashuk, M., & Taerum, T. (1980). Differences in attitude toward the concepts "male," "female," "male athlete," and "female athlete." *Research Quarterly for Exercise and Sport, 51,* 407-416.

Purpose: To assess attitudes toward the concepts *male, female, male athlete,* and *female athlete.*

Description: Participants respond to each of the four concepts (e.g., male athlete) using the semantic differential technique. A total of 14 bipolar adjective pairs are presented requiring a 7-point ordinal scale response for each pair.

Construction: The adjective pairs were selected based on a review of factor analytic studies of the dimensions of the semantic differential technique.

Reliability: Kuder Richardson-21 internal consistency coefficients ($n=132$ male and 132 female athletes) ranged from .75 for the term female to .82 for the term female athlete.

Validity: Analyses of variance supported differences between male and female participants on the evaluative and activity-potency dimensions identified through factor analyses. For example, females (but not males) perceive the concepts female athlete and male to be similar in the activity-potency dimension.

Norms: Not reported. Psychometric data were cited for 132 male and 132 female athletes representing independent samples of grades 7, 10, and university students.

Availability: Contact Joan Vickers, Faculty of Kinesiology, University of Calgary, 2500 University Drive, N. W., Calgary, Alberta, Canada, T2N 1N4. (Phone # 403-220-3420; FAX # 403-289-9117; E-mail: vickers@acs.ucalgary.ca)

82 *[Attitudes Toward Skiing Questionnaire] [ATSQ]

Yannis Theodorakis, Marios Goudas, and Haris Kouthouris

Source: Theordorakis, Y., Goudas, M., & Kouthouris, H. (1992). Change of attitudes toward skiing after participation in a skiing course. *Perceptual and Motor Skills, 75,* 272-274.

Purpose: To assess attitudes toward the sport of skiing.

Description: The ATSQ is a semantic differential test in which subjects respond using 12 bipolar adjective pairs (e.g., good-bad, exciting-calming, and so forth) to the stem "Participating in skiing is..."

Construction: Not discussed.

Reliability: A Cronbach alpha internal consistency coefficient of .74 was reported.

Validity: Construct validity was supported in that college students (N=50) evidenced increased positive attitudes toward skiing after completing a 5-week skiing module. Further, they had more positive attitudes toward skiing, based on ATSQ scores, than did students (N=34) who did not elect to participate in the skiing course.

Norms: Not cited. Psychometric data were reported for 84 college students.

**Availability: Contact Yannis Theodorakis, Department of Physical Education and Sports Sciences, Democritos University of Thrace, 69100, Komotini, Greece. (Phone # 0531 27192; FAX # 0531 33582).

83 [Attitudes Toward the Receipt of an Athletic Scholarship Questionnaire] [ARASQ]
Sharon A. Mathes, Shirley J. Wood, Charlene E. Christensen, and James E. Christensen

Source: Mathes, S. A., Wood, S. J., Christensen, C. E., & Christensen, J. E. (1979). An exploratory analysis of the attitudinal impact of awarding athletic scholarships to women. *Research Quarterly, 50,* 422-428.

Purpose: To assess the attitudes of female athletes toward receiving or not receiving an athletic scholarship.

Description: The questionnaire contains 86 items. Participants respond to each item using a 5-point Likert scale.

Construction: The items were derived from a literature review on cognitive dissonance theory.

Reliability: Alpha reliability coefficients (n=61 female athletes) of .84, .77, and .80 were reported for three derived factors.

Validity: Factor analysis led to the retention of three factors that centered on (a) effect of scholarships on the sport, (b) athletes' attitudes toward their coaches, and (c) athletes' attitudes about team relationships and individual performances.

Norms: Not cited. Psychometric data were reported for 61 female athletes representing 10 teams at one midwestern university.

Availability: Contact Sharon Mathes, Health and Human Performance, Iowa State University, 253 PEB, Ames, IA 50010. (Phone # 515-294-8766; FAX # 515-294-8740; E-mail: e2.sam@isumvs)

84 [Attitudes Toward the Referee Questionnaire] [ATRQ]

Jacques H. A. Van Rossum, C. R. Van der Togt, and H. A. Gootjes

Source: Van Rossum, J. H. A., Van der Togt, C. R., & Gootjes, H. A. (1984). The acceptance of referees' decisions in field hockey. *International Journal of Sports Medicine, 5* (Suppl. 1), 212-213.

Purpose: To examine the opinions held by referees and players regarding the practices of the referee in field hockey.

Description: The ATRQ contains 106 items. Cluster analysis identified 22 items (Cluster 1) focusing on "the degree to which the referee could be influenced" (p. 212) and 11 items (Cluster 2) focusing on "the influence of the referee" (p. 212) on the course of the game.

Construction: Not discussed.

Reliability: Kuder-Richardson (Formula 20) internal consistency coefficients were .75 and .69, for clusters 1 and 2, respectively.

Validity: Not cited.

Norms: Not presented. Psychometric data were based on the responses of 169 male and 47 female field hockey referees, and 154 male and 153 female field hockey players representing all levels of nationally organized field hockey competition in The Netherlands.

**Availability: Contact Jacques H. A. van Rossum, Vrije Universiteit, Faculty of Human Movement Sciences, Department of Movement Behavior, Van der Boechorststraat 9, 1081 BT Amsterdam, The Netherlands. (Phone # +31-20-444 8540; FAX # +31-20-444 5867)

[Attitudes Toward Women's Athletic Competition Scale] [AWACS]
Bea Harres

Source: Harres, B. (1968). Attitudes of students toward women's athletic competition. *Research Quarterly, 39,* 278-284.

Purpose: To examine the attitudes of male and female undergraduate students toward the desirability of intensive athletic competition for girls and women.

Description: The attitude inventory contains 38 items subdivided into the areas of sociocultural, mental-emotional, physical, and personality. Individuals respond to each item using a 5-point Likert scale.

Construction: Previous attitude scales were the basis for the initial development of 62 items that were pilot tested using 113 undergraduate students. Using Flanagan's index of discrimination, 38 items were retained.

Reliability: A corrected split-half odd-even internal consistency coefficient of .92 was reported among 100 undergraduate students.

Validity: Not discussed.

Norms: Not reported. Descriptive and psychometric data were cited for 284 undergraduate students (*n*=131 males and *n*=153 females) attending the University of California at Santa Barbara.

Availability: Unknown. Test items are not identified in the *Source.*

Children's Attitudes Toward Female Involvement in Sport Questionnaire (CATFIS)
Rosemary Selby and John H. Lewko

Source: Selby, R., & Lewko, J. H. (1976). Children's attitudes toward females in sports: Their relationship with sex, grade, and sports participation. *Research Quarterly, 47,* 455-463.

Purpose: To measure grade school childrens' attitudes toward female involvement in sports.

Description: The CATFIS is a 20-item questionnaire. Children respond using a 5-point Likert scale.

Construction: Based on an item analysis of the responses of 40 third grade children to 60 items, the item pool was reduced to 20 items.

Reliability: A test-retest reliability coefficient of .81 was reported for 33 boys and girls in grades 3-6.

Validity: Construct validity of the CATFIS was supported in that 185 boys and 84 girls (grades 3-6) who participated in a YMCA-sponsored sports program for five months became more positive in their attitudes toward female involvement in sport than those boys (n=126) and girls (n=168) who did not participate in the program.

Norms: Psychometric data were cited for 709 children in grades 3-9.

Availability: Contact John H. Lewko, Child and Development Studies, Laurentian University, Sudbury, Ontario, Canada P3E 2C6.

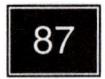 **87** ## *Coaches' Attitudes Toward Players With Disabilities Questionnaire (CATPD)
Terry L. Rizzo, Paul Bishop, Jimmy Huang, and Chris Grenfell

Source: Rizzo, T. L., & Bishop, P. (1995). Will everybody play? Attitudes of soccer coaches toward players with mild mental retardation [Abstract]. *Research Quarterly for Exercise and Sport, 66* (Suppl.), A-87.

Purpose: To assess the attitudes of youth sport soccer coaches toward coaching a player with mild mental retardation.

Description: The CATPD contains 22 items and three subscales: belief, normative belief, and motivation to comply. Coaches respond to each item using an 8-point semantic differential scale. Also included is a section measuring selected attributes of youth sport coaches.

Construction: The CATPD is based on the Theory of Reasoned Action (Ajzen & Fishbein, 1980). Nine experts in adapted physical education, psychology, and special education evaluated the items of the CATPD for content validity.

Reliability: Cronbach alpha internal consistency coefficients (N=82) were .79, .86, and .87 for the belief, normative belief, and motivation to comply subscales, respectively.

Validity: Not discussed.

Norms: Not cited. Psychometric data were reported for 82 youth soccer coaches residing in a suburban Southern California city.

**Availability: Contact Terry L. Rizzo, Physical Education Department, California State University, San Bernardino, CA 94207 (Phone # 909-880- 5355; FAX # 909-880-7085; E-mail: trizzo@wiley.csusb.edu)

References

Ajzen, I., & Fishbein, M. (1980). *Understanding attitudes and predicting social behavior.* Englewood Cliffs, NJ: Prentice-Hall.

*Rizzo, T. L., Bishop, P., & Grenfell, C. (1995). Attributes of soccer coaches affecting beliefs, attitudes and intentions toward coaching players with mild mental retardation [Abstract]. *Research Quarterly for Exercise and Sport, 66* (Suppl.), A-87.

88 *Coaching Behavior Questionnaire (CBQ)
Laura J. Kenow and Jean M. Williams

Source: Kenow, L. J., & Williams, J. M. (1992). Relationship between anxiety, self-confidence, and evaluation of coaching behaviors. *The Sport Psychologist, 6,* 344-357.

Purpose: To assess athletes' perceptions and evaluations of coaching behaviors in basketball.

Description: The CBQ contains 28 items designed to examine four behavioral categories: (a) athletes' perceptions/evaluations of the coach's ability to communicate, (b) the confidence the coach displays in his or her players, (c) the coach's composure and emotional control, and (d) how the coach's arousal level and behavior affect the player. Athletes respond to each item on a 4-point Likert scale ranging from 1 (*strongly disagree*) to 4 (*strongly agree*). For example, athletes are asked to respond to "My coach displays confidence in me as a player." There are seven filler items that are not scored.

Construction: Items and conceptual categories were based on the coaching and sport psychology experiences of the authors and on previous literature. Items were modified, based upon evaluations by six coaches, for item clarity and relevance.

Reliability: A Cronbach alpha reliability coefficient ($N=11$) of .90 was reported for the 21 items.

Validity: Not discussed.

Norms: Not cited. Psychometric data were reported for 11 female collegiate basketball players from a southwest NCAA Division III program.

**Availability: Contact Laura J. Kenow, Department of Health, Human Performance and Athletics, Linfield College, McMinnville, OR 97128-6894. (Phone # 503-434-2580; FAX # 503-434-2453; E-mail: lkenow@linfield.edu)

References

*Kenow, L. J. & Williams, J. M (1992). Factor structure of Coaching Behavior Questionnaire and its relationship to anxiety and self-confidence [Abstract]. *Journal of Sport & Exercise Psychology, 15* (Suppl.), S45.

*Kenow, L. J., & Williams, J. M. (1994). Perception of coaching behavior: Is compatibility the real issue? [Abstract]. *Journal of Sport & Exercise Psychology, 16,* (Suppl.), S70.

89 | Coaching Outcome Scale (COS)
Rainer Martens and Daniel Gould

Source: Martens, R., & Gould, D. (1979). Why do adults volunteer to coach children's sports? In G. C. Roberts & K. M. Newell (Eds.),

Psychology of motor behavior and sport-1978 (pp. 79-89). Champaign, IL: Human Kinetics Publishers.

Purpose: To assess volunteer youth sport coaches' preferences for the outcomes of winning, having fun, and socialization for children involved in youth sport.

Description: The COS contains three items, with each item having three response alternatives (i.e., the three outcomes). Coaches are asked to indicate their most and least preferred alternatives for each item.

Construction: Based on a content analysis of the youth sport literature, and from interviews and observations of coaches, the three outcome categories were developed. The content validity of the COI was verified by 12 prominent sport psychologists with 100% confirmation that the alternatives for each item correctly assessed the intended outcomes.

Reliability: Test-retest reliability coefficients across a one-week interval were .89 (winning), .77 (fun), and .77 (socialization).

Validity: Not presented.

Norms: Not cited. Descriptive data were presented for 423 youth sport coaches representing eight sports in communities of three different sizes in Illinois and Missouri.

Availability: Contact Rainer Martens, Human Kinetics Publishers, 1607 North Market Street, P. O. Box 5076, Champaign, IL 61825-5076. (Phone # 217-351-5076; FAX # 217-351-2674; E-mail: rainer@hkusa.com)

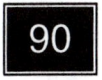

90 *Community Impact Scale (CIS)
James J. Zhang, Dale G. Pease, and Sai C. Hui

Source: Zhang, J. J., Pease, D. G., & Hui, S. C. (1996). Value dimensions of professional sport as viewed by spectators. *Journal of Sport & Social Issues, 21,* 78-94.

Purpose: To evaluate "the value dimensions of professional sport to the community as perceived by the spectators" (p. 78).

Description: The CIS contains eight subscales and 45 items: Community Solidarity (e.g., "Brings up community image versus takes down community image"); Public Behavior (e.g., "Encourages discipline versus discourages discipline"); Pastime Ecstasy (e.g, "Provides entertainment versus provides tension"); Excellence Pursuit (e.g., "Encourages achievement and success versus discourages achievement and success"); Social Equity (e.g., "Increases racial equality versus increases racial inequality"); Health Awareness (e.g., "Encourages exercise versus discourages exercise"); Individual Quality (e.g., "Promotes character building versus degrades character building"); Business Opportunity ("Attracts tourists/visitors versus hampers tourists/visitors"). Spectators' perceptions of professional sport are evaluated through "...a blend of semantic differential and Likert-type 5-point scales with bipolar statements..."(p. 81).

Construction: Based on a review of the research literature on critical theory, with the merits of functional and conflict theory also considered, 70 value areas of professional sport to the community were identified, and test items were developed. Five professors with expertise in sport sociocultural studies established content validity for the CIS by (a) evaluating items for relevancy, adequacy, representativeness, and accuracy of phrasing and (b) evaluating the appropriateness of the test format. Based on the criterion of 80% agreement among experts, a total of 66 items were retained.

The items (in questionnaire format) were then administered to a random sample (N=224) of professional basketball spectators. Exploratory principal component factor analysis followed by varimax rotation led to the retention of eight factors accounting for 57.10% of the variance in participants' responses to the CIS.

Reliability: Cronbach alpha internal consistency coefficients (N=224) ranged from .46 (Business Opportunity) to .85 (Community Solidarity); the authors reported an alpha coefficient of .95 for the total CIS scale.

Validity: Criterion-related validity was supported in that there were positive relationships reported (r ranged from .25 to .63) between spectators' frequency of attendance at professional basketball games and their composite scores for each subscale of the CIS; thus, spectators who had more positive perceptions about professional sport attended more games.

Norms: Not cited. Psychometric data were reported for 134 male and 90 female spectators, ranging in age from 15 to 70 years (M age= 31.78 years; SD= 11.50), who were randomly selected from six 1993 to 1994 season home games of a National Basketball Association Western Conference team in a major southern United States city.

**Availability: Contact James J. Zhang, Department of Health and Human Performance, University of Houston, Houston, TX 77204-5331. (Phone # 713-743-9869; FAX # 713-743-9860; E-mail: educ1b@jetson.uh.edu)

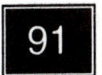

Game Orientation Scale [GOS]
Annelies Knoppers

Source: Knoppers, A., Schuiteman, J., & Love, B. (1986). Winning is not the only thing. *Sociology of Sport Journal, 3,* 43-56.

Purpose: To assess professional and play orientations toward sport.

Description: The GOS contains two contrasting scenarios: participation in a recreational sport situation and participation in a competitive situation. Participants are asked to rate each scenario in terms of how important they feel it is to win, to play fairly, to play well, and to have fun. Participants respond to each area using a 5-point Likert scale.

Construction: The GOS is a modification of Webb's (1969) Professionalization Scale.

Reliability: Alpha internal consistency coefficients were .77 for the recreational sport situation and .82 for the competitive sport situation. Test-retest reliability coefficients were .56 and .60 for the recreational sport situation and the competitive sport situation, respectively.

152

Validity: Exploratory factor analysis indicated that both scenarios produced similar constructs varying only in the amount of explained variance.

Norms: Descriptive data were cited, categorized by race, gender, and athletic status for 910 high school students representing nine schools in Missouri and six schools in Texas.

Availability: Last known address: Annelies Knoppers, Health and Physical Education Department, 131 IM Sports Circle, Michigan State University, East Lansing, MI 48824. (Phone # 517-355-4731)

References

*Greer, D., & Lacy, M. (1989). On the conceptualization and measurement of attitudes toward play: The Webb scale and the GOS. *Sociology of Sport Journal, 6,* 380-390.

*Knoppers, A., Zuidema, M., & Meyer, B. B. (1989). Playing to win or playing to play? *Sociology of Sport Journal, 6,* 70-76.

*Lacy, M. G., & Greer, D. L. (1992). Conceptualizing attitudes toward play: The Game Orientation Scale and the context modified Webb Scale. *Sociology of Sport Journal, 9,* 286-294.

Webb, H. (1969). Professionalization of attitudes toward play among adolescents. In G. S. Kenyon (Ed.), *Aspects of contemporary sport sociology* (pp. 161-187). Chicago, IL: Athletic Institute.

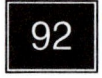 **92**

*General Sports Orientation Questionnaire [GSOQ]
Randy O. Frost and Katherine J. Henderson

Source: Frost, R. O., & Henderson, K. J. (1991). Perfectionism and reactions to athletic competition. *Journal of Sport & Exercise Psychology, 13,* 323-335.

Purpose: To assess "...general attitudes toward athletics and athletic competition" (p. 326).

Description: The GSOQ contains three subscales: 18 items focus on personal performance that emphasizes success and accomplishment; 17 items deal with failure or mistakes in athletic performance; and 11 items address athletes' perceptions of what other important people may think about their athletic performance. Athletes respond to each item on a scale ranging from 1 (*not at all*) to 5 (*extremely*).

Construction: Not discussed.

Reliability: Cronbach alpha reliability coefficients were reported as .89 (success orientation subscale), .91 (failure orientation subscale), and .83 (focus-on-others orientation subscale).

Validity: Convergent validity (*N*=40) was supported in that participants with high success orientations on the GSOQ exhibited high personal standards as assessed by the Multidimensional Perfectionism Scale (Frost, Marten, Lahart, & Rosenblate, 1990). Conversely, participants' failure orientation scores on the GSOQ were correlated with their scores on the Concern Over Mistakes and Doubts About Actions subscales of the Multidimensional Perfectionism Scale. It should be noted that the investigators reported that two of the subscales of the GSOQ (i.e., failure orientation and focus-on-others subscales) were highly correlated (.85).

Norms: Not cited. Psychometric data were reported for 40 females participating in five Division III varsity sports.

Availability: Contact Randy O. Frost, Department of Psychology, Smith College, 307 Bass Hall, Northampton, MA 01063. (Phone # 413-585-3911; FAX # 413-585-3786; E-mail: rfrost@smith.edu)

References
Frost, R. O., Marten, P., Lahart, C., & Rosenblate (1990). The dimensions of perfectionism. *Cognitive Therapy and Research, 14*, 449-468.

93	Orientations Toward Play Scale [OTP] Harry Webb

Source: Webb, H. (1969). Professionalization of attitudes toward play among adolescents. In G. S. Kenyon (Ed.), *Aspects of contemporary sport sociology* (pp. 161-187). Chicago, IL: Athletic Institute.

Purpose: To assess attitudes toward playing a game in terms of skill, fairness, and success.

Description: The OTP contains three items focusing on subject perceptions of skill, fairness, and success in sport. Participants respond on a 3-point ordinal scale to whether they feel playing as well as you can, beating the other player or team, or playing the game fairly is most important.

Construction: Not discussed.

Reliability: Test-retest reliability coefficients were above .90 among 920 public and 354 parochial students.

Validity: Not discussed.

Norms: Descriptive and psychometric data are cited for 920 public and 354 parochial male and female students, stratified by grade level (grades 3,6,8,10,12), from Battle Creek, Michigan.

Availability: OTP items can be found in the *Source*.

References
Albinson, J. G. (1974). Professionalized attitudes of volunteer coaches toward playing a game. *International Review of Sport Sociology, 9*(2), 77-87.

*Greer, D., & Lacy, M. (1989). On the conceptualization and measurement of attitudes toward play: The Webb scale and the GOS. *Sociology of Sport Journal, 6*, 380-390

Hoffman, S. J., & Luxbacher, J. A. (1983). Competitive attitude and religious belief [Abstract]. In *Psychology of motor behavior and sport* (p. 120). Proceedings of the North American Society for the Psychology of Sport and Physical Activity annual convention, East Lansing, MI.

*Lacy, M. G., & Greer, D. L. (1992). Conceptualizing attitudes toward play: The Game Orientation Scale and the context modified Webb Scale. *Sociology of Sport Journal, 9*, 286-294.

McElroy, M. (1983). Parents as significant others: Behavioral involvement and children's sport orientations [Abstract]. In *Psychology of motor behavior and sport* (p. 136). Proceedings of the North American Society for the Psychology of Sport and Physical Activity annual convention, East Lansing, MI.

*McElroy, M. A., & Kirkendall, D. R. (1980). Significant others and professionalized sport attitudes. *Research Quarterly for Exercise and Sport, 51*, 645-653.

*Snyder, E. E., & Spretzer, E. (1979). Orientations toward sport: Intrinsic, normative, and extrinsic. *Journal of Sport Psychology, 1*, 170-175.

 **94** ***Personal Meaning of Racquetball Participation** [PMRP]
Robert Rocco Battista

Source: Battista, R. R. (1990). Personal meaning: Attraction to sports participation. *Perceptual and Motor Skills, 70*, 1003-1009.

Purpose: To assess "...the personal meanings people attach to their participation in racquetball" (pp. 1004-1005).

Description: Participants are asked to rank 24 items (e.g., enjoyment, competition, challenge) for their importance in racquetball and whether the item illustrates a positive or negative experience.

Construction: Items were developed by reviewing previous literature on motives and attitudes toward sports, by consulting scholars in physical education, and via a pilot study.

Reliability: Reliability estimates ranged from .69 to .75. A Cronbach alpha reliability coefficient of .73 was reported.

Validity: Not discussed.

Norms: Not cited. Psychometric data were reported for 50 female and 48 male racquetball players (*M* age=30.1 years).

Availability: Last known address: Contact Robert R. Battista, 73 Hickory Road, Port Washington, NY 11050.

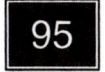 **95** ***Physical Activity Stereotyping Index** [PASI]
Arlene A. Ignico

Source: Ignico, A. A. (1989). Development and verification of a gender-role stereotyping index for physical activities. *Perceptual and Motor Skills, 68*, 1067-1075.

Purpose: To evaluate gender-labeling of physical activities.

Description: The PASI contains 24 androgynous stick-figure items depicting 8 female, 8 male, and 8 gender-neutral physical activities. For the children's version, five response alternatives are shown in picture form. For one response alternative, for example, a large box with a girl inside is shown to the subject to indicate that the activity is "a lot more for girls." For the adult version of the PASI, the response choices are just written. Scores on the PASI range from 0 (reflecting a gender-neutral response pattern) to 32 (reflecting a high degree of gender-role stereotyping). However, for a revised scoring system, see Ignico (1991).

Construction: Based on a review of the literature, five female physical activity characteristics (e.g., expression) and nine male activity characteristics (e.g., competition) were developed. Also, based on a literature review, a list of 15 male, 15 female, and 15 gender-neutral physical activities was established. Twelve experts in the motor or psychosocial development of children rated these activities according to the degree to which each activity involved each of the 14 research-based gender-specific physical activity characteristics. A total of 24 activities (8 male, 8 female, and 8 gender-neutral physical activities) were retained to form the preliminary questionnaire.

Reliability: Test-retest reliability coefficients (among parents, teachers, and children) across a 3-day interval ranged from .70 to .95.

Validity: Not discussed.

Norms: See Ignico (1991).

**Availability: Contact Arlene A. Ignico, School of Physical Education, Ball State University, Muncie, IN 47306-0270 (Phone # 317-285-5169; FAX # 317-285-8254; E-mail: 00aaignico@bsuvc.bsu.edu)

References
*Ignico, A. (1990). The influence of gender-role perception on activity preferences of children. *Play and Culture, 3*(4), 302-311.

*Ignico, A (1991). Revised scoring system and norms for the Physical Activity Stereotyping Index. *Perceptual and Motor Skills, 73*, 384-386.

*Ignico, A. A., & Mead, B. J. (1990). Children's perceptions of the gender-appropriateness of physical activities. *Perceptual and Motor Skills, 71*, 1075-1081.

*Mead, B. J., & Ignico, A. A. (1992). Children's gender-typed perceptions of physical activity: Consequences and implications. *Perceptual and Motor Skills, 75*, 1035-1042.

*Pellett, T. L., & Ignico, A. A. (1993). Relationship between children's and parents' stereotyping of physical activities. *Perceptual and Motor Skills, 77,* 1283-1289.

 ***[Psychosocial Functions of Sport Scale] [PFSS]**
Elmer Spreitzer and Eldon E. Snyder

Source: Spreitzer, E., & Snyder, E. E. (1975). The psychosocial functions of sport as perceived by the general population. *International Review of Sport Sociology, 10*(3-4), 87-93.

Purpose: To assess individuals' perceptions of the importance of sport for society and to themselves.

Description: The PFSS contains 15 items that participants respond to on a 5-point Likert Scale with the anchorings *strongly agree* to *strongly disagree*. For example, participants respond to "Sports are a good way for me to relax" or "Sports are valuable because they teach youngsters self discipline."

Construction: Items were developed from earlier qualitative research on the functions of sports.

Reliability: Not discussed.

Validity: Principal components factor analysis (varimax rotation) among 510 participants verified two factors labeled "societal" and "individual" that accounted for 93% of the variance. Furthermore, participants with higher levels of education had more positive attitudes toward the values of sport. Surprisingly, individuals who were less involved in sport (in terms of less active participation, fewer subscriptions to sports magazines, and less vicarious involvement) had more positive values toward the values of sport for society and for the individual than did those individuals who were more involved in sport.

Norms: Descriptive statistics (frequency distribution of responses) was presented for 510 residents of Toledo, Ohio, who were solicited via systematic probability sampling (*M* age=42 years; 49%=female; 75%=urban residents).

Availability: Contact Eldon E. Snyder, Department of Sociology, Bowling Green State University, Bowling Green, OH 43403-0231. (Phone # 419-353-3963; FAX # 419-372-8306; E-mail: esnyder@bgnet.bgsu.edu)

References

*Grove, S. J., & Dodder, R. A. (1979). A study of the functions of sport: A subsequent test of Spreitzer and Snyder's research. *Journal of Sport Behavior, 2,* 83-91.

*Martin, D. E., & Dodder, R. A. (1993). A reassessment of the Psychosocial Functions of Sport Scale. *Sociology of Sport Journal, 10,* 197-204.

97 Purposes of Sport Questionnaire [PSQ]
Joan L. Duda

Source: Duda, J. L. (1989). Relationship between task and ego orientation and the perceived purpose of sport among high school athletes. *Journal of Sport & Exercise Psychology, 11,* 318-335.

Purpose: To assess athletes' perceptions of the purposes of sport.

Description: Participants read the stem "A very important thing sport should do" and then respond to 60 items (e.g., "make us loyal" or "make us mentally tough"). Participants respond to each item using a 5-point Likert scale with the anchorings *strongly disagree* to *strongly agree*.

Construction: Items were developed by modifying relevant questions in the Purposes of Schooling Questionnaire (Nicholls, Patashnick, & Nolan, 1985), by reviewing the literature on the values and benefits of youth sport involvement, and through open-ended responses provided by high school students in a pilot investigation. Principal components factor analyses ($n=322$) followed by both varimax and oblique rotations resulted in the retention of seven factors accounting for 81% of the variance. These factors were labeled Mastery/Cooperation, Physically Active Lifestyle, Good Citizen, Competitiveness, High Status Career, Enhance Self-Esteem, and Enhance Social Status.

Reliability: Cronbach alpha internal consistency coefficients ($n=321$) ranged from .75 to .83 across the seven factors.

Validity: Discriminant validity was supported in that male students believed competitiveness, social status, and high-status career opportunities to be more important purposes of sport participation than did female students; conversely, female students perceived mastery/cooperation to be a more important purpose of sport than did males.

Norms: Not cited. Psychometric data were reported for 128 male and 193 female varsity interscholastic athletic participants from six high schools in a midwestern community. The students were in the 11th or 12th grades, and participated in sports such as basketball, track and field, tennis, and softball.

**Availability: Contact Joan L. Duda, Department of HKLS, 113 Lambert Hall, Purdue University, Lafayette, IN 47907-1362. (Phone # 317-494-3172; FAX # 317-496-1239; E-mail: lynne@vm.cc.purdue.edu)

References

Nicholls, J., Patashnick, M., & Nolan, S. B. (1985). Adolescents' theories of education. *Journal of Educational Psychology, 77,* 683-692.

*Walling, M. D., & Duda, J. L. (1995). Goals and their associations with beliefs about success in and perceptions of the purposes of physical education. *Journal of Teaching in Physical Education, 14,* 140-156.

98 *Purposes of Sport Scale [PSS]
Darren C. Treasure and Glyn C. Roberts

Source: Treasure, D. C., & Roberts, G. C. (1994). Cognitive and affective concomitants of task and ego goal orientations during the middle school years. *Journal of Sport & Exercise Psychology, 16,* 15-28.

Purpose: To examine children's beliefs about the purposes of sport.

Description: The PSS contains 15 items and three subscales: (a) Enhance Social Status (e.g., "Make me look and feel important in front of other people"); (b) Lifetime Health (e.g., "Motivate me to keep fit throughout my life"); and (c) Personal Development (e.g., "Teach me to respect authority"). Children respond to the stem "A very important thing sport does for me is..." using a 5-point Likert scale with the anchorings 1 (*strongly agree*) and 5 (*strongly disagree*).

Construction: Not discussed

Reliability: Cronbach alpha coefficients (N=330) ranged from .79 to .82 for the Enhance Social Status subscale, .80 to .84 for the Personal Development subscale, and .82 for the Lifetime Health subscale.

Validity: Exploratory principal axis factor analysis (using both orthogonal and oblique rotations) supported the hypothesized three-factor subscale structure.

Norms: Not cited. Psychometric data were summarized for 330 children attending a large comprehensive school in a major city in Great Britain. A total of 96 children attended the first year of the school (n=48 females, n=48 males; M age=11.3 years); 156 children attended the third year of the school (n=78 females, n=78 males; M age=13.4 years); and 77 children attended the fifth year of the school (n=44 females, n=34 males; M age=15.3 years).

Availability: Contact Darren Treasure (E-mail: dtreasur@eniac.ac.siue.edu) or Glyn C. Roberts, Department of Kinesiology, University of Illinois, Louise Freer Hall, 906 South Goodwin Avenue, Urbana, IL 61801. (Phone # 217-333-6563; FAX # 217-244-7322; E-mail: glync@staff.uiuc.edu)

99 | *Satisfaction in Sport Scale [SS]
Darren C. Treasure and Glyn C. Roberts

Source: Treasure, D. C., & Roberts, G. C. (1994). Cognitive and affective concomitants of task and ego goal orientations during the middle school years. *Journal of Sport & Exercise Psychology, 16,* 15-28.

Purpose: To assess children's beliefs concerning the reasons they experience satisfaction by participating in sport.

Description: The Satisfaction in Sport scale contains 11 items and three subscales reflecting commonly experienced sport-related outcomes: (a) Mastery Experiences (e.g., "Learn new skills"); (b) Social Approval (e.g., "Please your friends"); and (c) Normative Success (e.g., "Do better than others"). Children respond to the stem "In your sport how much satisfaction do you feel when you..." using a 5-point Likert scale with the anchorings 1 (*little*) and 5 (*a lot*).

Construction: Not discussed.

Reliability: Cronbach alpha coefficients (*N*=330) ranged from .69 to .81 for the Mastery Experiences subscale, from .74 to .85 for the Social Approval subscale, and from .62 to .65 for the Normative Success subscale.

Validity: Exploratory principal axis factor analysis (*N*=330), using both orthogonal and oblique rotations, supported the hypothesized three-factor subscale structure.

Norms: Not cited. Psychometric data were summarized for 330 children attending a large comprehensive school in a major city in Great Britain. A total of 96 children attended the first year of the school (*n*=48 females, *n*=48 males; *M* age=11.3 years); 156 children attended the third year of the school (*n*=78 females, *n*=78 males; *M* age=13.4 years); and 77 children attended the fifth year of the school (*n*=44 females, *n*=34 males; *M* age=15.3 years).

Availability: Contact Darren Treasure (E-mail: dtreasu@eniac.ac.siue.edu) or Glyn C. Roberts, Department of Kinesiology, University of Illinois, Louise Freer Hall, 906 S. Goodwin Ave., Urbana, IL 61801. (Phone # 217 333-6563; FAX # 217-244-7322; E-mail: glync@staff.uiuc.edu)

100 Sport Attitude Questionnaire (SAQ)
Robert J. Smith, Donn W. Adams, and Elaine Cork

Source: Smith, R. J., Adams, D. W., & Cork, E. (1976). Socializing attitudes toward sport. *The Journal of Sports Medicine and Physical Fitness, 16,* 66-71.

Purpose: To evaluate and compare Little League athletes with nonparticipants in terms of attitudes toward organization/authority, parental influence, aggression, the group experience, and other socializing factors.

Description: The SAQ contains 46 items. Children respond on a 7-point Likert scale.

Construction: Four researchers wrote a number of items pertinent to how they felt participants and nonparticipants would value differentially the Little League experience. The items were modified to enhance their clarity and meaningfulness to preadolescents. A total of 86 items were administered to nine participants and eight nonparticipants of organized youth sport. Item analyses led to the retention of 15 items, the revision of 6 items, and the addition of 25 new items (based on 100% agreement among the four researcher-judges).

Reliability: Not discussed.

Validity: The SAQ discriminated between 52 male participants and 40 male nonparticipants, particularly in terms of items intuitively labeled as "organization/authority." The nonparticipants consistently were opposed to adult-managed sport and preferred friendly, informal games controlled by the players.

Norms: Not cited. Psychometric data were based on the responses of 52 male participants of organized youth sport leagues and 40 nonparticipants (*M* age= 10.75 years). These individuals resided in an American community, located in West Berlin, Germany.

Availability: Unknown

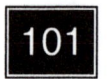 **101** *Sport Interpersonal Relationships Questionnaires (SIRQ)
Paul Wylleman, Paul De Knop, Yves Vanden Auweele, Hedwig Sloore, and K. De Martelaer

Source: Wylleman, P., De Knop, P., Vanden Auweele, Y., Sloore, H., & De Martelaer, K. (1995). Elite young athletes, parents and coaches: Relationships in competitive sports. In F. J. Ring (Ed.), *Children in Sport: Proceedings of the 1st Bath Sports Medicine Conference* (pp. 124-133). Bath, United Kingdom: University of Bath Centre for Continuing Education.

Purpose: To evaluate young elite athletes' perceptions of the socio-emotional aspects of their relationships with their father and mother, with their coach, and their perceptions of the parent-coach relationship.

Description: There are two SIRQs. One questionnaire examines young elite athletes' perceptions of their relationships with their mother and father (e.g., ("I want to please my father/mother") and with their coach (e.g., "The coach respects my personal opinion"). The other questionnaire examines young elite athletes' perceptions of the parent-coach relationship (e.g., "My father/mother asserts his/her personal point of view to the coach"). Each questionnaire contains 40 items. Participants respond to each item on a 5-point ordinal scale with the anchorings 1 (*never*) to 5 (*always*).

Construction: Items for the SIRQ are derived from existing instruments that assess the parent-child relationship. Items were reformulated and made sport-specific based on "...content-analysis of interviews with, and essays written by young athletes on how they experience the relationships in the athletic triangle" (p. 125). Further, interviews were conducted with parents and coaches, and items were also evaluated by two sport psychologists and one physical educator for appropriateness in assessing young athletes' perceptions of a particular relationship within the athletic triangle (Wylleman, Vanden Auweele, De Knop, & Sloore, 1995). Items were also piloted tested, and small modifications were made with regard to the layout of the final form.

Exploratory factor analysis ($N=260$) with varimax rotation produced "Thirty-five (35) factorial scales or dimensions with acceptable inter-scale correlations..." (p. 127).

Reliability: Cronbach alpha internal consistency coefficients ($N=260$) all exceeded .60 and ranged from .62 to .93. Test-retest reliability coefficients ($N=58$) across a 4-week interval ranged from .63 to .83 for the SIRQ-Athlete-Coach (Wylleman et al., 1995).

Validity: Convergent validity was supported (Wylleman et al., 1995) in that participants' ($N=89$) responses to the SIRQ-Athlete-Coach correlated, as hypothesized, with their responses to various scales of the Leadership Scale for Sports.

Norms: Not cited. Descriptive and psychometric data were reported for

260 young elite athletes, ages 12 to 29 years (*M* age= 17.5 years; *SD*= 3.6; 51.4% = male), competing at the national or international level in various sports. Convergent validity and test-retest reliability data were reported for a second sample of 89 17- to 23-year-old students (*M* age=18.4 years; 46.6% female) in physical education or physiotherapy who had been competing in various sports at the subnational, national, or international levels.

Availability: Contact Paul Wylleman, Faculty of Movement and Sport Sciences-HILOK, Vrije Universiteit, Pleinlaan 2, B1050 Brussel, Belgium. (Phone # 02/629.27.65-27.45; FAX # 02/629.28.99; E-mail: pwyllema@vnet3.vub.ac.be)

References
*Wylleman, P., De Knop, P., Sloore, H., & Vanden Auweele, Y. (1995). Parents-coach relationship: The young athlete's point of view [Abstract]. In A. Hantzi & M. Solman (Eds.), *Abstract of the IV European Congress of Psychology* (pp. 194-195). Athens, Greece: Ellinika Grammata.
*Wylleman, P., De Knop, P., Vanden Auweele, Y.,& Sloore, H. (1994). The development of a questionnaire to assess elite young athletes' perceptions of the parents-coach relationship. In M. Audiffren & G. Minvielle (Eds.), *Psychologie des pratiques physiques et sportives* (pp. 79-80). Poitiers, France: A.P.S de l'Universite de Poitiers.
*Wylleman, P., Vanden Auweele, Y., De Knop, P., & Sloore, H. (1995). The athlete-coach relationship within the context of the athletic triangle. In R. Vanfraechem-Raway & Y. Vanden Auweele (Eds.), *Proceedings of the IXth European Congress of Sport Psychology* (pp. 597-604). Belgium: ATM.

102   *Sport Socialization Questionnaire [SSQ]
Thomas G. Power and Christi Woolger

Source: Power, T. G., & Woolger, C. (1994). Parenting practices and age group swimming: A correlational study. *Research Quarterly for Exercise and Sport, 65,* 59-66.

Purpose: To assess the attitudes and behaviors of parents towards their parenting practices with respect to their children's participation in swimming.

Description: The SSQ contains 51 items and four subscales: Support (e.g., "After a meet, no matter how poorly my child performed, I try to point out something positive he/she did"); Directiveness (e.g., "Before a meet, I remind my child of what he/she needs to work on"); Performance Goals (e.g., "I believe my child should be one of the best athletes in his/her age group"); and Modeling (e.g., "participate in swimming meets without your child"). Parents respond to each item using a 5-point Likert scale.

Construction: Items were developed through a review of the literature and by interviews with parents, children, and college athletes.

Reliability: Cronbach alpha internal consistency coefficients ($N=88$) ranged from .56 (Modeling) to .86 (Performance Goals).

Validity: Parental support was moderately correlated (Mean $r=.46$) with their children's enthusiasm for swimming. Also, children who reported more enthusiasm for swimming had fathers who reported moderate levels of directiveness and performance outcome goals.

Norms: Not cited. Psychometric data were reported for 40 fathers (M age=40.3 years; $SD=44.4$) and 43 mothers (M age=38.4 years; $SD=4.3$) of children, ages 6 to 14 years participating in competitive swimming.

Availability: Contact Thomas G. Power, Department of Psychology, University of Houston, Houston, TX 77204-5341. (Phone # 713-743-8574; E-mail: tpower@uh.edu)

103 Sport Socialization Subscale (SSS)
Rainer Martens and Daniel Gould

Source: Martens, R., & Gould, D. (1979). Why do adults volunteer to coach children's sports? In G. C. Roberts & K. M. Newell (Eds.), *Psychology of motor behavior and sport-1978* (pp. 79-89). Champaign, IL: Human Kinetics Publishers.

Purpose: To examine the degree to which youth sport coaches emphasized the physical, psychological, and social outcomes of youth sport for children.

Description: The SSS contains three items, with each item having three response alternatives (i.e., the three outcomes). Coaches are asked to indicate their most and least preferred alternatives for each item.

Construction: Based on a content analysis of the youth sport literature, and from interviews and observations of coaches, socialization outcomes were derived. The content validity of the SSS was verified by 12 prominent sport psychologists with 100% confirmation that the alternatives for each item correctly assessed the intended outcomes.

Reliability: Test-retest reliability coefficients across a one-week interval were .70 (physical), .51 (psychological), and .76 (social).

Validity: Not presented.

Norms: Not cited. Descriptive data were presented for 423 youth sport coaches representing eight sports in communities of three different sizes in Illinois and Missouri.

Availability: Contact Rainer Martens, Human Kinetics Publishers, 1607 North Market Street, P. O. Box 5076, Champaign, IL 61825-5076. (Phone # 217-351-5076; FAX # 217-351-2674; E-mail: rainer@hkusa.com)

104 *Sport Stereotype Inventory (SSI)
Candice E. Cates Zientek

Source: Zientek, C. (1992). Development of an inventory to identify stereotypes of success in sport. *Clinical Kinesiology, 46* (1), 16-21.*

Purpose: To examine the extent to which individuals identify themselves as stereotypical "winners" or "losers" in sport.

Description: The SSI is a 20-item inventory in which participants are asked to evaluate themselves in terms of: being envied; praised; disappointed*; feeling things are against you*; skilled at sport; apathetic*; believes in your own ability; disillusioned*; jubilant; frustrated*; confident; has a difficult time in sport*; proud; apologetic*; admired;

*Note: This summary was adapted from a summary prepared by the test author (C. E. C. Zientek, personal communication, April 13, 1996)

depressed*; has good sports ability; embarrassed*; successful; and hesitant*. Participants respond to these 20 items using a 5-point Likert scale with the anchorings 1 (*not a lot*) to 5 (*a lot*). (*Items were recoded.)

Construction: Items were generated from four open-ended questions developed in an attempt to assess stereotypes of those who normally win and those who normally lose in sport. Fifty-two undergraduate students were asked to complete the questionnaire. The questions included What characteristics do .you associate with (a) sports participants, (b) those who normally participate in sport, (c) those who normally win at sport, and (d) those who normally lose at sports?

Additional items were selected from newspaper sports pages. For 3 weeks, six daily London newspapers were read, and adjectives were compiled. This list of characteristics was then added to the list compiled through the use of the questionnaire.

An alphabetical list of 309 characteristics was compiled forming a second questionnaire. A second group of 76 undergraduate students were then asked to complete a 10-minute, forced-choice questionnaire, rating the 309 items according to how true each characteristic was of people who normally win, and then of people who normally lost in sport. The Likert scale was anchored from 1 (*never*) to 7 (*always*).

Independent *t*-tests were carried out to determine on which characteristics winners and losers significantly differed. In order to have a total of 20 items, mean difference was chosen as a selection criterion. Based on the mean differences, 10 items were chosen from the rank ordering of characteristics describing winners, and 10 were chosen from the rank ordering of losers.

Reliability: Cronbach alpha internal consistency coefficients of .83 (N=76) and .84 (N=206) were reported. A test-retest reliability coefficient of .70 (N=206) was reported across a 2-month interval (Zientek, 1990).

Validity: Exploratory factor analysis (varimax rotation) produced four factors accounting for 53.60% of the variance. Factor 1 (27% accountable variance) comprised all 20 items (Zientek, 1990).

Discriminant validity was supported in that both disabled sports participants and nondisabled sports participants scored higher on the SSI than did nondisabled nonparticipants. Gender also mediated participants' responses to the SSI; males scored higher on the SSI than did females.

Norms: Not cited. Psychometric data were reported for 12 members of the team representing the United States in the 5th World Nordic Disabled Ski Championships, 150 undergraduate students from a large, midwestern university, and 44 undergraduate students enrolled in a small, eastern university.

**Availability: Contact Candice E. Cates Zientek, Department of Physical Education, Shippensburg University, 1871 Old Main Drive, Shippensburg, PA 17257. (Phone # 717-532-1274; FAX # 717-532-1273; E-mail: cezien@ark.ship.edu)

References

*Zientek, C. (1990). *U.S. disabled Nordic skiers' identification with stereotypes of success.* Paper presented at the 5th annual conference of the Association for the Advancement of Applied Sport Psychology, San Antonio, TX.

*Zientek, C. (1991). Think your way to success. In G. Breakwell (Ed.), *The Marshall Cavendish encyclopedia of personal relationships. Vol. 17. Shaping your life* (pp. 2088-2096). New York: Marshall Cavendish.

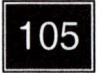

105 [Sportsmanship Attitude Scales] [SAS]
Marion Lee Johnson

Source: Johnson, M. L. (1969). Construction of sportsmanship attitude scales. *Research Quarterly, 40*, 312-316.

Purpose: To assess sportsmanship attitudes of boys and girls in grades 7-9.

Description: Alternative forms A and B each contains 21 items.

Construction: The scale-discrimination technique was used to evaluate an initial set of 152 items descriptive of ethically critical sportsmanship behavior. These items were treated with the equal-appearing interval, summated rating, and scale analyses methods. Unidimensional scale rankings of the items were made by judges. Item analysis of half of the items judged least ambiguous were made among 208 junior high school boys and girls. Scale analysis led to the retention of 42 items, which were divided in half as alternative forms of the same test. A correlation coefficient ($n=102$ 7th- to 9th-grade boys and girls) of .86 was reported among these equivalent forms.

Reliability: Not reported.

Validity: Correlation coefficients of .19 and .42 were reported when contrasting the composite scores of two groups of female junior high school students on the scale with their corresponding sportsmanship behavior as assessed by their instructors. However, correlation coefficients of -.01 and .16 were reported among male junior high school basketball players using the same criterion.

Norms: Not reported.

Availability: Last known address: Health & Physical Education Department, College of Education, Southeastern Louisiana University, Box 670, Hammond, LA 70402.

 ## Sportsmanship Attitudes in Basketball Questionnaire [SABQ]
Joan L. Duda, Linda K. Olson, and Thomas J. Templin

Source: Duda, J. L., Olson, L. K., & Templin, T. J. (1991). The relationship of task and ego orientation to sportsmanship attitudes and the perceived legitimacy of injurious acts. *Research Quarterly for Exercise and Sport, 62,* 79-87.

Purpose: To evaluate individuals' views regarding sportsmanship in basketball.

Description: The SABQ contains 22 items reflecting "unsportsmanlike" (e.g., faking an injury to stop the clock) and prosocial (e.g., helping a player up from the floor) behaviors. Participants respond on a 5-point Likert scale with the anchorings *strongly disapprove* to *strongly approve*.

Construction: The SABQ is a basketball sport-specific version of Lakie's (1964) Competitive Attitude Scale. Four experts, with extensive experience in high school level basketball as players, coaches, and referees, developed the basketball-specific items. A principal component factor analysis with oblique rotation (n=56 male and n=67 female inter-scholastic basketball players) identified three factors accounting for 81.1% of the variance. These factors were labeled Unsportsmanlike Play/Cheating, Strategic Play, and Sportsmanship.

Reliability: Cronbach alpha internal consistency coefficients (n=123) were .80 (Unsportsmanlike Play/Cheating), .60 (Strategic Play), and .62 (Sportsmanship).

Validity: Discriminant validity was supported in that males scored higher than females on Unsportsmanlike Play/Cheating and Strategic Play, whereas females scored higher on Sportsmanship. Furthermore, canonical analysis revealed that a strong, negative emphasis on task orientation and a moderate, positive emphasis on ego orientation were correlated (r=.49) with an endorsement of unsportsmanlike play/cheating, thus supporting the concurrent validity of the SABQ.

Norms: Not available. Psychometric data were cited for 56 male and 67 female interscholastic basketball players representing five high schools in a midwestern community.

**Availability: Contact Joan L. Duda, Department of HKLS, 113 Lambert Hall, Purdue University, West Lafayette, IN 47907-1362. (Phone # 317-494-3172; FAX # 317-496-1239; E-mail: lynne@vm.cc.purdue.edu)

Reference

Lakie, W. (1964). Expressed attitudes in various groups of athletes toward athletic competition. *Research Quarterly, 35,* 479-503.

107 Survey of Values in Sport [SVS]
Dale D. Simmons and R. Vern Dickinson

Source: Simmons, D. D., & Dickinson, R. V. (1986). Measurement of values expression in sports and athletics. *Perceptual and Motor Skills, 62,* 651-658.

Purpose: To measure the role of personal values in sport.

Description: The SVS contains 14 sports-related values including Time-Out, Energy Release, Rewards, Being in a Good Place, Cooperation, Expressing Feelings, Reaching Personal Limits, Group Coordination, Winning, Physical Pleasure, Being a Good Sport, Risk, Competition, and Maintaining Good Health. Respondents are asked to rank order the 14 values for a given sport and then rate the importance of each value on a 14-point ordinal scale. A score for each value is derived by multiplying the rank times the rating.

Construction: Not discussed.

Reliability: Test-retest reliability coefficients (n=41 male and 54 female undergraduate students) ranged from .51 (Time-Out) to .82 (Competition) over a 2-week interval with an average coefficient of .65 reported across the 14 values.

Validity: A principal component factor analysis (n=95) of the SVS resulted in the retention of five factors accounting for 62.50% of the variance.

Norms: Not reported. Psychometric data were cited for 95 undergraduate students plus 21 female collegiate athletes representing two sports.

Availability: Contact Dale D. Simmons, Professor Emeritus, Department of Psychology, Oregon State University, Corvallis, OR 97331-5303. (Phone # 541-737-3524; E-mail: simmonsd@cla.orst.edu)

Chapter 7

Attributions

Tests in this chapter assess the explanations sport participants give for their successes and failures in sport and related physical activities.

108 *Attribution Style for Physical Activity Scale (ASPAS)

Eric Cooley, Robert Ayres, and James Beaird

Source: Cooley, E., Ayres, R., & Beaird, J. (1991). Construct validity of the Attributional Style for Physical Activity Scale [Abstract]. *Proceedings of the Association for the Advancement of Applied Sport Psychology annual convention* (p. 33). Savannah, GA.

Purpose: To evaluate respondents' attributions for success or failure in a physical activity.

Description: Participants respond on a 5-point rating scale to the relative importance of ability, effort, and external factors for explaining the outcomes of 22 situations involving success or failure in physical activity. The ASPAS contains three 10-item scales for success outcomes and three 12-item scales for failure outcomes.

Construction: Not discussed.

Reliability: Cronbach alpha reliability coefficients ranged from .65 to .82 with a mean alpha reliability coefficient of .72 (N=158).

Validity: Convergent validity was partially supported in that participants' (N=158) scores on the failure scales of the ASPAS correlated negatively, as hypothesized, with physical self-concept (Physical Self-Perception Profile); however, no statistically significant correlation coefficients were reported with the Health Locus of Control Scale.

Norms: Not provided.

Availability: Contact Eric Cooley, Department of Psychology, Western Oregon State College, Monmouth, OR 97361. (Phone # 503-838-8331)

Reference
*Cooley, E. (1990). The Attributional Style for Physical Activity Scale: Preliminary scale analysis [Abstract]. *Proceedings of the Association for the Advancement of Applied Sport Psychology annual convention* (p. 32). San Antonio, TX.

109 | *Beliefs About the Causes of Success [BCS]
Jeffrey J. Seifriz, Joan L. Duda, and Likang Chi

Source: Seifriz, J. J., Duda, J. L., & Chi, L. (1992). The relationship of perceived motivational climate to intrinsic motivation and beliefs about success in basketball. *Journal of Sport & Exercise Psychology, 14,* 375-391.

Purpose: To assess the degree to which basketball athletes feel that success in sport stems from ability or motivation/exerted effort.

Description: The BCS contains 12 items and two subscales (Motivation/Effort and Ability Beliefs). Basketball players are asked "What do you think is most likely to help players do well or succeed on this basketball team?" Participants respond to each item on a 5-point Likert scale with the anchorings 1 (*strongly disagree*) and 5 (*strongly agree*).

Construction: The BCS was developed from the previous theoretical and assessment literature on attributions.

Reliability: Cronbach alpha internal consistency coefficients (*N*=105) of .81 (Motivation/Effort) and .70 (Ability Beliefs) were reported.

Validity: Athletes' task orientations were shown to be predictive of the belief that effort causes success, whereas their ego orientations were predictive of the belief that ability causes success.

Norms: Not cited. Psychometric data were reported for 105 male high school basketball players from nine teams in midwestern America.

**Availability: Contact Dr. Joan Duda, Department of Health, Kinesiology, and Leisure Studies, Purdue University, Lambert 113, West Lafayette, IN 47907. (Phone # 317-494-3172; FAX # 317-496-1239; E-mail: lynne@vm.cc.purdue.edu)

References
*Duda, J. L., Fox, K. R., Biddle, S. J. H., & Armstrong, N. (1992). Children's achievement goals and beliefs about success in sport. *British Journal of Educational Psychology, 62,* 313-323.

*Duda, J. L., & Nicholls, J. G. (1992). Dimensions of achievement motivation in schoolwork and sport. *Journal of Educational Psychology, 84*, 290-299.

*Duda, J. L., & White, S. A. (1992). The relationship of goal perspectives to beliefs about success among elite skiers. *The Sport Psychologist, 6*, 334-343.

*Guest, S. M., & White, S. A. (1995). The role of goal orientations and beliefs about the causes of success in predicting gender and level of sport involvement in sport participants [Abstract]. *Journal of Applied Sport Psychology, 7* (Suppl.), S67.

*Guivernau, M., & Duda, J. L. (1995). The generality of goals, beliefs, interest and perceived ability across sport and school: The case of Spanish student-athletes [Abstract]. *Journal of Sport & Exercise Psychology, 17* (Suppl.), S6.

*Guivernau, M., & Duda, J. L. (1995). Psychometric properties of a Spanish version of the Task and Ego Orientation in Sport Questionnaire (TEOSQ) and Beliefs about the Causes of Success inventory. *Revista de Psicologia del Deporte, 5*, 31-51.

*Hall, H. K., & Earles, M. (1995). Motivational determinants of interest, and perceptions of success in school physical education [Abstract]. *Journal of Sport & Exercise Psychology, 17* (Suppl.), S57.

*Newton, M., & Duda, J. L. (1993). Elite adolescent athletes' achievement goals and beliefs concerning success in tennis. *Journal of Sport & Exercise Psychology, 15*, 437-448.

*Newton, M. L., & Walling, M. D. (1995). Goal orientations and beliefs about the causes of success among Senior Olympic Games participants [Abstract]. *Journal of Sport & Exercise Psychology, 17* (Suppl.), S81.

*Walling, M. D., & Duda, J. L. (1995). Goals and their associations with beliefs about success in and perceptions of the purpose of physical education. *Journal of Teaching in Physical Education, 14*, 140-156.

*White, S. A., & Duda, J. L. (1993). Dimensions of goals-beliefs about success among disabled athletes. *Adapted Physical Activity Quarterly, 10*, 125-136.

 *Causal Attributions in Team Sports Questionnaire (CATSQ)

Bruce G. Klonsky and Jack S. Croxton

Source: Croxton, J. S., & Klonsky, B. G. (1982). Sex differences in causal attributions for success and failure in real and hypothetical sport settings. *Sex Roles, 8*, 399-409.

Purpose: To assess causal attributions made about success and failure in team sports.

Description: The CATSQ is a 48-item attribution questionnaire constructed to provide as wide a range of potential causal attributions for the outcome of the game as possible. Each potential causal explanation is rated on a 10-point ordinal scale with the anchorings 1 (*not at all important*) to 10 (*extremely important*). The wording of the items on the questionnaire differs for winning and losing teams. An example of a winning questionnaire item is "You have a great deal of natural ability," whereas the comparable losing questionnaire item would be "You have very little natural ability."

Construction: The CATSQ was based primarily on Elig and Frieze's (1979) three-dimensional classification scheme that characterized attributions as either internal or external, stable or unstable, and intentional or unintentional. Because in team sports there are three major potential attributional targets (oneself, one's own team, and the opposing team), the authors thus expanded the Elig and Frieze (1979) model to include 12 attribution categories. The authors felt that "such a model provides a more comprehensive framework for classifying causal attributions and also gives individuals more flexibility as they seek to explain their performance outcomes" (p. 402).

Reliability: Not reported.

Validity: Construct validity was supported in that college varsity basketball athletes ($N=22$) rated (a) stable and intentional characteristics as more important than unstable and unintentional characteristics in determining basketball outcomes, and (b) team and self characteristics as most important for a win and opponent characteristics as most important for a loss. It was also noted (B. Klonsky, personal communication, July, 19, 1995) that sex differences in causal attributions for success and failure in sport situations obtained with the CATSQ were generally consistent with those reported in earlier research in athletic and other achievement situations (e.g., males being more inclined to avoid responsibility for negative outcomes).

Norms: Descriptive data were obtained after intrasquad scrimmages for 10 members of a women's college varsity basketball team and 12 members of a men's college varsity basketball team, as well as from 54 undergraduate students (24 males; 30 females) after being asked to imagine they had either just won or lost as part of a basketball team.

**Availability: Contact Bruce G. Klonsky, Department of Psychology Department, State University of New York, College at Fredonia, Thompson Hall W339, Fredonia, NY 14063. (Phone # 716-673-3225; FAX # 716-673-3332; E-mail: klonsky@fredonia.edu)

References

*Croxton, J. S., & Klonsky, B. G. (1980, October). *Causal attributions as a function of sports participation, performance outcome and sex of participant.* Paper presented at the 1st annual meeting of the North American Society for the Sociology of Sport, Denver, CO.

*Croxton, J. S., & Klonsky, B. G. (1981). Causal attributions of college athletes as a function of performance and sex of participant. In S. L. Greendorfer & A. Yiannakis (Eds.), *Sociology of sport: Diverse perspectives* (pp. 67-76). West Point, NY: Leisure Press.

Elig, T., & Frieze, I. H. (1979). Measuring causal attributions for success and failure. *Journal of Personality and Social Psychology, 37,* 621-634.

*Klonsky, B. G., & Croxton, J. S. (1981, April). *Causal attributions in sport situations as a function of sex, performance outcome, and athletic ability and experience.* Paper presented at the meeting of the Eastern Psychological Association, New York, NY.

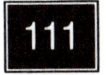

*Causes of Success in Sport Scale [CSS]
Darren C. Treasure and Glyn C. Roberts

Source: Treasure, D. C., & Roberts, G. C. (1994). Cognitive and affective concomitants of task and ego goal orientations during the middle school years. *Journal of Sport & Exercise Psychology, 16,* 15-28.

Purpose: To assess childrens' beliefs about the causes of success in sport.

Description: The CSS contains 15 items and 3 subscales: (a) Motivation/Effort (e.g., "They try hard"); (b) Ability (e.g., "They are talented"); and (c) External Factors (e.g., "They dress right"). Children respond to the stem: "What is most likely to help someone do well in sport?" using a 5-point Likert scale with the anchorings 1 (*strongly disagree*) and 5 (*strongly agree*).

Construction: Not discussed.

Reliability: Cronbach alpha coefficients (N=330) ranged from .61 to .88 for the Motivation/Effort subscale and from .70 to .71 for the External Factors subscale; an internal consistency coefficient of .78 was reported for the Ability subscale.

Validity: Results of a principal axis factor analysis (N=330), using both orthogonal and oblique rotations, supported the hypothesized three-factor structure.

Norms: Not cited. Psychometric data were reported for 330 children attending a large comprehensive school in a major city of Great Britain. A total of 96 children (n=48 females, n=48 males; M age= 11.3 years) were in enrolled the first year of school, 156 children (n=78 females, n=78 males; M age=13.4 years) were enrolled in the third year, and 78 children (n=44 females, n=34 males; M age=15.3 years) were in their fifth year of enrollment.

Availability: Contact Darren C. Treasure (E-mail: dtreasu@eniac.ac. siue.edu) or Glyn C. Roberts, Department of Kinesiology, University of Illinois, Louise Freer Hall, 906 South Goodwin Avenue, Urbana, IL 61801. (Phone #217-333-6563; FAX # 217-244-7322; E-mail: glync@staff.uiuc.edu)

112 | Performance Outcome Survey (POS)
Larry M. Leith and Harry Prapavessis

Source: Leith, L. M., & Prapavessis, H. (1989). Attributions of causality and dimensionality associated with sport outcomes in objectively evaluated and subjectively evaluated sports. *International Journal of Sport Psychology, 20,* 224-234.

Purpose: To assess causal attributions athletes give to explain their successes and failures when competing in sport.

Description: The POS assesses the attributional dimensions of controllability, locus of control, and stability. Athletes are asked to recall vividly one successful and one unsuccessful athletic performance. They respond to three items per attributional dimension using a 7-point Likert scale.

Construction: The POS is a sport-specific version of Russell's (1982) Causal Dimensional Scale.

Reliability: Cronbach alpha internal consistency coefficients of .63 (controllability), .74 (locus of control) and .83 (stability) were reported.

Validity: Not discussed.

Norms: Not cited. Psychometric data were based on the responses of 52 male and female athletes (ages 14 to 17 years) enrolled in an academic program for gifted athletes in a secondary school in Toronto, Canada.

**Availability: Contact Larry Leith, School of Physical and Health Education, University of Toronto, 320 Huron Street, Toronto, Canada M5S 1A1. (Phone # 416-978-3448; FAX # 416-978-4384; E-mail: leith@phe.utoronto.ca).

Reference

Russell, D. (1982). The Causal Dimension Scale: A measure of how individuals perceive causes. *Journal of Personality and Social Psychology, 42,* 1137-1145.

113 Softball Outcomes Inventory (SOI)
A. Craig Fisher and J. A. Soderlund

Source: Fisher, A. C., & Soderlund, J. A. (1985). Causal attributions to success and failure sport situations with self-confidence as a mediating factor [Abstract]. *Proceedings of the Canadian Society of Psychomotor Learning and Sport Psychology annual convention* (pp. 51-52). Montreal, Canada.

Purpose: To assess college female softball athletes' attributions for their success and failure in softball situations.

Description: The SOI presents athletes with 16 softball situations, each with varying degrees of success and failure. The athletes are asked to rate nine attributions (typical ability, task difficulty, effort expended, quality of opponents, ability expended, luck, typical effort, coaching, psychological state) on a scale of 1 to 5, indicating the degree to which each attribution accounted for each situation's outcome.

Construction: Not discussed.

Reliability: Not indicated.

Validity: Construct validity was supported in that ANOVA analyses indicated that athletes tend to attribute their successes to internal factors, while attributing their failures to external factors. However, individual

182

differences scaling produced results that were not as conclusive. Furthermore, little relationship was found between athletes' responses to the SOI and their level of self-confidence.

Norms: Not presented. Psychometric data were based on the responses of 65 college female softball athletes.

**Availability: Contact A. Craig Fisher, Department of Exercise and Sport Sciences, Ithaca College, Ithaca, NY 14850. (Phone # 607-274-3112; FAX # 607-274-1943; E-mail: cfisher@ithaca.edu)

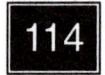 ***Sport Attributional Style Questionnaire (SASQ)**
Zenong Yin, John Callaghan, and Jeff Simons

Source: Yin, Z., Callaghan, J., & Simons, J. (1992). The development and preliminary validation of the Sport Attributional Style Questionnaire [Abstract]. *Proceedings of the Association for the Advancement of Applied Sport Psychology* (p. 139). Colorado Springs, CO.

Purpose: To evaluate athletes' causal explanations regarding negative sport situations.

Description: Athletes provide causal explanations for 13 statements regarding negative sport situations. The dimensional properties of these causal attributions are assessed in relation to Internality, Stability, Globality, and Controllability. Athletes respond to a structured alternative format using a 7-point ordinal scale.

Construction: The content validity of 20 initial statements was examined through expert evaluation.

Reliability: The author reported (Z. Yin, personal communication, May 17, 1996) the following reliability coefficients: Internality (.65); Stability (.79); Globality (.76); and Controllability (.71).

Validity: The factor analysis of athletes' ($N=617$) responses to the SASQ supported the construct validity of a 12-item SASQ.

Norms: Not cited. Psychometric data were cited for 617 athletes of NCAA Division I and Division II programs.

**Availability: Contact Zenong Yin, Kinesiology and Health Department, University of Texas, 6900 North Loop 1604 West, San Antonio, TX 78249-0654. (Phone # 210-458-5642; FAX # 210-458-5848; E-mail: zyin@pclan.utsa.edu)

115 Sport Attributional Style Scale (SASS)
Stephanie J. Hanrahan and J. Robert Grove

Source: Hanrahan, S. J, & Grove, J. R. (1990). Further examination of the psychometric properties of the Sport Attributional Style Scale. *Journal of Sport Behavior, 13,* 183-193.

Purpose: To assess attributional style in sport, based on subjective interpretations of success and failure in sport.

Description: The SASS uses 7-point bipolar scales to measure the causal dimensions of stability, internality, controllability, globality, and intentionality. Separate attribution responses arerequired for eight positive and eight negative events. For each event, participants are asked to vividly imagine themselves in the situation, to decide the single most likely cause of the event, and then they are asked to respond to questions about the cause and about the event. An example of a positive event presented is "You perform well in a competition"; an example of a negative event is "You are not selected for the starting team in an important competition." The positive and negative events are matched for content.

Construction: Not discussed.

Reliability: A mean alpha reliability coefficient (n=164 male and n=124 female college students) of .73 was reported, with alpha reliability coefficients at acceptable levels for all subscales (Hanrahan, 1988). Test-retest reliability coefficients (n=41) across a 5-week interval ranged from .54 to .63 for the positive events (mean reliability coefficient=.60), and from .46 to .80 for the negative events (mean reliability coefficient=.60).

Validity: Confirmatory factor analysis verified the hypothesized factor structure, supporting the construct validity of the SASS. Participants' (n=288) scores on the SASS were also predictive of their scores on scales measuring achievement motivation and physical self-esteem (Hanrahan, 1988). Convergent validity was supported in that participants' (n=55) responses to the SASS were correlated with their responses to the more global Attributional Style Questionnaire; these correlation coefficients ranged from .24 to .61 across dimensional subscales, with a mean coefficient of .42.

Norms: Not reported. Psychometric data were cited for 288 college students representing 40 different sports and all levels of participation, as well as 37 male and 59 female physical education undergraduate students.

**Availability: Contact Stephanie J. Hanrahan, Department of Human Movement Studies, University of Queensland, Queensland 4072, Australia. (Phone 61-7-3365-6240; FAX # 61-7-3365-6877; E-mail: steph@hms01.hms.uq.oz.au)

References

*Hanrahan, S. J. (1988). The development of a tool to measure attributional style in sport [Abstract]. In *Psychology of motor behavior and sport* (p. 13). Proceedings of the North American Society for the Psychology of Sport and Physical Activity annual convention, Knoxville, TN.

Hanrahan, S. (1993). Attributional style, intrinsic motivation, and achievement goal orientations. *Proceedings of the Eighth World Congress of Sport Psychology* (pp. 846-850). Lisbon, Portugal.

*Hanrahan, S. J., & Grove, J. R. (1989). Intrinsic motivation and attributional style in sport: Does a relationship exist? In *Sport Psychology and human performance* (pp. 89-90). Proceedings of the 7th World Congress in Sport Psychology, Singapore.

*Hanrahan, S. J., & Grove, J. R. (1989). Psychometric properties of a measure of sport-related attributional style. In *Sport psychology and human performance* (pp. 89-90). Proceedings of the 7th World Congress in Sport Psychology, Singapore.

*Hanrahan, S. J., & Grove, J. R. (1990). A short form of the Sport Attributional Style Scale. The *Australian Journal of Science and Medicine in Sport, 22,* 97-101.

*Hanrahan, S. J., Grove, J. R., & Hattie, J. A. (1989). Development of a questionnaire measure of sport-related attributional style. *International Journal of Sport Psychology, 20,* 114-134.

Sellars, C., & Biddle, S. (1994). Attributional style and the coach [Abstract]. *Journal of Sports Sciences, 12,* 209.

116 Wingate Sport Achievement Responsibility Scale (WSARS)

Gershon Tenenbaum, David Furst, and Gilad Weingarten

Source: Tenenbaum, G., Furst, D., & Weingarten, G. (1984). Attribution of causality in sport events: Validation of the Wingate Sport Achievement Responsibility Scale. *Journal of Sport Psychology, 6,* 430-439.

Purpose: To assess an athlete's enduring attitudes or expectations in attributing success and failure in sport.

Description: The WSARS includes two versions: one for team sport athletes and one for individual sport athletes. Each version is divided into successful (11 items) and unsuccessful (11 items) events. The items represent a wide range of negative and positive events in sport settings, such as interactions with coach, teammates, and audience, and perceived successful and unsuccessful athletic performance. Each item contains two alternatives: external or internal. For example, respondents are asked if "good results in sport are usually a result of luck or uncontrollable factors" or "the personal efforts invested by the participants." Athletes are asked to respond to each item on a 5-point ordinal scale, ranging from 0 (*externality*) to 5 (*internality*).

Construction: A total of 44 items (22 for successful and 22 for unsuccessful events) were developed from interactions with coaches, athletes, and sport psychologists, and the responses typically given for success and failure. Using the probabilistic Rasch model and estimates of internal consistency, the pool of items was reduced to 22 items.

Reliability: Internal consistency coefficients, based on testing 107 adult athletes (69 participating in team sports and 39 in individual sports) from the Wingate School of Coaching in Israel, were reported as greater than .70 for each subscale (i.e., successful and unsuccessful events) for each test version (i.e., team sports versus individual sports).

Validity: Concurrent validity was supported in that low but statistically significant correlation coefficients were reported between athletes'

186

(n=107) responses to the WSARS and the more general Rotter I-E scale.

Norms: Not reported. Psychometric data were reported for 107 adult athletes residing in Israel.

**Availability: Contact Gershon Tenenbaum, Department of Psychology, University of Southern Queensland, Toowoomba, Queensland, Australia 4350. (Phone # 76-31-1703; FAX # 76-31-2721; E-mail: tenenbau@zeus.usq.edu.au)

Reference

*Tenenbaum, G., & Furst, D. (1985). The relationship between sport achievement responsibility, attribution and related situational variables. *International Journal of Sport Psychology, 16*, 254-269.

Chapter 8

Body Image

Tests in this chapter assess the attitudes of individuals toward their body appearance and structure, and confidence in movement. Tests assessing individual differences in body esteem and body satisfaction are also prominent. The chapter concludes with a test to determine the extent to which people become anxious when others observe or evaluate their physiques.

117 Body Attitude Scale (BAS)
Richard M. Kurtz

Source: Kurtz, R. M. (1969). Sex differences and variations in body attitudes. *Journal of Consulting and Clinical Psychology, 33*(5), 625-629.

Purpose: To assess an individual's general, overall global attitude or feeling about the outward form and appearance of his or her body.

Description: Three separate body attitudes (Evaluation, Potency, and Activity) are measured using a semantic differential technique. Individuals respond to 30 body concepts using nine bipolar 7-point adjective scales.

Construction: The BAS is a modification of Osgood's (Osgood, Suci, & Tannenbaum, 1957) Semantic Differential.

Reliability: Not discussed.

Validity: The BAS discriminated among 89 male and 80 female undergraduate students. The females liked their bodies better than did the males and had a more clearly differentiated idea of what they liked and disliked about their bodies. The males viewed their bodies as more potent and more active than did the female students.

Norms: Not cited. Psychometric data were reported for 89 male and 89 female undergraduate Caucasians from predominantly middle-class backgrounds.

Availability: Contact Richard M. Kurtz, Department of Psychology, Campus Box 1125, Washington University, One Brookings Drive, St. Louis, MO 63130. (Phone # 314-935-6520; E-mail: rmkurtz @artsci.wustl.edu)

References
*Collingwood, T. R., & Willett, L. (1971). The effect of physical training upon self-concept and body attitude. *Journal of Clinical Psychology, 27*, 411-412.
*Kurtz, R. M. (1971). Body attitude and self-esteem [Summary]. *Proceedings of the 79th annual convention of the American Psychological Association, 6*, 467-468.
*Kurtz, R., & Hirt, M. (1970). Body attitude and physical health. *Journal of Clinical Psychology, 26*, 149-151.

Osgood, C., Suci, G., & Tannenbaum, P. (1957). *The measurement of meaning.* Urbana, IL: University of Illinois Press.

*Van Denburg, E. J., & Kurtz, R. M. (1989). Changes in body attitude as a function of posthypnotic suggestions. *The International Journal of Clinical and Experimental Hypnosis, 37,* 15-30.

Body Consciousness Questionnaire [BCQ]
Lynn C. Miller, Richard Murphy, and Arnold H. Buss

Source: Miller, L. C., Murphy, R., & Buss, A. H. (1981). Consciousness of body: Private and public. *Journal of Personality and Social Psychology, 41,* 397-406.

Purpose: To assess individual differences in the awareness of internal body sensations and the external appearance of the body.

Description: The BCQ contains three subscales: Private Body Consciousness [PBC], Public Body Consciousness [PBCS], and Body Competence [BC]. The BCQ contains 15 items. For example, participants are asked to respond to the item "I'm capable of moving quickly" (Body Competence). Participants are asked to respond to each item on a 4-point ordinal scale with the anchorings *extremely uncharacteristic* to *extremely characteristic.*

Construction: Items were selected at face value that dealt with either the public or private aspects of the body. After pilot research, the final form was administered to 561 college men and 720 college women. Factor analysis of all participants' responses revealed three factors (see subscales labeled above) accounting for 46% of the variance. These results were replicated among two new samples of 460 and 680 college students. Low intercorrelation coefficients (n=628) were observed across the three defined factors.

Reliability: Test-retest reliability coefficients (n=130) over a 2-month interval were .69 (PBC), .73 (PBCS), and .83 (BC).

Validity: In terms of concurrent validity, the BCQ subscales generally evidenced low correlation coefficients (n=275 males, n=353 females) with the Self-Consciousness Inventory, but were not related to measures of social anxiety, hypochondriasis, or emotionality. Construct validity was evident, because college students who scored higher on the PBC subscale were more aware of the stimulating effects of caffeine than were low-scoring individuals.

Norms: Norms were presented for 568 college men and 731 college women on each of the three subscales.

Availability: Lynn C. Miller, GFS Hall, School of Communications, University of Southern California, Los Angeles, CA 91107. (Phone #213- 740-3938; FAX # 213-740-0014; E-mail: lmiller@rcf.usc.edu)

References

Nelson, T. R., Kearney-Cooke, A., & Lansky, L. M. (1990). Body image and body-beautification among female college students. *Perceptual and Motor Skills, 71,* 281-289.

Robertson, K. S., Mellors, S., Hughes, M., Sanderson, F. H., & Reilly, T. (1990). Psychological health status of squash players of differing standards [Abstract]. *Journal of Sports Sciences, 8,* 71-72.

*Skrinar, G. S., Bullen, B. A., McArthur, J. W., Check, J. M., & Vaughan, L. K. (1986). Effects of endurance training on body-consciousness in women. *Perceptual and Motor Skills, 62,* 483-490.

*Skrinar, G. S., Williams, N. I., Bullen, B. A., McArthur, J. W., & Mihok, N. (1992). Changes in body consciousness relate to regularity of exercise training. *Perceptual and Motor Skills, 75,* 696-698.

 ## Body Esteem Scale [BES]
Stephen L. Franzoi and Stephanie A. Shields

Source: Franzoi, S. L., & Shields, S. A. (1984). The Body Esteem Scale: Multidimensional structure and sex differences in a college population. *Journal of Personality Assessment, 49,* 173-178.

Purpose: To examine individual differences in perceptions of body esteem.

Description: The BES contains 35 items focusing on such factors as perceived upper body strength and physical attractiveness in men, and perceived attractiveness and weight control in women. Individuals respond to each item using a 5-point Likert scale.

Construction: Principal component factor analyses of the responses of 366 female and 257 male undergraduate students to the Body Cathexis Scale led the authors to the conclusions that body esteem is multidimensional and that there are gender differences in the factor structure of the Body Cathexis Scale. The BES was then constructed from 23 Body Cathexis Scale items and 16 new items reflective of the derived factor structures within gender. A second principal component factor analysis was conducted with another sample of 483 undergraduate students (n=301 females; n=182 males). This analysis led to the retention of 35 items accounting for 39% (males) and 36 % (females) of the variance in the three-factor solution models derived.

Reliability: Alpha reliability coefficients of .81 (Attractiveness factor), .85 (Upper Body Strength factor), and .86 (General Physical Condition factor) were reported for 331 male undergraduate students. Similarly, alpha coefficients of .78 (Attractiveness), .87 (Weight Concerns), and .82 (General Physical Condition) were reported for 633 female undergraduate students.

Validity: Convergent validity was demonstrated when correlating the responses of 44 male and 78 female undergraduate students to the BES with Rosenberg's Self-Esteem Scale. Discriminant validity was demonstrated in that anorexic women scored higher on the BES weight concern factor than did nonanorexic women. Similarly, 39 male weightlifters scored higher on the factor of perceived upper body strength than did 41 male nonweightlifters.

Norms: Presented for 331 males and 633 female undergraduate students for each of the three derived factors.

Availability: Contact Stephen Franzoi, Department of Psychology, Marquette University, Milwaukee, WI 53233. (Phone # 414-224-1650; E-mail: 6771franzois@vms.csd.mu.edu)

References
*Caruso, C. M., & Gill, D. L. (1992). Strengthening physical self-perceptions through exercise. *The Journal of Sports Medicine and Physical Fitness, 32,* 416-427.

*DiNucci, J. M., Finkenberg, M. E., McCune, S. L., McCune, E. D., & Mayo, T. (1994). Analysis of body esteem of female collegiate athletes. *Perceptual and Motor Skills, 78,* 315-319.

*Eklund, R. (1995). Self-esteem and social physique anxiety [Abstract]. *Journal of Sport & Exercise Psychology, 17* (Suppl.), S49.

*Finkenberg, M. E., DiNucci, J. M., McCune, S. L., & McCune, E. D. (1993). Body esteem and enrollment in classes with different levels of physical activity. *Perceptual and Motor Skills, 76,* 783-792.

*Martin, J., Wirth, J. C., & Engels, H. J. (1993). The relationship among self-esteem, social physique anxiety, and body-esteem in adolescent elite female figure skaters [Abstract]. *Proceedings of the Association for the Advancement of Applied Sport Psychology annual convention* (p. 95). Montreal, Canada.

*Martin, J., Wirth, J. C., & Engels, H. J. (1994). Self and bodily perceptions of elite female soccer players [Abstract]. *Journal of Sport & Exercise Psychology, 16* (Suppl.), S85.

*Silberstein, L. R., Striegel-Moore, Timko, C., & Rodin, J. (1988). Behavioral and psychological implications of body dissatisfaction: Do men and women differ? *Sex Roles, 19,* 219-232.

Body-Esteem Scale [For Children] [BES-C]
Beverley Katz Mendelson and Donna Romano White

Source: Mendelson, B. K., & White, D. R. (1982). Relation between body-esteem and self-esteem of obese and normal children. *Perceptual and Motor Skills, 54,* 899-905.

Purpose: To assess children's affective evaluations of their bodies.

Description: The BES-C currently contains 20 items reflecting how children evaluate their appearance and body, and how they feel they are evaluated by others. Children respond yes or no to items such as "I wish I were thinner" and "Kids my own age like my looks."

Construction: Not discussed.

Reliability: A split-half odd-even internal consistency coefficient of .85 was reported among 36 children (*n*=15 males and *n*=21 females), ages 7.5 to 12 years.

Validity: Concurrent validity was supported in that a correlation coefficient of .67 was obtained between these children's (*n*=36) scores on the BES-C and their corresponding scores on the Physical Appearance and Attributes component of the Piers-Harris Children's Self-concept Scale.

Norms: Not reported. Psychometric data were cited for 20 normal and 16 obese children residing in Montreal, Canada.

194

**Availability: Contact Donna Romano White, Center for Research in Human Development, Concordia University, 7141 Sherbrooke St., West, PY-170, Montreal, Quebec, Canada H4B 1R6. (Phone # 514-848-7542; FAX # 514-848-2815; E-mail: dwhite@vax2.concordia.ca)

References

*Mendelson, B. K., & White, D. R. (1985). Development of self-body-esteem in over-weight youngsters. *Developmental Psychology, 21,* 90-96.

Mendelson, B. K., & White, D. R. (1995). Children's global self-esteem predicted by body-esteem but not by weight. *Perceptual and Motor Skills, 80,* 97-98.

*Mendelson, B. K., White, D. R., & Mendelson, M. J. (in press). Self esteem and body-esteem: Effects of sex, age, and weight. *Journal of Applied Developmental Psychology.*

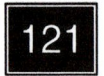

Body-Image Distortion Questionnaire [BIDQ]
Harriett M. Mable, Williams D. G. Balance, and Richard J. Galgan

Source: Mable, H. M., Balance, W. D. G., Galgan, R. J. (1986). Body-image distortion and dissatisfaction in university students. *Perceptual and Motor Skills, 63,* 907-911,

Purpose: To assess participants' perceptions of their body size.

Description: Participants are asked to indicate the point that they thought represented their body size on a line ranging from "50% under-weight" to "50% overweight," with the halfway point designated as "just right." Questions center on height, weight, and body build.

Construction: Not discussed.

Reliability: Test-retest reliability coefficients across a 3-week interval were .83 ($n=40$ males), .89 ($n=41$ females), and .92 (the combined sample) (from Mable, Balance, & Galgan, 1988).

Validity: Concurrent validity was supported in that a correlation coefficient of .89 was obtained between participants' ($n=81$) responses to the BIDQ and their actual body size (from Mable et al., 1988).

Norms: Not cited. Psychometric data were based on the responses of 40 male and 41 female undergraduate students.

Availability: Contact Williams D. G. Balance, Department of Psychology, 186 Windsor South Hall, University of Windsor, 401 Sunset Avenue, Windsor, Ontario, Canada N9B 3P4. (Phone # 519-253-4232, ext. 2227)

References

Loosemore, D. J., Mable, H. M., Galgan, R. J., Balance, W. D. G., & Moriarty, R. J. (1989). Body image disturbance in selected groups of men. *Psychology: A Journal of Human Behavior, 26*(2/3), 56-59.

*Mable, H. M., Balance, W. D. G., & Galgan, R. J. (1988). Reliability and accuracy of self-report of a new body-image measure. *Perceptual and Motor Skills, 66*, 861-862.

Body-Image Identification Test [BIIT]
Eleanor G. Gottesman and Willard E. Caldwell

Source: Gottesman, E. G., & Caldwell, W. E. (1966). The body-image identification test: A quantitative projective technique to study an aspect of body image. *The Journal of Genetic Psychology, 108*, 19-33.

Purpose: To measure feelings of masculinity-femininity as they relate to body image.

Description: The BIIT is a projective technique containing seven silhouette drawings of the human figure. Each participant is asked to choose which body and body part seem most like his or hers, and which body and body part he or she would prefer to have. The figures were scaled from 1 (*most masculine*) to 7 (*most feminine*).

Construction: In developing the figures, "the artist tried to incorporate some of the essential differentiating qualities between masculine and feminine attributes. . . ." (pp. 22-23).

Reliability: Not reported.

Validity: The BIIT discriminated among normal, disturbed, and slow learning individuals.

196

Norms: Not cited. Psychometric data were based on 21 female and 21 male slow learners (ages 13 to 17), 30 disturbed males (ages 8 to 11), and 31 normal males (ages 8 to 11).

Availability: Last known address: Contact Willard E. Caldwell, Apt. #316, 1101 New Hampshire Ave., NW, Washington, DC 20037. (Phone # 202-223-0223, Ext. 316)

References
Darden, E. (1972). A comparison of body image and self-concept variables among various sport groups. *Research Quarterly, 43,* 7-15.

*Darden, E. (1972). Masculinity-femininity body rankings by males and females. *The Journal of Psychology, 80,* 205-212.

123 Body-Image Questionnaire [BIQ]
Marilou Bruchon-Schweitzer and Florence Cousson

Source: Bruchon-Schweitzer, M. (1987). Dimensionality of the body-image: The Body-image questionnaire. *Perceptual and Motor Skills, 65,* 887-892.

Purpose: To assess perceptions, feelings, and attitudes induced by one's body, in terms of Favourable Body Image (FBI).

Description: The BIQ is a 19-item questionnaire in which participants respond to bipolar adjective pairs using a 5-point Likert format.

Construction: A total of 65 male and 72 female high school students were interviewed, and 300 words related to the body image were elicited. These words were grouped into 13 large categories containing antonyms and synonyms. Each category was illustrated by one or two items resulting in a 19-item questionnaire.

Reliability: The average test-retest reliability coefficient of the 19 items was .67 for a 10-day interval ($N=89$ male or female French students). A Cronbach alpha reliability coefficient ($N=393$ female French adults) of .86 was reported by the first author (M. Bruchon-Schweitzer, personal communication, April 22, 1996) on the FBI revised score.

Validity: A principal factor analysis of the responses of 245 male and 374 female respondents (ages 10 to 40 years) to the French version of the BIQ (with communalities in the diagonals) yielded four axes (with 84.60% accountable variance). The first one was identified as Favourable Body Image (with 29.21% accountable variance). Varimax rotations were carried out resulting in four meaningful factors. These factors were labeled Accessibility/ closeness, Satisfaction/dissatisfaction, Activity/passivity, and Relaxation/tension.

The first author noted (M. Bruchon-Schweitzer, personal communication, April 22, 1996) that in 1996 a principal axis analysis was conducted on the responses of 393 females on the same 19 items. The first axis was identified again as Favourable Body Image (with 25.72 accountable variance). With the 16 items having the greater loadings on this axis, the authors calculated the FBI revised score (14 of the 16 items are the same in the original and in the new score). The solutions obtained after varimax rotations were unclear, and further research is necessary to verify the four-factor solution originally reported.

The first author also reported (M. Bruchon-Schweitzer, personal communication, April 22, 1996) that the discriminant validity of the BIQ was supported in that 211 hospitalized patients (when compared to 200 healthy individuals) had more unfavorable body image scores. Furthermore, the FBI original score of the hospitalized patients was positively related ($r=.22$ for male patients; $r=.43$ for female patients) to the somatic outcome rated by the medical staff at the end of the hospitalization. Favorable body image scores predicted a better recovery, especially for female patients.

Norms: Normative data were presented for 245 male and 374 female students, ages 10-40, residing in France. Additional normative data are available from the first author for 393 French female adults on the original and revised FBI scores.

**Availability: Contact Marilou Bruchon-Schweitzer, Department of Psychology, Universite' de Bordeaux II, 3 Place de la Victoire, 33076 Bordeaux Cedex, France. (Phone # (33) 57 57 18 11; FAX # (33) 56 31 42 11)

Reference
*Bruchon-Schweitzer, M., Quintard, B., Paulhan, I., Nuissier, J., & Cousson, F. (1995). Psychological adjustment to hospitalization: Factorial structure, antecedents and outcome. *Psychological Reports, 76,* 1091-1100.

124 *Body-Image Questionnaire [BIQ]
D. Craig Huddy

Source: Huddy, D. C., Nieman, D. C., & Johnson, R. L. (1993). Relationship between body image and percent body fat among college male varsity athletes and nonathletes. *Perceptual and Motor Skills, 77,* 851-857.

Purpose: To assess negative and positive feelings toward one's body image.

Description: The BIQ contains 20 items (e.g., "I feel good about body image"). Participants respond to each item using three response alternatives: agree, undecided, or disagree. Total scores on the BIQ can range from 20 (least favorable body image) to 60 (most favorable body image).

Construction: Not discussed.

Reliability: The author reports that a Cronbach alpha internal consistency coefficient of .72 was obtained.

Validity: Participants' (*N*=45) scores on the BIQ correlated negatively (.51) with scores on skinfold measurements to assess percent of body fat.

Norms: Not cited. Psychometric data were reported for 15 sedentary male students, 15 varsity football athletes, and 15 male varsity swimmers attending a large midwestern university.

**Availability: Contact D. Craig Huddy, Department of Health, Leisure, and Exercise Science, Appalachian State University, Boone, NC 28608. (Phone # 704-262-2935; FAX # 704-262-3138). Items are listed in the *Source.*

125 *Body Image Satisfaction Questionnaire (BIS)

Maijaliisa Rauste-von Wright

Source: Rauste-von Wright, M. (1989). Body image satisfaction in adolescent girls and boys: A longitudinal study. *Journal of Youth and Adolescence, 18,* 71-83.

Purpose: To assess participants' satisfaction with various parts of their bodies.

Description: Individuals are asked on the BIS to rate 17 body parts (e.g., nose, legs) on a 5-point ordinal scale with the anchorings 1 (*dissatisfied*) to 5 (*satisfied*).

Construction: Not discussed.

Reliability: Cronbach alpha reliability coefficients of .82 ($N=105$), .85 ($N=100$), .91 ($N=95$), and .92 ($N=90$) were reported for samples of 11- to 12-year-old children, 13- to 14-year-old children, 15- to 16-year-old adolescents, and 18- to 19-year-old young adults, respectively.

Validity: Participants' scores on the BIS were positively correlated to experienced attractiveness, and negatively correlated to anxiety and frequency of psychosomatic symptoms.

Norms: Not cited. Psychometric data were reported for four age groups of children and adolescents residing in Helsinki, Finland, who were tested over a 7-year period.

**Availability: Contact Maijaliisa Rauste-von Wright, Department of Education, University of Helsinki, PL 38, Fin 00014, Helsinki, Finland. [Phone # (358-0) 492373; FAX # (358-0) 497274]

126 Body Parts Satisfaction Scale (BPSS)
Ellen Berscheid, Elaine Waltser, and George Bohrnstedt

Source: Berscheid, E., Walster, E., & Bohrnstedt, G. (1973). The happy American body: A survey report. *Psychology Today, 7*(6), 119-123, 126-131.

Purpose: To assess an individual's satisfaction with his or her body.

Description: The BPSS contains a list of 25 body parts and characteristics. Participants rate their satisfaction/dissatisfaction with each body part and characteristic using a 6-point ordinal scale with the anchorings 0 (*extremely dissatisfied*) to 5 (*extremely satisfied*). Seven subscores plus a total score are derived.

Construction: Not discussed.

Reliability: Cronbach alpha internal consistency coefficients ranged from .66 to .82 for the subscores for females; .74 to .84 for male participants. Total scores reliability estimates were .86 for females and .89 for males (G. Bohrnstedt, personal communication, March 26, 1996).

Validity: Participants' (*n*=2,000) responses on the total score BPSS correlated positively (.45 for females; .44 for males) with the Janis-Fiel-Eagley Self-Esteem Scale supporting convergent validity. It was also noted (G. Bohrnstedt, personal communication, March 26, 1996) that the total score BPSS correlated -.21 (females) and -.28 (males) with comfort in interacting with members of the opposite sex.

Norms: Presented for 1,000 males and 1,000 females categorized by three age groups--under 24, 25-44, and 45+ years.

**Availability: Contact George W. Bohrnstedt, American Institutes for Research, P. O. Box 1113, 1791 Arastradero Road, Palo Alto, CA 94302-1113. (Phone # 415-493-3550; FAX # 415-858-0958; E-mail: gbohrnstedt@air-ca.org)

References

*Butters, J. W., & Cash, T. F. (1987). Cognitive-behavioral treatment of women's body-image dissatisfaction. *Journal of Consulting and Clinical Psychology, 55,* 889-897.

Gutherie, S. R., Ferguson, C., & Grimmett, D. (1994). Elite women bodybuilders: Ironing out nutritional misconceptions. *The Sport Psychologist, 16,* 271-286.

Petrie, T. A. (1993). Disordered eating in female collegiate gymnasts: Prevalence and personality/attitudinal correlates. *Journal of Sport & Exercise Psychology, 15,* 424-436.

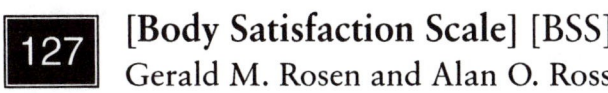

127   [Body Satisfaction Scale] [BSS]
Gerald M. Rosen and Alan O. Ross

Source: Rosen, G. M., & Ross, A. O. (1968). Relationship of body image to self-concept. *Journal of Consulting and Clinical Psychology, 32,* 100.

Purpose: To evaluate a person's satisfaction with his or her physical appearance.

Description: The BSS contains a list of 24 body parts. Participants are asked to indicate, using a 6-point Likert scale, how satisfied they are with the appearance of each body part and how important that body part is to them.

Construction: Not discussed.

Reliability: Not cited.

Validity: Concurrent validity was supported in that the correlation coefficient between participants' (n=82) responses to the BSS and the Gough Adjective Check List was .52, indicating a positive but low relationship between satisfaction with one's body image and satisfaction with one's self-concept.

Norms: Not cited. Psychometric data were based on the responses of 82 undergraduate students.

Availability: Last known address: Gerald M. Rosen, Cabrina Medical Tower, 901 Boren Ave., Suite 1910, Seattle, WA 98104. (Phone # 206-343-9474). Also can be obtained from ADI Auxiliary Publications Project, No. 9756, Photoduplication Service, Library of Congress, Washington, DC 20540.

128 *Body Scale [BS]
Janet A. Wilkins, Fred J. Boland, and John
Albinson

Source: Wilkins, J. A., Boland, F. J., & Albinson, J. (1991). A comparison of male and female university athletes and nonathletes on eating disorder indices: Are athletes protected? [Abstract]. *Proceedings of the Association for the Advancement of Applied Sport Psychology annual conference* (p. 133). Savannah, GA.

Purpose: To provide "...a measure of the respondent's self-confidence regarding his/her body and its ability to move and perform" (p. 133).

Description: The BS contains eight items, and was described as an exploratory scale.

Construction: Not discussed.

Reliability: A Cronbach alpha coefficient of .61 was reported for a university sample.

Validity: Not discussed.

Norms: Not cited. Psychometric data were reported for 295 university students (n=99 male athletes; n=78 female athletes; n=39 male nonathletes; and n=78 female nonathletes). Note that nonathletes were defined as individuals who did not compete beyond the intramural level of competition.

Availability: Contact John Albinson, School of Physical Education and Health Education, Queen's University, Kingston, Ontario, Canada K7L 3N6. (Phone # 613-545-6283; FAX # 613-545-2009; E-mail: albinson@knot.queensu.ca)

129 Body Self-Relations Questionnaire (BSRQ)
Thomas F. Cash and Barbara A. Winstead

Source: Cash, T. F., Winstead, B. A., & Janda, L. H. (1986). The great American shape-up. *Psychology Today, 20*(4), 30-34, 36-37.

Purpose: To assess feelings and attention paid toward one's appearance, health, and physical fitness, as well as how one rates the importance of various aspects of body image.

Description: The BSRQ is an attitudinal measure of body image that produces data on the attitudinal components of evaluation, attention/importance, and activity for the somatic domains of appearance, fitness, and health. The BSRQ also provides a sexuality evaluation score. Participants respond to 140 items using a 5-point Likert scale.

Construction: Not discussed.

Reliability: Cronbach alpha coefficients of .88 and .80 were reported for the Appearance Evaluation scale and the Body Areas Satisfaction scale, respectively (Cash, 1989).

Validity: The BSRQ discriminated among 1,020 females and 980 males, in that females evaluated themselves more negatively than did the males across all body image areas.

Norms: Normative data were cited for 1,020 females and 980 males ranging in age from less than 20 to 75 years.

Availability: Contact Thomas Cash, Department of Psychology, Old Dominion University, Norfolk, VA 23529-0267. (Phone # 804-683-4213; E-mail: tfc100f@viper.mgb.odu.edu)

References
Adame, O. D., Johnson, T. C., Cole, S. P., Matthiasson, H., & Abbas, M. A. (1990). Physical fitness relation to amount of physical exercise, body image, and locus of control among college men and women. *Perceptual and Motor Skills, 70,* 1347-1350.

*Adame, O. D., Radell, S. A., & Johnson, T. C. (1991). Physical fitness, body image, and locus of control in college women dancers and nondancers. *Perceptual and Motor Skills, 71,* 91-95.

*Butters, J., W., & Cash, T. F. (1987). Cognitive-behavioral treatment of women's body-image dissatisfaction. Journal of Consulting and *Clinical Psychology, 55*, 889-897.

*Cash, T. F. (1989). Body-image affect: Gestalt versus summing the parts. *Perceptual and Motor Skills, 69*, 17-18.

*Cash, T. F. (1993). Body-image attitudes among obese enrollees in a commercial weight-loss program. *Perceptual and Motor Skills, 77*, 1099-1103.

*Cash, T. F. (1994). Body-image attitudes: Evaluation, investment, and affect. *Perceptual and Motor Skills, 78*, 1168-1170.

*Cash, T. F., & Green, G. K. (1986). Body weight and body image among college women: Perception, cognition, and affect. *Journal of Personality Assessment, 50*, 290-301.

*Cash, T. F., Wood, K. C., Phelps, K. D., & Boyd, K.(1991). New assessments of weight-related body image derived from extant instruments. *Perceptual and Motor Skills, 73*, 235-241.

Gutherie, S. R., Ferguson, C., Grimmett, D. (1994). Elite women bodybuilders: Ironing out nutritional misconceptions. *The Sport Psychologist, 8*, 271-286.

*Noles, S. W., Cash, T. F., & Winstead, B. A. (1985). Body image, physical attractiveness, and depression. *Journal of Consulting and Clinical Psychology, 53*, 88-94.

*Pasman, L., & Thompson, J. K. (1988). Body image and eating disturbance in obligatory runners, obligatory weightlifters, and sedentary individuals. *International Journal of Eating Disorders, 7*, 759-769.

Radell, S. A., Adame, D. D., & Johnson, T. C. (1993). Dance experiences associated with body-image and personality among college students: A comparison of dancers and nondancers. *Perceptual and Motor Skills, 77*, 507-513.

130 [Movement Satisfaction Scale] [MSS]
Barbara A. Nelson and Dorothy J. Allen

Source: Nelson, B. A., & Allen, D. J. (1970). Scale for the appraisal of movement satisfaction. *Perceptual and Motor Skills, 31*, 795-800.

Purpose: To assess an individual's satisfaction or dissatisfaction with his or her movement ability.

Description: The MSS contains 50 items focusing on time, force, flow, the quality of movement, and the use of space (e.g., "ability to walk with poise," "ability to produce sudden movement"). Participants describe the strength of their feelings about each item on a 5-point scale, with responses ranging from *strong negative feelings* to *strong positive feelings*.

Construction: A total of 129 items were developed based on Laban's elements of movement. These items were evaluated by eight experts in psychology and in physical education in terms of item clarity, content relevance, and appropriateness for high school and college age groups. A total of 75 items were retained, which were then administered to 176 males and females, ages 18-21 years. Item analyses led to the retention of 50 items.

Reliability: An internal consistency coefficient (based on the Kuder-Richardson formula) of .95 was obtained among 359 men and 518 women.

Validity: The MSS discriminated between males (n=359) and females (n=518) in that males had greater satisfaction than did females. Older individuals (18-21 years) responded with more dissatisfaction regarding movement ability than did younger individuals (14-17 years).

Norms: Descriptive and psychometric data reported were based on the responses of 359 males and 518 females (ages 14-21 years) who were enrolled in either one of three high schools, one junior high school, or at The Ohio State University.

Availability: Order document NAPS-01152 from ASIS National Auxiliary Publication Service, c/o CCM Information Corporation, 909 Third Ave., 21st floor, New York, NY 10022.

Reference

*Burton, E. C. (1976). Relationship between trait and state anxiety, movement satisfaction, and participation in physical education activities. *Research Quarterly, 47*, 326-331.

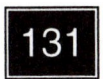 ## My Body Index [MBI]
Carol Cutler Riddick and Robin Stanger Freitag

Source: Riddick, C. C., & Freitag, R. S. (1984). The impact of an aerobic fitness program on the body image of older women. *Activities, Adaptation & Aging, 6*(1), 59-70.

Purpose: To examine perceived body image among older women.

Description: The MBI contains 13 pairs of bipolar adjectives. For each pair of adjectives, participants indicate how they feel about their bodies by responding to a 6-point semantic differential continuum.

Construction: Four academics in recreation (2 males and 2 females) were instructed to identify, for each pair of adjectives, the adjective that would more likely be construed as negative (in relation to body image) among women 50 years of age or older.

Reliability*: A Cronbach alpha reliability coefficient of .96 (n=26) was reported.

Validity: Construct validity was supported in that females 50 years of age or older (n=6) had higher MBI scores after participation in an 8-week aerobic fitness program than did control subjects (n=8).

Norms: Not cited. Psychometric data were reported for 14 females, 50 years of age or older, who were enrolled in an aerobic exercise program in Laurel, Maryland.

Availability: Last known address: Carol Cutler Riddick, Department of Physical Education and Recreation, Gallaudet University, 800 Florida Ave. NE, Washington, DC 20002-3625. (Phone # 202-651-5510)

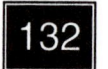 Perceived Somatotype Scale (PS)
Larry A. Tucker

Source: Tucker, L. A. (1982). Relationship between perceived somatotype and body cathexis of college males. *Psychological Reports, 50,* 983-989.

Purpose: To assess males' perceptions of their actual versus ideal body build.

Description: The scale contains a lineup of seven male figures representing seven different somatotypes. Participants select the figure most representative of their own body build. They are also asked to select their ideal body figure, that is, the body build they would like to have as their own.

Construction: Figures were drawn from photographs and sketches of Sheldon's (1954) classification of somatotypes.

Reliability: Test-retest reliability coefficients ($n=63$ males) were reported as .96 (perceived body image) and .94 (ideal body image) across a 2-week time interval.

Validity: Not discussed. The author noted, however, (L. A. Tucker, personal communication, March 6, 1990) that "indirect validation of the Perceived Somatotype Scale is supported by a number of studies in which PS scores were strongly related to body image, global self-concept, neuroticism, extroversion, and physical fitness levels."

Norms: Not cited. Psychometric data were reported for 63 male college students.

Availability: Contact Larry A. Tucker, College of Physical Education, 212 Richards Building, Brigham Young University, Provo, UT 84602. (Phone # 801-378-4927; E-mail: larry_tucker@byu.edu)

References

*Davis, L. L. (1985). Perceived somatotype, body-cathexis, and attitudes toward clothing among college females. *Perceptual and Motor Skills, 61,* 1199-1205.

Sheldon, W. H. (1954). *Atlas of men.* New York: Harper.

*Tucker, L. A. (1983). Self-concept: A function of self-perceived somatotype. The *Journal of Psychology, 113,* 123-133.

*Tucker, L. A. (1984). Physical attractiveness, somatotype, and the male personality: A dynamic interactional perspective. *Journal of Clinical Psychology, 40,* 1226-1234.

Tucker, L. A. (1985). Physical, psychological, social, and lifestyle differences among adolescents classified according to cigarette smoking intention status. *Journal of School Health, 55,* 127-131.

133 Social Physique Anxiety Scale (SPAS)
Elizabeth A. Hart, Mark R. Leary, and W. Jack Rejeski

Source: Hart, E. A., Leary, M. R., & Rejeski, W. J. (1989). The measurement of social physique anxiety. *Journal of Sport & Exercise Psychology, 11,* 94-104.

Purpose: To assess the extent to which people become anxious when others observe or evaluate their physiques.

Description: The SPAS is a 12-item self-report scale focusing on anxiety arising as a result of others' evaluations of one's body. Participants respond to each item using a 5-point Likert scale.

Construction: A pool of 30 self-report items that dealt with physique anxiety were reviewed by experts in body movement, psychology, or exercise science for item clarity, content validity, and appropriateness for both sexes. Based on their evaluation, the pool was reduced to 22 items. Factor analysis of 195 undergraduate students' (n=97 females; n=98 males) responses to the 22 items led to the retention of 11 items loading greater than .60 on a single unrotated factor. An additional item was added to the test. Similar factor loadings emerged when a principal component analysis was then applied to the responses of 46 females and 43 males on this 12-item test.

Reliability: An alpha reliability coefficient of .90 was reported (n=89). An 8-week test-retest reliability coefficient for this sample was .82.

Validity: Concurrent validity was demonstrated by showing that participants' (93 women and 94 men) responses to the SPAS correlated with measures that relate to general concerns with others' evaluations. The SPAS also correlated with public self-consciousness and measures of body cathexis and body esteem. Discriminant validity was evident by lack of correlation with a social desirability measure and by the failure of these participants' scores on the SPAS to relate to a measure of private self-consciousness.

Further support for criterion-related validity was evident by demonstrating that women (n=56 undergraduate women) who scored high on the SPAS were heavier and had a higher percentage of body fat than did low scorers on the SPAS. Furthermore, high scorers reported greater anxiety than low scorers during an actual evaluation of their physiques.

Norms: Not reported. Psychometric data were presented for 195 women and 137 men.

Availability: Contact W. Jack Rejeski, Department of Health and Sport Science, Campus Box 7234, 309 Gymnasium, Wake Forest University, Winston-Salem, NC 27109. (Phone # 910-759-5837; E-mail: rejeski@wfu.edu)

References

*Cramer-Hammann, B., Lutter, C., Cornelius, A., Piontek, K., & Hardy, C. J. (1993). Examining the factor structure of the Social Physique Anxiety Scale [Abstract]. *Proceedings of the Association for the Advancement of Applied Sport Psychology annual convention* (p. 34). Montreal, Canada.

*Crawford, S., & Eklund, R. C. (1994). Social physique anxiety, reasons for exercise, and attitudes toward exercise settings. *Journal of Sport & Exercise Psychology, 16,* 70-82.

*Diehl, N., & Petrie, T. (1995). A longitudinal investigation of the effects of different exercise modalities on social physique anxiety [Abstract]. *Journal of Applied Sport Psychology, 7* (Suppl.), S55.

*Eklund, R. (1995). Self-esteem and social physique anxiety [Abstract]. *Journal of Sport & Exercise Psychology, 17* (Suppl.), S49.

*Eklund, R. C., & Crawford, S. (1994). Active women, social physique anxiety, and exercise. *Journal of Sport & Exercise Psychology, 16,* 431-448.

*Hart, E. (1991). The influence of exercise experience on social physique anxiety and exercise behavior [Abstract]. *Proceedings of the Association for the Advancement of Applied Sport Psychology annual convention* (p. 63). Savannah, GA.

*Isogai, H. (1995). Gender differences in social physique anxiety [Abstract]. *Journal of Sport & Exercise Psychology, 17* (Suppl.), S63.

*Jackson, C., Kambis, K., & Jackson, C. (1991). Cross-validation of the Social Physique Anxiety Scale [Abstract]. *Proceedings of the Association for the Advancement of Applied Sport Psychology annual convention* (p. 72). Savannah, GA.

*Johnson, C., Diehl, N., Petrie, T., & Rogers, R. (1995). Social physique anxiety and eating disorders: What's the connection? [Abstract]. *Journal of Applied Sport Psychology, 7* (Suppl.), S76.

*Lantz, C., Hardy, C., & Ainsworth, B. (1991). The effects of social physique anxiety, gender, age and depression on exercise behavior [Abstract]. *Proceedings of the Association for the Advancement of Applied Sport Psychology annual convention* (p. 91). Savannah, GA.

*Martin, J., Wirth, J. C., & Engles, H. J. (1993). The relationships among self-esteem, social physique anxiety, and body-esteem in adolescent elite female figure skaters [Abstract]. *Proceedings of the Asssociation for the Advancement of Applied Sport Psychology annual convention* (p. 95). Montreal, Canada.

*Martin, J., Wirth, J. C., & Engles, H. J. (1994). Self and bodily perceptions of elite female soccer players [Abstract]. *Journal of Sport & Exercise Psychology, 16* (Suppl.), S85.

*Petrie, T. A., Diehl, N. S., Rogers, R., & Johnson, C. L. (1995). The Social Physique Anxiety Scale: Reliability and construct validation [Abstract]. *Journal of Applied Sport Psychology, 7* (Suppl.), S99.

*Reel, J. J., & Gill, D. L. (1995). Psychosocial factors related to eating disorders among high school and college female cheerleaders [Abstract]. *Journal of Applied Sport Psychology, 7* (Suppl.), S103.

*Remington, L., Hardy, C., & Ainsworth, B. (1991). Exploring the physical activity of socially physique anxious subjects [Abstract]. *Proceedings of the Association for the Advancement oaf Applied Sport Psychology annual convention* (p. 128). Savannah, GA.

Spink, K. S. (1992). Relation of anxiety about social physique to location of participation in physical activity. *Perceptual and Motor Skills, 74,* 1075-1078.

Van Raalte, J. L., Schmelzer, G., & Brewer, B. W. (1995). Social physique anxiety and body esteem of competitive male rowers [Abstract]. *Journal of Applied Sport Psychology, 7* (Suppl.), S118.

Chapter 9

Cognitive Strategies

Tests in this chapter assess the cognitive skills athletes employ prior to and during sport competition. These strategies include self-talk, coping with anxiety, imagery, association/dissociation, and concentration. Tests also assess thoughts during running, coping strategies athletes employ to adjust to pain, task-irrelevant cognitions, and thoughts that occur following mistakes during athletic competition.

Chapter 9. Cognitive Strategies — 211

134 *[Associative/Dissociative Scales for Triathlon Athletes] [ADSTA]

Frank C. Bakker, Richard J. A. van Diesen,
Marielle C. Spekreijse, and J. Rob Pijpers

Source: Bakker, F. C., van Diesen, R. J. A., Spekreijse, M. C., & Pijpers, J. R. (1993). Cognitive strategies of elite and non-elite triathlon participants. *Proceedings of the Eighth World Congress of Sport Psychology* (pp. 332-336). Lisbon, Portugal.

Purpose: To examine the frequency of associative and dissociative thoughts reported by elite and nonelite triathlon participants directly following the finish of a race.

Description: The ADSTA contains five items that focus on the frequency of associative thoughts and five items that focus on the frequency of dissociative thoughts. Separate scales exist for swimming, cycling, and running. Participants indicate the frequency of thoughts with the anchorings 1 (*not at all*) to 5 (*very often*).

Construction: Not discussed.

Reliability: Cronbach alpha coefficients (*N*=55) ranged from .56 to .72.

Validity: Not discussed.

Norms: Not cited. Psychometric data were reported for 31 male European Middle Distance participants and 24 male Long Distance triathlon participants. The mean age of participants was 29.5 years (*SD*=6.2).

Availability: Last known address: Frank C. Bakker, Faculty of Human Movement Sciences, Free University, Amsterdam, The Netherlands.

135 Cognitive Activity During Competition (CADC)

Eric J. Cooley

Source: Cooley, E. J. (1987). A process study of cognitions during competition [Abstract]. *Proceedings of the Association for the Advancement of Applied Sport Psychology annual conference* (p. 43). Newport Beach, CA.

Purpose: To examine the cognitive patterns relating to competitive sport performance.

Description: The CADC contains 58 items describing possible thoughts occurring immediately before (10 minutes) and during the event. For example, participants are asked to respond to the item "I analyzed the appearance and behavior of my competition." Participants respond to each item using a 5-point Likert Scale in which items are rated for frequency of occurrence.

Construction: Not discussed.

Reliability: Not reported.

Validity: Athletes' responses to the CADC were correlated with self-rated performance outcome. Good performance was associated with self-confidence, strategic thinking, positive self-talk, and lower levels of self-criticism.

Norms: Not cited. Psychometric data were reported for 32 male and 22 female intercollegiate track athletes.

Availability: Contact Eric J. Cooley, Department of Psychology, Western Oregon State University, Monmouth, OR 97361. (Phone # 503-838-8331)

Reference

Cooley, E. (1988). A process approach to cognitions during competition [Abstract]. *Proceedings of the Association for the Advancement for Applied Sport Psychology annual conference*. Nashua, NH.

136 *Cognitive Style in Sport Inventory (CSSI)
Mark H. Anshel, L. R. T Williams, and J. J. Quek

Source: Anshel, M. H., Williams, L. R. T., & Quek, J. J. (1992). Development of the Cognitive Style in Sport Inventory [Abstract]. *Proceedings of the North American Society for the Psychology of Sport and Physical Activity annual convention* (p. 130). Pittsburgh, PA.

Purpose: To assess an athlete's disposition or preference to perceive, process, and respond to information in the competitive sport environment.

Description: The CSSI contains 63 items and five primary dimensions that assess cognitive style: Social, Affect, Coping with Stress, Sensory Perception, and Motor Skill Reception. Participants respond on a 5-point Likert scale with the anchorings *strongly agree* to *strongly disagree.*

Construction: Initially, a total of 143 items were administered to 806 athletes in Australia and Singapore. Item analyses led to the retention of 63 items.

Reliability: For the Australian sample ($N=395$), an overall Hoyt coefficient of .71 and a Cronbach alpha coefficient of .59 were reported. For the Singapore sample ($N=411$), a Hoyt coefficient of .70 and a Cronbach alpha coefficient of .57 were reported.

Validity: There was little support for construct validity in that only 27.9% of the variance in participants' responses to the 63 items could be accounted for based on the factor analytic model employed.

Norms: Not cited. Psychometric data were reported for 395 Australian ($n=186$ females; $n=209$ males) and 411 Singapore ($n=246$ females; $n=165$ males) athletes ages 11 to 18 years.

**Availability: Contact Mark H. Anshel, Department of Psychology, University of Wollongong, P. O. Box 1144, Wollongong, New South Wales, Australia 2522. (Phone # 61-42-213732; FAX # 61-42-214163; E-mail: m.anshel@uow.edu.au).

137 Diving Questionnaire [DQ]

Pamela S. Highlen and Bonnie B. Bennett

Source: Highlen, P. S., & Bennett, B. B. (1983). Elite divers and wrestlers: A comparison between open- and closed-skilled athletes. *Journal of Sport Psychology, 5,* 390-409.

Purpose: To identify cognitive and behavioral strategies used by divers when preparing for and engaging in major competitive events.

Description: The DQ contains five subscales and a total of 65 items representing these subscales. The five subscales include Thoughts, Coping With Anxiety, Positive-Negative Thoughts, Attributions for Better Performance, and Imagery. Divers respond to each item on an 11-point interval scale.

Construction: An initial pool of 110 items were placed into 14 factors if they appeared conceptually related. These items were derived from previous research on elite wrestlers and discussions with one college diving coach. The DQ was pilot tested with several collegiate divers. An item analysis led to the retention of 65 items.

Reliability: Alpha internal consistency coefficients (n=44 elite divers) were .82 (Thoughts), .78 (Coping With Anxiety), .75 (Positive-Negative Thoughts), .68 (Attributions), and .64 (Imagery).

Validity: The DQ discriminated between eventual qualifiers (n=8) versus nonqualifiers (n=36) to Canada's diving team at the Pan-American Games. The qualifiers scored higher on self-confidence, concentration, and the use of imagery.

Norms: Not reported. Psychometric data were cited for 44 elite Canadian divers.

**Availability: Contact Pamela S. Highlen, 142 Townshend Hall, Department of Psychology, The Ohio State University, 1885 Neil Avenue Mall, Columbus, OH 43210-1222. (Phone # 614-422-5308; FAX # 614 292-4537; E-mail: phighlen@magnus.acs.ohio-state.edu)

138 *Mental Attributes of Performance Scale (MAPS)

Lynette Evans and Chris Madden

Source: Evans, L., & Madden, C. (1993). Strategies related to performance in sport. *Proceedings of the Eighth World Congress of Sport Psychology* (pp. 348-351). Lisbon, Portugal.

Purpose: To assess the mental coping strategies used by athletes.

Description: The MAPS contains 48 items that assess nine factors related to strategies used in competition: (a) Attention and Energy Control, (b) Preparation and Problem-Focused Coping, (c) Arousal Control and Concentration, (d) Communication and Perceptual Abilities, (e) Self Control and Orientation to Others, (f) Effort, (g) Task Focus, (h) Risk Taking and Determination, and (i) Self-Assurance under Pressure. Athletes are asked to recall the last game they played, and respond to each item on a 4-point Likert scale with the anchorings 1 (*not at all*) to 4 (*very often*).

Construction: The items were derived from the sport psychology literature, and "... were selected on the basis of their representing strategies used by athletes to enhance their performance or cope with the demands of competition" (p. 349).

Reliability: Not reported.

Validity: Discriminant validity was supported in that all nine factors on the MAPS distinguished high- from low-performing athletes. Performance assessments were based on Australian football athletes' (*N*=38) self ratings of their performances in a previous game. The largest differences indicated that high- performing athletes used Arousal Control and Concentration, Self-Control and Orientation to Others, Effort, and Task Focus more frequently than did low-performing athletes.

Norms: Not cited. Psychometric data were reported for 38 Australian Rules football players (*M* age=21 years).

Availability: Contact Chris Madden, Department of Behavioural Health Sciences, Carlton Campus, 625, La Trobe University, Swanston Street, Carlton, Victoria 3053, Australia. (Phone # 03 9479 1741)

Reference
Madden, C., & Evans, L. (1993). Mental Attributes of Performance in Sport (MAPS). *Proceedings of the Eighth World Congress of Sport Psychology* (pp. 463-466). Lisbon, Portugal.

*Reactions to Mistakes During Competition Scale (RMDC)

Randy O. Frost and Katherine J. Henderson

Source: Frost, R. O., & Henderson, K. J. (1991). Perfectionism and reactions to athletic competition. *Journal of Sport & Exercise Psychology, 13,* 323-335.

Purpose: To assess thoughts that occur following mistakes during athletic practice or competition.

Description: The RMDC contains 16 items, 7 of which were combined to form a social concerns subscale (e.g., "My teammates are judging me"). Nine other items are analyzed separately.

Construction: Not discussed.

Reliability: A Cronbach alpha internal consistency coefficient ($N=40$) of .94 was reported for the social concerns subscale.

Validity: Convergent validity was supported in that participants' ($N=40$) reactions to mistakes during athletic performance were positively correlated with their scores on the Concern Over Mistakes and Doubts About Actions subscales of the Multidimensional Perfectionism Scale (Frost, Marten, Lahart, & Rosenblate, 1990).

Norms: Not cited. Psychometric data were reported for 40 females participating in five Division III varsity sports.

Availability: Contact Randy O. Frost, Department of Psychology, Smith College, 307 Bass Hall, Northampton, MA 01063. (Phone # 413-585-3911; FAX # 413-585-3786; E-mail: rfrost@smith.edu)

Reference

Frost, R. O., Marten, P., Lahart, C., & Rosenblate, A. (1990). The dimensions of perfectionism. *Cognitive Therapy and Research, 14,* 449-468.

 ## Running Styles Questionnaire [RSQ]
John M. Silva and Mark Appelbaum

Source: Silva, J. M., & Appelbaum, M. (1983). Association- dissociation patterns of contestants at the 1980 United States Olympic Marathon Trials [Abstract]. In *Psychology of motor behavior and sport-1983* (p.70). Proceedings of the North American Society for the Psychology of Sport and Physical Activity annual convention. Michigan State University, East Lansing.

Purpose: To assess association-dissociation cognitive strategies employed by elite long-distance runners.

Description: The RSQ contains 12 multiple-choice items and 6 open-ended type questions.

Construction: A panel of experts from collegiate track and field programs, sport psychology, and psychology were used to establish the content validity of the RSQ (J. M. Silva, personal communication, March 19, 1990).

Reliability: An intraclass correlation coefficient of .73 was obtained among 43 males (who were enrolled in either a long- distance running class or who were members of a collegiate cross- country team) across a one-week interval.

Validity: Runners (*n*=32) less or more successful at the 1980 United States Olympic Marathon Trials could successfully be differentiated on the basis of their responses to the RSQ.

Norms: Not cited. Psychometric data were reported for 32 male partic-

220

ipants in the Olympic marathon trials and for 43 male undergraduate students.

Availability: Contact John M. Silva, Department of PESSS, CB #8700, 203 Fetzer Gym, University of North Carolina, Chapel Hill, NC 27599-8700. (Phone # 919-962-5176; FAX # 919-962-0489; E-mail: usilva@uncmvs.oit.unc.edu)

References

*Menickelli, J., & McPherson, S. L. (1995). Associative and dissociative cognitive strategies utilized by male and female collegiate mile runners during performance [Abstract]. *Journal of Sport & Exercise Psychology, 17* (Suppl.), S80.

*Smith, A. L., Gill, D. L., Crews, D. J., Hopewell, R., & Morgan, D. W. (1995). Attentional strategy use by experienced distance runners: Physiological and psychological effects. *Research Quarterly for Exercise and Sport, 66*(2), 142-150

141 *[Self-Regulation Questionnaire] [SRQ]
Mark H. Anshel

Source: Anshel, M. H. (1995). An examination of self-regulatory cognitive-behavioural strategies of Australian elite and non-elite competitive male swimmers. *Australian Psychologist, 30,* 78-83.

Purpose: To describe and evaluate the self-regulatory thoughts and strategies used by elite and nonelite athletes.

Description: The SRQ contains 100 items and five subscales: Problem Identification, Commitment, Execution, Environmental Management, and Generalisation. Participants respond to each item using a 5-point Likert type scale with the anchorings 1 (*very much like me*) to 5 (*not at all like me*).

Construction: Items and subscales for the questionnaire are based on the components of Kirschenbaum and Wittrock's (1984) self-regulation model. Five swim coaches, 10 competitive swimmers, 2 postgraduate students, and 1 sport psychology researcher were interviewed. These individuals were provided with definitions and examples of the application of the self-regulation model. The "interviewees were asked to describe psychological characteristics and behaviours that were consistent with each component. Survey items were then constructed for comprehension by athletes with a minimum reading level of Grade 7" (p. 80). Content validity was established in a pilot study with nonelite athletes.

Reliability: Cronbach alpha internal consistency coefficients (*N*=125) of .72 (Problem Identification, .83 (Commitment), .89 (Execution), .69 (Environment), and .46 (Generalisation) were reported.

Validity: Discriminant validity was supported in that elite athletes (*n*=77) differed from nonelite athletes (*n*=48) on Commitment and Execution. Generally, it was found that elite athletes engaged in self-regulatory behaviours more extensively than did nonelite athletes.

Norms: Not cited. Psychometric data were reported for 77 elite male competitive swimmers, ages 17.4 to 22.3 years, and 48 nonelite male competitive swimmers, ages 17.1 to 19.6 years. The elite swimmers were identified by Australia's national competitive swimming organization as members of their national team, whereas nonelite swimmers were members of local swim clubs in New South Wales, Australia.

Availability: Contact Mark H. Anshel, Department of Psychology, University of Wollongong, P. O. Box 1144, Wollongong, New South Wales, Australia 2522. (Phone #61-42-213732; FAX #61-42-214163; E-mail: m.anshel@uow.edu.au)

142 Self-Statement Questionnaire (SSQ)
Gerry Larsson and I. Anderzen

Source: Larsson, G., & Anderzen, I. (1987). Appraisal, coping, catecholamine excretion and psychomotor performance during calm and stressful conditions. *Scandinavian Journal of Sports Sciences, 9,* 47-51.

Purpose: To assess competition-specific cognitive coping.

Description: The SSQ contains 36 items. Respondents are asked to indicate (on a 3-point ordinal scale) the extent to which they use positive self-talk (18 items) or negative self-talk (18 items) during competition. An example of a positive self-talk item is "You can handle the pressure, just take one shot at a time." An example of a negative self-talk item is "I'll probably make a mistake right at the beginning."

Construction: Not discussed.

Reliability: Not presented.

Validity: The construct validity of the SSQ was supported in that 14 Swedish elite male golfers reduced the amount of negative self-talk (when compared to a control group of 14 Swedish elite male golfers) after being exposed to a stress inoculation training program (Larsson, Cook, & Starrin, 1988).

Norms: Not presented. Psychometric data were based on the responses of 28 Swedish elite male golfers, ages 16-17 years.

**Availability: Contact Gerry Larsson, Centre for Public Health Research, Box 9104, S-650 09 Karlstad, Sweden. (Phone # +46-54-885522; FAX # +46-54-885523; E-mail: gerry.larsson@hks.se)

Reference

Larsson, G., Cook, C., & Starrin, B. (1988). A time and cost efficient stress inoculation training program for athletes: A study of junior golfers. *Scandinavian Journal of Sports Sciences, 10,* 23-28.

143 [Sport Cognitive Interference Questionnaire] [SCIQ]
Peter Schwenkmezger and Lothar Laux

Source: Schwenkmezger, P., & Laux, L. (1986). Trait anxiety, worry, and emotionality in athletic competition. In C. D. Spielberger & R. Diaz-Guerrero (Eds.), *Cross-cultural anxiety* (Vol. 3, pp. 65-78). Washington, DC: Hemisphere Publishing Corporation.

Purpose: To assess task-irrelevant cognitions experienced by elite athletes in handball.

Description: The SCIQ contains 10 items. Athletes respond to items such as "I thought about things unrelated to the game" or "I was concerned about previous mistakes" using a 5-point ordinal scale.

Construction: An initial set of 18 items were formed by modifying Sarason's (1978) Cognitive Interference Questionnaire. Experts (coaches and players) in handball were asked to evaluate which items were relevant to occurrences during handball competition and were related to deteriorations in performance. Based on the experts' evaluations, 10 items were retained.

Reliability: The author (P. Schwenkmezger, personal communication, March 26, 1996) reported a Cronbach alpha coefficient of .86 in a sample of elite German handball players.

Validity: Construct validity was supported in that elite female handball athletes (n=35) high on trait anxiety experienced an increase in task-irrelevant cognitions in handball competition versus handball practice, whereas low-trait-anxiety athletes experienced no change in task-irrelevant cognitions under these two conditions. Concurrent validity was partially supported in that there was some evidence of a relationship between participants' (n=42 male and female elite handball athletes) scores on the SCIQ and their corresponding scores on Spielberger's (1970) trait anxiety scale. Predictive validity was supported in that these athletes' postcompetition scores on the SCIQ were related to two experts' evaluations of their game performance based on videotaped assessments.

Norms: Not cited. Psychometric data were reported for 35 elite female handball athletes (M age=22.5 years), two additional groups of 10 male and 10 female members of the German national handball team, and 22 male and female youth elite handball athletes also residing in the Federal Republic of Germany.

**Availability: Contact Peter Schwenkmezger, Department of Psychology, University of Trier, P. B. 3825, 54286 Trier, Germany. (Phone # 0651-201-2889; FAX # ++49/651/201-3812; E-mail: schwenkm@pcmail.uni-trier.de)

Reference

Sarason, I. G. (Ed.). (1978). The test anxiety scale: Concept and research. In C. D. Spielberger & I. G. Sarason (Eds.), *Stress and anxiety* (Vol. 5). Washington, DC: Hemisphere Publishing Corporation.

144 *[Sport-Specific Task-Irrelevant Cognitions Scale] [SSTICS]

Frantisek Man, Iva Stuchlikova, and Pavel Kindlmann

Source: Man, F., Stuchlikova, I, & Kindlmann, P. (1995). Trait-state anxiety, worry, emotionality, and self-confidence in top-level soccer players. *The Sport Psychologist, 9*, 212-224.

Purpose: To assess among players task-irrelevant cognitions that occur during sport competition.

Description: The SSTICS contains 10 items (e.g., "I ruminated about previous mistakes" and "I thought about the referee being prejudiced"). Participants respond to each item using a 5-point ordinal scale with the anchorings 1 (*never*) to 5 (*very often*).

Construction: Eighteen items were derived from previous scales assessing sport-specific task-irrelevant cognitions. Soccer coaches and players evaluated each item for content validity and relevance to performance deterioration. Based on their evaluations, a total of 10 items were retained.

Reliability: A Cronbach alpha internal consistency coefficient of .70 was reported.

Validity: Elite soccer athletes' (*N*=45) scores on the SSTICS were not related to their corresponding competitive state anxiety scores.

Norms: Not cited. Psychometric data were reported for 45 elite male soccer players (ages 18-30 years) residing in the Czech Republic.

Availability: Last known address: Frantisek Man, Faculty of Education,

University of South Bohemia, Jeronymova 10, 371 15 Ceske Budejovice, Czech Republic. The items are also listed in the *Source*.

145 | *Sports Inventory for Pain (SIP)
Michael C. Meyers, Anthony E. Bourgeois, and Arnold LeUnes

Source: Meyers, C., Bourgeois, A. E., Stewart, S., & LeUnes, A. (1992). Predicting pain responses in athletes: Development and assessment of the Sports Inventory for Pain. *Journal of Sport & Exercise Psychology, 14*, 249-261.

Purpose: To identify and predict an athlete's capability to cope with pain and to identify beneficial and detrimental coping strategies employed to adjust to pain.

Description: The SIP contains 25 items and a total of five subscales: Coping (8 items); Cognitive (5 items); Avoidance (4 items); Catastrophizing (4 items); and Body Awareness (4 items). Athletes are asked to respond on a 5-point Likert scale to items such as "Tell myself to be tough and carry on" (Coping), "Often feel I can't stand it anymore" (Catastrophizing), and "Seldom notice minor injuries" (Body Awareness).

Construction: An initial pool of 44 items was derived from a survey of 20 injured high school or college athletes, and from existing nonsport psychometric pain inventories. Written statements were derived from the injured athletes and were categorized as either sensory-discriminative, affective-motivational, coping, or cognitive-evaluative statements of pain. Principal components factor analysis (varimax rotation) of the responses of 449 college students led to the retention of 25 items within a five-factor structure that accounted for 77.44% of the variance.

Reliability: Cronbach alpha coefficients (N=449) ranged from .61 (Avoidance) to .88 (Coping). Test-retest reliability coefficients (2-week interval) ranged from .69 (Catastrophizing) to .88 (Coping).

Validity: The Coping and Cognitive subscale scores, as well as a compositive score, significantly increased with the number of reported sport injuries (*N*=449), years of sport participation, and number of sports played. In other words, participants reporting more sport-related injuries "have learned to cope with pain rather than to avoid potential pain producing situations" (p. 255).

The first author (M. C. Meyers, personal communication, April 12, 1996) also reported that scores on the SIP were not related to social desirability bias (because correlation coefficients with the Marlowe Crowne Social Desirability Scale ranged from -.16 to .22).

Norms: Not cited. Psychometric data were reported for 210 male and 239 female college students. *T*-score normatives are available from the authors (*N*=2,500; 10 sports).

**Availability: Contact Michael C. Meyers, Department of Health & Human Development, Montana State University, Bozeman, MT 59717. (Phone # 406-994-6324; FAX # 406-994-6314; E-mail: uhdmm@msu.oscs.montana.edu)

References

*Meyers, M. C., Bourgeois, A. E., LeUnes, A. D., Erick, A., & Havelka, P. (1992). Relationship between pain coping styles and athletic performance in top versus bottom-ranked college athletes [Abstract]. *Proceedings of the Association for the Advancement of Applied Sport Psychology annual convention* (p. 73). Colorado Springs, CO.

Raaum, K., Bourgeois, A. E., Meyers, M. C., & LeUnes, A. D. (1992). The relationship of psychological response to pain to sex-role orientation and attitudes toward physical activity [Abstract]. *Proceedings of the Association for the Advancement of Applied Sport Psychology annual convention* (p. 84). Colorado Springs, CO.

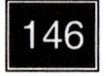

*Thoughts During Running Scale (TDRS)
Kathryn T. Goode and David L. Roth

Source: Goode, K. T., & Roth, D. L. (1993). Factor analysis of cognitions during running: Association with mood change. *Journal of Sport & Exercise Psychology, 15,* 375-389.

Purpose: To examine the thought patterns of runners experienced during typical training runs.

Description: The TDRS contains 38 items. Runners indicate the prevalence to which thoughts such as "my job," "how my body feels," and "family problems" occur while running. Runners respond on a 5-point ordinal scale with the anchorings *never* to *very often*.

Construction: The results of interviews with experienced runners and a review of previous research were the basis for the development of an initial pool of 32 items. A total of 533 undergraduate students (who sometimes went for a run or brisk walk) were asked to respond to the 32 items plus list other thoughts that occurred while running. Exploratory principal components factor analysis (varimax rotation) produced a five factor solution with 46.3% accountable variance. All 32 items were retained plus 6 new items were added that reflected additional thoughts the participants experienced while running. Confirmatory factor analysis produced a five-factor model. These factors were labeled Associative, External Surroundings, Interpersonal Relationships, Daily Events, and Spiritual Reflection.

Reliability: Cronbach alpha internal consistency coefficients ($N=150$) ranged from .77 (Associative; External Surroundings) to .85 (Daily Events).

Validity: Concurrent validity was examined by correlating runners' ($N=150$) TDRS scores with their scores on the Profile of Mood States (POMS), and variables pertaining to their running histories and training runs. It was found that increases in Vigor (POMS) were significantly correlated with External Surroundings, Interpersonal Relationships, and Daily Events; however, the reported correlation coefficients were low. Similarly, there was a statistically significant but low relationship between the runners' responses to the External Surroundings subscale and the time and distance of their run.

Norms: Not reported. Psychometric data were cited for 150 male or female runners (M age=31.7 years; SD=10.6). Participants averaged 7 years of regular running and 19 miles per week running.

Availability: Contact Kathryn T. Goode, Department of Psychology, University of Alabama, Campbell Hall, Birmingham, AL 35294. (Phone # 205-934-3850)

Chapter 10

Cohesion

Tests in this chapter assess attraction to the group, interpersonal interactions, group integration, and team unity across sport team members and coach.

147 Group Environment Questionnaire (GEQ)
Albert V. Carron, W. Neil Widmeyer, and Lawrence R. Brawley

Source: Carron, A. V., Widmeyer, W. N., and Brawley, L. R. (1985). The development of an instrument to assess cohesion in sport teams: The Group Environment Questionnaire. *Journal of Sport Psychology, 7,* 244-266.

Purpose: To assess the task and social aspects of an individual's perceptions of a sport group as a totality and the individual's attraction to the group, as they relate to the development and maintenance of group cohesion.

Description: The GEQ is an 18-item, four-scale measure of group cohesion. The four subscales are Individual Attractions to Group-Task (ATGT), Individual Attractions to Group-Social (ATGS), Group Integration-Task (GIT), Group Integration-Social (GIS). Participants are asked to respond to each item using a 9-point Likert format.

Construction: The perceptions of independent samples of active sport group members and a review of the literature on cohesion formed the conceptual basis for item development. An initial item pool was generated by four investigators and a senior research assistant.

Item-trimming was based on subarea representation, item clarity, lack of ambiguity, and other factors. Items were further evaluated by five experts in the area of group dynamics. The reduced 53-item pool was placed in questionnaire format and administered to 212 male and female athletes representing 20 intercollegiate and adult municipal association sport teams. Based on item analyses and estimates of internal consistency, the GEQ was reduced to 24 items.

This decision was supported by a replication study involving 247 athletes representing 26 different sport teams. Factor analyses of subjects' (n=212) responses and further item analyses (n=247) led to the retention of an 18-item GEQ.

Reliability: For ATGT, ATGS, GIT, and GIS, alpha reliability coefficients (n=247) were .75, .64, .70, and .76, respectively.

Validity: Content validity was demonstrated during the test construction process. Construct validity was demonstrated by factor analysis of participants' (n=212) responses to the 24-item GEQ in which the hypothesized four factors emerged. Carron noted that further research (see reference list) has supported the concurrent and predictive validity of the GEQ (A. V. Carron, personal communication, March 14, 1990).

Norms: Psychometric data are reported for independent samples (n=212; n=247) of male and female athletes representing intercollegiate and and municipal association sport teams.

Availability: Contact Albert V. Carron, Faculty of Kinesiology, University of Western Ontario, London, Ontario, Canada N6A 3K7. (Phone # 519-679-2111, Ext. 5475; FAX # 519-661-2008; E-mail: bert.carron@uwo.ca)

References

*Allain, M. (1995). Team building through experiential learning [Abstract]. *Journal of Applied Sport Psychology, 7* (Suppl.), S36.

Boone, K., Kuhlman, J., & Beitel, P. (1995). Goal orientation and its influence on cohesion [Abstract]. *Journal of Sport & Exercise Psychology, 17* (Suppl.), S29.

*Boone, K., Kuhlman, J, & Beitel, P. A. (1995). Interrelationships of perceptions of performance and perceived cohesion [Abstract]. *Journal of Applied Sport Psychology, 7* (Suppl.), S42.

*Brawley, L. R., Carron, A. V., & Widmeyer, W. N. (1987). Assessing the cohesion of teams: Validity of the Group Environment Questionnaire. *Journal of Sport Psychology, 9,* 275-294,

*Brawley, L. R., Carron, A. V., & Widmeyer, W. N. (1988). Exploring the relationship between cohesion and group resistance to disruption. *Journal of Sport & Exercise Psychology, 10,* 199-213.

*Brawley, L. R., Carron, A. V., & Widmeyer, W. N. (1993). The influence of the group and its cohesiveness on perceptions of group goal-related variables. *Journal of Sport & Exercise Psychology, 15,* 245-260.

*Brawley, L., Carron, A., Widmeyer, N., & Martin, K. (1995). Social cohesion as a predictor of the magnitude of group importance in leisure time sport [Abstract]. *Journal of Sport & Exercise Psychology, 17* (Suppl.), S32

*Brawley, L. R., Carron, A. V., Widmeyer, W. N., & Spink, K.S. (1994). Symposium: A decade of research with the GEQ: Theory, instrument development and correlates of cohesion [Abstract].*Journal of Sport & Exercise Psychology, 16* (Suppl.), S7-S9.

*Carron, A. V., Prapavessis, H., & Carron, A. V. (1994). Group effects and self-handicapping. *Journal of Sport & Exercise Psychology, 16,* 246-257.

*Carron, A. V., & Ramsey, M. C. Internal consistency of the Group Environment Questionnaire modified for university residence settings. *Perceptual and Motor Skills, 79,* 141-142.

*Carron, A. V., & Spink, K. S. (1992). Internal consistencyof the Group Environment

Questionnaire modified for an exercise setting. *Perceptual and Motor Skills, 74,* 304-306.

Carron, A. V., & Spink, K. S. (1993). Team building in an exercise setting. *The Sport Psychologist, 7,* 8-18.

*Carron, A. V., Widmeyer, W. N., & Brawley, L. R. (1988). Group cohesion and individual adherence to physical activity. *Journal of Sport & Exercise Psychology, 10,* 127-138.

*Chi, L., & Lu, S-E. (1995). The relationships between perceived motivational climates and group cohesiveness in basketball [Abstract]. *Journal of Sport & Exercise Psychology, 17* (Suppl.), S41.

*Cogan, K. D., & Petrie, T. A. (1995). Sport consultation: An evaluation of a season-long intervention with female collegiate gymnasts. *The Sport Psychologist, 9,* 282-296.

*Copeland, B. W., Bonnell, R. J., & Reider, L. R. (1995). Introducing team cohesion and relaxation skills with junior U.S. national luge trainees [Abstract]. *Journal of Applied Sport Psychology, 7* (Suppl.), S50.

*Copeland, B. W., & Peinkofer, B. (1995). Exploring team cohesion and perceptions of learning motor skills [Abstract]. *Research Quarterly for Exercise and Sport, 66* (Suppl.), A-75.

*Copeland, B., & Straub, W. F. (1993). The relevance of cohesion in co-acting teams [Abstract]. *Proceedings of the Association for the Advancement of Applied Sport Psychology annual convention* (p. 29). Montreal, Canada.

*Courneya, K. S., & McAuley, E. (1995). Reliability and discriminant validity of subjective norm, social support, and cohesion in an exercise setting. *Journal of Sport & Exercise Psychology, 17,* 325-337.

*Dorsch, K. D., Widmeyer, W. N., Paskevich, D. M., & Brawley, L. R. (1995). Collective efficacy: Its measurement and relationship to cohesion in ice hockey [Abstract]. *Journal of Applied Sport Psychology, 7* (Suppl.), S56.

*Eichas, T. M., & Krane, V. (1993). Relationships among perceived leadership styles, member satisfaction, and team cohesion in high school basketball players [Abstract]. *Research Quarterly for Exercise and Sport, 64* (Suppl.), A-101-102.

Everett, J. J., Smith, R. E., & Williams, K. D. (1992). Effects of team cohesion and identifiability on social loafing in relay swimming performance. *International Journal of Sport Psychology, 23,* 311-324.

Frierman, S., & Gill, D. (1994). The influence of individual and team goals on cohesion and performance in youth bowling [Abstract]. *Journal of Sport & Exercise Psychology, 16* (Suppl.), S54.

*Frierman, S. H., & Weinberg, R. S. (1989). The relationship between cohesion and performance in competitive bowling teams [Abstract]. *Psychology of motor behavior and sport* (p. 138). Kent, OH: Proceedings of the North American Society for the Psychology of Sport and Physical Activity annual convention.

Glenday, L., & Widmeyer, W. N. (1993). Describing and explaining gender differences in the cohesion of athletic teams [Abstract]. *Proceedings of the Association for the Advancement of Applied Sport Psychology annual convention* (p. 51). Montreal, Canada.

*Hausenblas, H. A., & Carron, A. V. (1995). Relationship between group cohesion and eating disorders [Abstract]. *Journal of Applied Sport Psychology, 7* (Suppl.), S69.

*Hoar, S. D., Widmeyer, W. N., & Hardy, C. (1993). Social support-cohesion relationships in athletic teams [Abstract]. *Proceedings of the Association for the Advancement of Applied Sport Psychology annual convention* (p. 71). Montreal, Canada.

*Iordanoglou, D. (1993). The relationship between team ability, team cohesion and team performance in professional soccer teams. *Proceedings of the Eighth World Congress of Sport Psychology* (pp. 850-855). Lisbon, Portugal.

*Kim, M., & Sugiyama, Y. (1992). The relation of performance norms and cohesiveness for Japanese School Athletic teams. *Perceptual and Motor Skills, 74,* 1096-1098.

*Kozub, S. A. (1994). Exploring the relationship between team cohesion and player leadership [Abstract]. *Journal of Sport & Exercise Psychology, 16* (Suppl.), S73.

*Kozub, S. A. (1995). Investigating the determinants of team cohesion [Abstract]. *Journal of Applied Sport Psychology, 7* (Suppl.), S82.

*Krane, V., Deifendeifer, K., & Yothers, A. (1995). Relationships among intrinsic motivation and task and social cohesion [Abstract]. *Journal of Applied Sport Psychology, 7* (Suppl.), S83.

*Li, F., & Harmer, P. A. (1994). Construct validation of the Group Environment Questionnaire: First and higher order factor models [Abstract]. *Research Quarterly for Exercise and Sport, 65* (Suppl.), A-58.

*Matheson, H., Mathes, S., & Murray, M. (1994). Changes in group cohesion of female intercollegiate coacting and interacting teams across a competitive season [Abstract]. *Journal of Sports Sciences, 12,* 200-201.

Pease, D. G., & Kozub, S. A. (1994). Perceived coaching behaviors and team cohesion in high school girls basketball teams [Abstract]. *Journal of Sport & Exercise Psychology, 16* (Suppl.), S93.

*Remers, L., Widmeyer, W. N., Williams, J. M., & Myers, L. (1995). Possible mediators and moderators of the class size-member adherence relationship in exercise. *Journal of Applied Sport Psychology, 7,* 38-49.

*Schutz, R. W., Eom, H. J., Smoll, F. L., & Smith, R. E. (1994). Examination of the factorial validity of the Group Environment Questionnaire. *Research Quarterly for Exercise and Sport, 65,* 226-236.

*Shields, D. L. L., Bredemeier, B. J. L., Gardner, D. E., & Bostrom, A. (1995). Leadership, cohesion, and team norms regarding cheating and aggression. *Sociology of Sport Journal, 12,* 324-336.

*Spink, K. S. (1990). Group cohesion and collective efficacy of volleyball teams. *Journal of Sport & Exercise Psychology, 12,* 301-311.

*Spink, K. S. (1995). Cohesion and intention to participate of female sport team athletes. *Journal of Sport & Exercise Psychology, 17,* 416-427.

*Spink, K. S. (1995). Cohesion and leadership behaviors as predictors of athlete satisfaction [Abstract]. *Journal of Applied Sport Psychology, 7* (Suppl.), S111.

*Spink, K. S., & Carron, A. V. (1992). Group cohesion and adherence in exercise classes. *Journal of Sport & Exercise Psychology, 14,* 78-86.

*Swain, A. B. J., Thorpe, S. E., & Martin, R. (1994). Relationships between perceptions of ability on specific team performance factors and group cohesion in interactive sports teams [Abstract]. *Journal of Sports Sciences, 12,* 212-213.

*Swain, A. B. J., Thorpe, S. E., & Parfitt, G. (1995). Self-efficacy, collective efficacy and performance: The mediating role of group cohesion [Abstract]. *Journal of Sports Science, 13,* 75-76.

*Twardochleb, T., & Spink, K. S. (1995). Actual and perceived leadership behaviors as predictors of cohesion in exercise classes [Abstract]. *Journal of Applied Sport Psychology, 7* (Suppl.), S118.

*Westre, K. R., & Weiss, M. (1991). The relationship between perceived coaching behaviors and group cohesion in high school football teams. *The Sport Psychologist, 5,* 41-54.

*Widmeyer, W. N., Brawley, L. R., & Carron, A. V. (1985). *The measurement of cohesion in sport teams: The Group Environment Questionnaire*. London, Ontario: Spodym Publishers.

*Widmeyer, W. N., Carron, A. V., & Brawley, L. R. (1993). The cohesion performance outcome relationship with teams as the units of analysis [Abstract]. *Journal of Sport & Exercise Psychology, 15* (Suppl.), S90.

*Williams, J. M., & Widmeyer, W. N. (1991). The cohesion-performance outcome relationship in a coacting sport. *Journal of Sport & Exercise Psychology, 13*, 364-371.

*Zimmerman, T., & DeVoe, D. (1993). As assessment of family systems therapy (consultation) for female collegiate basketball players [Abstract]. *Research Quarterly for Exercise and Sport, 66* (Suppl.), A-106.

148 Howe Sport Behaviour Scale-I [HSBS]
Bruce L. Howe and P. Zachary

Source: Howe, B. L., & Zachary, P. (1986). Revision and validation of the Howe Sport Behavior Scale [Abstract]. *Proceedings of the Canadian Association of Sport Sciences annual convention,* Ottawa, Canada.

Purpose: To examine achievement and affiliation orientations in sport.

Description: The questionnaire contains two subscales-- Achievement and Affiliation, each containing 15 items. For example, participants are asked to respond to the item "I am loyal to my team members" (Affiliation). Participants respond to each item using a 5-point ordinal scale.

Construction: Based on item analyses (*n*=426 high school and university students) of the original 25-item scale (Howe, 1976), a total of 15 items were retained.

Reliability: Internal consistency coefficients (*n*=426) were .78 (Achievement) and .68 (Affiliation). Test-retest reliability coefficients (*n*=74) over a one-week period were .86 and .81 for Achievement and Affiliation, respectively. Over a 6-month period, test-retest reliability coefficients (*n*=31) were .80 (Achievement) and .82 (Affiliation).

Validity: The authors indicated that the discriminant validity of the HSBS-I was supported in that males scored lower on affiliation and higher on achievement than did females.

236

Norms: Not cited. Psychometric data were cited for 426 university and high school students.

Availability: Contact Bruce L. Howe, School of Physical Education, Box 3015, University of Victoria, 131 McKinnon, Victoria, British Columbia, Canada V8W 3N4. (Phone # 604-721-8383; E-mail: blhowe@uvic.ca)

References

Howe, B. L. (1976). Validating a new scale of personality traits important in sport performance. In J. Broekhoff (Ed.), *Physical education, sports and the sciences* (pp. 346-352). Eugene, OR: College of Health, Education, and Recreation Microform Publications.

McMorris, T., & Cobb, P. (1993). Motivation and field dependence of males and females engaging in team and individual sports. In J. R. Nitsch & R. Seiler (Eds.), *Motivation, emotion, stress* (pp. 86-90). Proceedings of the VIII European Congress of Sport Psychology (Volume 1). Sankt Augustin, Germany: Academia Verlag.

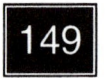 **Medford Player-Coach Interaction Inventory [MPCII]**
Pamela Medford and Jo Anne Thorpe

Source: Thorpe, J., & Medford, P. (1986). An inventory for measuring player-coach interaction. *Perceptual and Motor Skills, 63,* 267-270.

Purpose: To assess positive interactions of the coach with his or her team.

Description: Participants respond to 23 adjectives using a 7-point Likert scale. Two forms are available: a player's form and a coach's form.

Construction: The literature relevant to attitude inventories and inventories that dealt with interaction or interpersonal relations were reviewed. Following this review, adjectives and statements indicative of player-coach interactions were collected from five female coaches and two female former coaches. These adjectives were sorted by three judges (one linguist and two graduate faculty physical educators) into 20 synonyms in order to reduce redundancy by using a card-sorting technique. A total of 23 (out of 81) adjectives that seemed most indicative and easily understood were selected for the inventory.

Reliability: Test-retest reliability coefficients (n=55 female athletes) ranged from .50 to .83 over a one-week interval for each adjective; 60% of the adjectives were found reliable. A test-retest reliability coefficient, based on the total test score, was .87.

Validity: Content validity was examined by having players and coaches rate (using a 5-point scale) the predictive value for each adjective. Ratings were "high," indicating that the adjectives were appropriate predictors of player-coach interaction.

Norms: Not reported. Psychometric data were cited for 55 female collegiate athletes.

**Availability: Contact Jo Anne Thorpe, (Professor Emeritus, Southern Illinois University at Carbondale), 1012 East Emma Street, Tampa, FL 33603-4143. (Phone # 813-238-6226; FAX # 813-239-9298)

150 Multidimensional Sport Cohesion Instrument (MSCI)
David Yukelson, Robert Weinberg, and Allen Jackson

Source: Yukelson, D., Weinberg, R., & Jackson, A. (1984). A multidimensional group cohesion instrument for intercollegiate basketball teams. *Journal of Sport Psychology, 6,* 103-117.

Purpose: To assess group cohesion based on both task-related and social- related forces that presumably exist in intercollegiate basketball.

Description: The MSCI is a 22-item self-report test. Factor analyses indicated that four factors are discernable (accounting for 62% of the variance): Attraction to the Group, Unity of Purpose, Quality of Teamwork, and Valued Roles. Participants are asked to respond to each item (e.g., "How good do you think the teamwork is on your team?") using an 11-point ordinal scale.

Construction: Items for the MSCI were logically derived by (a) modifying items found in previous cohesion instruments, (b) synthesizing information from theoretical work on cohesion, (c) surveying research in the area of industrial and organizational psychology, and (d) interviewing coaches or other social scientists regarding their perceptions of group cohesion. An initial pool of 41 items (23 items were task-related items and 17 were social-related items), plus a 4-item lie scale, was administered and evaluated among 95 male and 101 female intercollegiate basketball players representing 16 colleges throughout Texas, Michigan, and California. The results of alpha and canonical factor analyses led to the retention of four meaningful factors (see test description above) representing 22 items.

Reliability: Alpha reliability coefficients ($n=196$) were .93 (total test), .88 (Attraction to the Group), .86 (Unity of Purpose), .86 (Quality of Teamwork), and .79 (Valued Roles).

Validity: Construct validity was supported by the retention of the four hypothesized factors based on factor analyses.

Norms: Not reported. Psychometric data were cited for 196 male and female intercollegiate basketball players residing in three states.

**Availability: Contact David Yukelson, Academic Support Center for Student Athletes, 328 Boucke Building, Pennsylvania State University, University Park, PA 16802. (Phone # 814-865-0407; FAX # 814-863-1539; E-mail: y39@psuvm.psu.edu)

References
*Foster, C., & McClure, B. (1987). The effects of membership in a personal growth group on group cohesiveness within a women's gymnastics team [Abstract]. *Proceedings of the annual conference of the Association for the Advancement for Applied Sport Psychology* (p. 76). Newport Beach, CA.

*Maynard, I. W., & Watson, J. C. (1995). Cohesion and performance in elite male basketball players [Abstract]. *Journal of Sports Sciences, 13,* 66-67.

*McClure, B. A., & Foster, C. D. (1991). Group work as a method of promoting cohesiveness within a gymnastics team. *Perceptual and Motor Skills, 73,* 307-313.

*Yukelson, D., Weinberg, R., & Jackson, A. (1983). Group cohesion in sport: A multidimensional approach [Abstract]. *Psychology of motor behavior and sport* (p. 127). Proceedings of the annual conference of the North American Society for the Psychology of Sport and Physical Activity, East Lansing, MI.

151	**[Sports Cohesiveness Questionnaire] [SCQ]** Rainer Martens and James A. Peterson

Source: Martens, R., & Peterson, J. A. (1971). Group cohesiveness as a determinant of success and member satisfaction in team performance. *International Review of Sport Sociology, 6,* 49-61.

Purpose: To assess various dimensions of group cohesiveness in sport.

Description: Seven questionnaire items focus on interpersonal attraction, contributions of members based on ability and enjoyment, influence (power) of each member, sense of belonging, value of membership, and perceptions of teamwork and how closely knit the sport group was. Participants are asked to respond to each item using a 9-choice alternative between two polarities.

Construction: Item selection was based on a review of literature on the theoretical basis of cohesiveness and assessment alternatives.

Reliability: Not reported.

Validity: When comparing successful to unsuccessful college intramural basketball teams, only members' (n=1,200 males) ratings of the cohesiveness of their team as a whole was a discriminating factor. However, the majority of cohesiveness items discriminated between satisfied and unsatisfied teams.

Norms: Psychometric data are cited for 1,200 male undergraduate students participating on 144 intramural basketball teams at the University of Illinois.

Availability: Contact Rainer Martens, Human Kinetics Publishers, P. O. Box 5076, 1607 North Market Street, Champaign, IL 61825-5076. (Phone # 217-351-5076; FAX # 217-351-2674; E-mail: rainer@hkusa.com)

References

*Carron, A. V., & Ball, J. R. (1977). An analysis of the cause-effect characteristics of cohesiveness and participation motivation in intercollegiate hockey. *International Review of Sport Sociology, 12* (2), 49-60.

*Carron, A. V., & Chelladurai, P. (1981). The dynamics of group cohesion in sport. *Journal of Sport Psychology, 3,* 123-139.

Hacker, C. M., & Williams, J. M. (1981). Cohesion, satisfaction, and performance in intercollegiate field hockey [Abstract]. In *Psychology of motor behavior and sport-1981* (p. 99). Proceedings of the North American Society for the Psychology of Sport and Physical Activity annual convention. Asilomar, CA.

*Peterson, J. A., & Martens, R. (1972). Success and residential affiliation as determinants of team cohesiveness. *Research Quarterly, 43,* 62-76.

*Widmeyer, W. N., & Martens, R. (1978). When cohesion predicts performance outcome in sport. *Research Quarterly, 49,* 372-380.

152   Team Climate Questionnaire [TCQ]
Robert R. Grand and Albert V. Carron

Source: Grand, R. R. & Carron, A. V. (1982). Development of a Team Climate Questionnaire. In L. M. Wankel & R. B. Wilberg (Eds.), *Psychology of sport and motor behavior: Research and practice* (pp. 217-229). Proceedings of the annual conference of the Canadian Society for Psychomotor Learning and Sport Psychology. Edmonton, Alberta, Canada.

Purpose: To assess role clarity, role acceptance, perceived role performance, conformity, task cohesion, and social cohesion in sport groups.

Description: The TCQ consists of 60 items pertaining to the six constructs above. Each construct is assessed by 10 items. Participants respond to each item using a 7-point Likert scale. In addition, a single, direct cohesion measure was included bringing the total number of items on the TCQ to 61.

Construction: Operationalization of the six constructs involved modifying some items from a number of psychological inventories and scales including Jackson's Personality Inventory, the Sport Cohesiveness Questionnaire, and the Role Conflict and Ambiguity Scale. Other items were developed based on the objectives of the study. A series of pilot studies followed in which item analyses and evaluations of internal consistency were made. Samples included 112 undergraduate students, 34 Canadian high school hockey players, and an additional 111 undergraduate students. The first pilot study involved an evaluation of 58 items, whereas the second pilot study involved a subanalysis of the most reliable 36 items. In the final stage of the pilot project, a revised version of the original questionnaire with 61 items was included for analyses, because it was found that the shorter version of the questionnaire was less reliable.

Reliability: Kuder-Richardson-20 internal consistency coefficients (n=75) ranged from .76 to .91.

Validity: Not discussed.

Norms: Not cited. Psychometric data are reported for 75 hockey players participating on five selected university and junior hockey teams in Canada.

Availability: Contact Albert V. Carron, Faculty of Kinesiology, University of Western Ontario, London, Ontario, Canada N6A 3K7. (Phone # 519-679-2111, Ext. 5475; FAX # 519-661-2008; E-mail: bert.carron@uwo.ca)

References
*Bolger, P., & Carron, A. V. (1984). The relationship of task and social cohesion to sex, starting status, participation level, and performance of high school and university basketball teams [Abstract]. *Proceedings of the annual conference of the Canadian Society of Psychomotor Learning and Sport Psychology* (p. 4). Kingston, Ontario, Canada.

*Brawley, L. R., Carron, A. V. & Widmeyer, W. N. (1987). Assessing the cohesion of teams: Validity of the Group Environment Questionnaire. *Journal of Sport Psychology, 9,* 275-294.

*Foster, C., & McClure, B. (1987). The effects of membership in a personal growth group on group cohesiveness within a women's gymnastic team [Abstract]. *Proceedings of the annual conference of the Association for the Advancement for Applied Sport Psychology* (p. 76). Newport Beach, CA.

*McClure, B. A., & Foster, C. D. (1991). Group work as a method of promoting cohesiveness within a gymnastics team. *Perceptual and Motor Skills, 73,* 307-313.

153 Team Cohesion Questionnaire [TCQ]
Joseph J. Gruber and Gary R. Gray

Source: Gruber, J. J., & Gray, G. R. (1981). Factor patterns of variables influencing cohesiveness at various levels of basketball competition. *Research Quarterly for Exercise and Sport, 52,* 19-30.

Purpose: To provide a measure of interpersonal working relationships, success obtained by the sport group, and personal forces attracting individuals to the sport group.

Description: The cohesiveness questionnaire contains 13 items. Participants are asked to respond to each item using a 9-point Likert scale.

Construction: Items were selected for inclusion in the questionnaire based on their frequency of use in previous investigations of sport cohesion, and their relevance to an hypothesized factor structure of sport cohesiveness.

Reliability: Intraclass correlation coefficients across a 2-week interval, computed by analysis of variance procedures, ranged from .73 to .94 among 89 varsity junior high school basketball players, and from .80 to .98 among 34 varsity small college basketball players.

Validity: Factor analyses of the responses of 515 male varsity basketball players, representing various educational levels, led to the retention of six factors. The factor of team performance satisfaction accounted for the majority of variance across all levels of competition, ranging from 51% to 65% accountable variance. (Additional information concerning discriminant validity can be found in the *Source*.)

Norms: Not reported. Psychometric data are cited for 92 elementary school basketball players from 8 school teams, 116 junior high school basketball players from 10 school teams, 110 senior high school basketball players from 9 school teams, 115 small college players from 10 teams, and 82 large college basketball players from 7 college teams.

Availability: Last known address: Joseph J. Gruber, Department of Health, Physical Education, and Recreation, Seaton Building 216, University of Kentucky, Lexington, KY 40506. (Phone # 606-257-3293)

References

*Gruber, J. J. (1981). Comparison of relationships among team cohesion scores and measures of team success in male varsity basketball teams. *International Review of Sport Sociology, 16*(4), 43-54.

*Gruber, J. J., & Gray, G. R. (1982). Responses to forces influencing cohesion as a function of player status and level of male varsity basketball competition. *Research Quarterly for Exercise and Sport, 53*, 27-36.

Chapter 11

Confidence (Exercise)

Tests in this chapter assess perceptions of movement competence, physical fitness capacities, and the physical self concept. The strength of perceived self-efficacy in relation to exercise participation and one's confidence in overcoming barriers toward exercising are also assessed.

154 *Exercise Identity Scale [EIS]
Dean F. Anderson and Charles M. Cychosz

Source: Anderson, D. F., & Cychosz, C. M. (1994). Development of an Exercise Identity Scale. *Perceptual and Motor Skills, 78,* 747-751.

Purpose: To assess the extent to which exercise is descriptive of one's concept of self.

Description: The EIS is a nine-item scale. Participants respond to items such as "I have numerous goals related to exercising" utilizing a Likert scale format with the anchorings 1 (*strongly disagree*) to 7 (*strongly agree*).

Construction: Utilizing the sociological tradition that assumes the reciprocal relationship between role identities and behavior, items for the EIS were derived from the research literature on the salience of role identity with blood donation, religious involvement, college retention, and sport involvement.

Reliability: A Cronbach alpha internal consistency coefficient ($N=51$) of .94 was reported. A stability coefficient of .93 was reported over a one week period. In a second study involving law enforcement personnel ($N=448$), the Cronbach alpha internal consistency coefficient was also .94 (Anderson, Cychosz, & Franke, 1996)

Validity: Participants' ($N=51$) scores on the EIS were correlated with their self-report data on the number of weeks exercising, frequency of exercise per week, and the duration and intensity of exercise experienced. For law enforcement personnel ($N=448$), scores on the EIS were correlated with their self-report data on the number of weeks exercising, duration and intensity of exercise, as well as physiological indicators of muscular endurance, percent body fat, and VO2 peak (Anderson, Cychosz, & Franke, 1996).

Norms: Not cited. Psychometric data were reported for 16 males and 35 females enrolled in two sections of an elective first aid class.

**Availability: Contact Dean F. Anderson, Department of Health and

246

Human Performance, Iowa State University, 235 P. E. Building, Ames, IA 50011. (Phone # 515-294-1425; FAX # 515-294-8740; E-mail: deanf@iastate.edu)

Reference
*Anderson, D. F., Cychosz, C., & Franke, W. (1996). Association of exercise identity with measures of exercise commitment and physiological indicators of fitness in a law enforcement cohort [Abstract]. *Research Quarterly for Exercise and Sport, 67,* A39.

*[Exercise-Specific Self-Efficacy Scale] [ESSES]
Edward McAuley

Source: McAuley, E. (1991). Efficacy, attributional, and affective responses to exercise participation. *Journal of Sport & Exercise Psychology, 13,* 382-393.

Purpose: To examine individuals' perceived capabilities to exercise in the face of barriers to participation.

Description: Participants are "... asked to indicate on a percentage rating scale their degree of confidence in being able to continue to exercise at their current level of frequency, duration, and intensity in the event that they had to overcome..." barriers or obstacles to exercise (p. 385). For example, they are asked to rate their ability to continue to exercise regularly if they are bored or self-conscious about their appearance.

Construction: Barriers to exercising were determined through attributional analysis of participants' (*N*=37 males; *N*=43 females) reasons for dropping out of exercise programs.

Reliability: A Cronbach alpha internal consistency coefficient of .85 was reported.

Validity: Exercise efficacy was positively correlated (*N*=80) with exercise frequency and positive-affective reactions.

Norms: Not cited. Psychometric data were reported for 37 males and 43 females (*M* age=53.7 years; *SD*=6.3) who were halfway through a 5-month structured exercise program.

Availability: Contact Edward McAuley, Department of Kinesiology, University of Illinois, 215 Freer Hall, 906 South Goodwin Avenue, Urbana, IL 61801. (Phone # 217-333-6487; FAX # 217-244-7322; E-mail: a-mc3@staff.uiuc.edu)

156 High-Risk Activity Inventory (HRAI)
Evan B. Brody, Bradley D. Hatfield, and Thomas W. Spalding

Source: Brody, E. B., Hatfield, B. D., & Spalding, T. W. (1988). Generalization of self-efficacy to a continuum of stressors upon mastery of a high-risk sport skill. *Journal of Sport & Exercise Psychology,* 10, 32-44.

Purpose: To assess an individual's strength of perceived self-efficacy in relation to high-risk physical activities.

Description: The HRAI is a 12-item test that requires an individual to report his or her degree of confidence of ability to perform the following activities: scuba diving, sky diving, hang gliding, mountain climbing, white-water rafting, rock climbing, downhill skiing, automobile racing, hot-air ballooning, white-water tubing, diving (swimming), and motorcycle racing.

Construction: Not stated.

Reliability: An alpha internal consistency coefficient of .88 was reported.

Validity: Not stated.

Norms: Not available

Availability: Contact Bradley D. Hatfield, Department of Kinesiology, University of Maryland, College Park, MD 20742. (Phone # 301-405-2489; FAX # 301-314-9167; E-mail: bh5@umail.umd.edu)

157 Motor Skill Perceived Competence Scale (MSPCS)

Mary E. Rudisill, Matthew T. Mahar, and Karen S. Meaney

Source: Rudisill, M. E., Mahar, M. T., & Meaney, K. S. (1989). The development of a motor skill perceived competence scale for children. *Research abstracts of the annual convention of the American Alliance for Health, Physical Education, Recreation, and Dance annual convention* (p. 193). Boston, MA.

Purpose: To assess children's (ages 9-12) perceptions of motor skill competence.

Description: The MSPCS is a semantic differential scale containing 18 items. Two parallel forms exist: Form A and Form B, each containing nine items. Each item is designed so that the child circles the number (5-point scale) between the two opposite statements that best represents his or her feelings about the sentence. For example, the child is asked to indicate along a 5-point continuum whether he or she cannot or can run fast. Imbedded in both forms is one item based on the child's general competence.

Construction: A 35-item Likert type scale was originally constructed. Results of the analysis of the original scale indicated that three items were not well understood by the students and were eliminated from the scale. The item analysis identified 11 additional items that could be eliminated without a significant reduction in scale reliability.

To increase the percentage of students responding to each item and to minimize social desirability response distortions, the remaining items were structured in a semantic differential scale format. The revised 21-item semantic differential type scale was administered to 300 children. Item analyses led to the retention of 18 items that were then administered to 929 students. Based on further item analyses, items with similar discrimination indexes were randomly assigned to either Form A or Form B.

Reliability: Internal consistency coefficients ($n=929$) were .78, .79, and .88, for Form A, Form B, and both forms combined, respectively. A test-retest reliability coefficient (*n*= 322 male and female children, ages 9-12 years) of .88 was reported across a 2-week interval.

Validity: Alpha factor analysis with oblique rotation resulted in the retention of one factor for both Forms A and B. Ratings of perceived motor skill competence correlated .34 to .42 with actual motor skill performance (*n*=929). Also, participants' responses to the MSPCS correlated .41 with teacher ratings of these subjects' motor skill performance.

Norms: Psychometric data were presented for 929 male and female children, ages 9-12.

Availability: Contact Mary E. Rudisill, Department of Health and Human Performance, University of Houston, Houston, TX 77204-5331 (Phone # 713-743-9852; FAX #713-743-9860)

References

Rudisill, M. E. (1990). The influence of various achievement goal orientations on children's perceived competence, expectations, persistence and performance for three motor tasks. *Journal of Human Movement Studies, 18,* 231-249.

*Rudisill, M. E., Mahar, M. T., & Meaney, K. S. (1989). A comparison of the Motor Skill Perceived Competence Scale and Harter's Physical Domain Perceived Competence Scale for predicting motor skill competence [Abstract]. *Psychology of motor behavior and sport* (p. 98). Kent, OH: Proceedings of the North American Society for the Psychology of Sport and Physical Activity annual convention.

*Rudisill, M. E., Mahar, M. T., & Meaney, K. S. (1993). The relationship between children's perceived and actual motor competence. *Perceptual and Motor Skills, 76,* 895-906.

158 Movement Confidence Inventory (MCI)
Norma S. Griffin, Jack F. Keogh, and Richard Maybee

Source: Griffin, N. S., Keogh, J. F., & Maybee, R. (1984). Performer perceptions of movement confidence. *Journal of Sport Psychology, 6,* 395-407.

Purpose: To assess individual perceptions of movement confidence based on competence, potential for enjoying movement sensations, and potential for harm. Movement confidence is defined as how sure a participant is of completing a movement task.

Description: The MCI is organized around 12 movement tasks (such as playing golf or jogging) and requires three different ratings for each movement-task situation. Participants are asked to rate their experience with each task situation (on a 5-point ordinal scale), their level of confidence in performing the task situation (on a 6-point ordinal scale), and to rate the extent to which 22 paired descriptor words contribute to the stated level of confidence in doing the imagined performance of the task.

Construction: Twelve movement tasks were selected in terms of the potential importance of the three confidence components (competence, enjoyment, and harm). Descriptor words (third rating component) were selected from a pool of words obtained by asking children and college students to select words that were important in describing their confidence in movement situations. Overall, the content and format of the MCI were determined by meetings and small-group interactive conferences with consultants.

Reliability: Alpha reliability coefficients obtained among 206 female and 146 male undergraduate students ranged on the subscale tasks from .83 (basketball) to .94 (skiing); an alpha coefficient of .90 was obtained for the composite MCI.

Validity: Partial support for construct validity was obtained through factor analyses ($n=352$), which indicated that the major contribution to perceived movement confidence is a personal feeling of competence.

Norms: Not reported. Psychometric data were cited for 352 undergraduate students from six colleges in four states.

Availability: Contact Norma S. Griffin, Department of Speech Education, 301 Barkley Center, University of Nebraska, Lincoln, NE 68588-0732. (Phone # 402-472-5486; E-mail: ngriffin@unlinfo.unl.edu)

Reference
*Crocker, P. R. E., & Leclerc, D. R. (1992). Testing the validity of the movement confidence model in a high-risk dive by novices. *Journal of Sport & Exercise Psychology,* 14, 159-168.

159 Perceived Physical Competence Scale [PPCS]
Taru Lintunen

Source: Lintunen, T. (1987). Perceived Physical Competence Scale for children. *Scandinavian Journal of Sports Sciences, 9,* 57-64.

Purpose: To assess cognitive appraisals of physical self among children, including perceptions of both physical performance capacity (physical fitness) and physical appearance.

Description: The child is asked to compare him- or herself to children of the same age and sex in terms of physical fitness, motor ability, anthropometric characteristics, and other physical attributes. The child responds to each of the 10 items on the PPCS using a 5-point scale in which a discrimination must be made between bipolar adjective descriptors.

*Construction: The items that compose the Perceived Fitness subscale were based on the Model of Physical Performance Capacity (Pitkanen, Komi, Nupponen, Rusko, and Tiainen, 1979) and cover a wide range of physical capacities. Furthermore, it was assumed that those factors associated with appearance are also important elements of perceived physical competence. Three items composing the Perceived Appearance subscale were derived from a review of literature on body image scales.

Exploratory principal component factor analysis yielded two factors (Perceived Fitness and Perceived Appearance) for children at age 10 (Lintunen, 1987) and for adolescents with disabilities (Lintunen, Heikinaro-Johansson, & Sherrill, 1995). Confirmatory factor analysis was used to study the stability and the unidimensionality of perceived fitness for 11- to 15-year-olds during a 4-year follow-up period (Lintunen, 1995). The factor of perceived fitness was found to be tenable and stable across 4 years among both boys and girls. However, perceived appearance was not a consistent factor during the follow-up period. The author recommends that the three items of the Perceived Appearance subscale be analyzed separately item by item.

*Reliability: Cronbach alpha internal consistency coefficients ($N=113$) for Perceived Fitness ranged from .57 to .78 for measurements taken annually across a 4-year period among children ages 11 to 15 years old

*Note: This section was extracted from a summary prepared by the author (T. Lintunen, personal communication, June 3, 1996).

(Lintunen, Leskinen, Oinonen, Salinto, & Rahkila, 1995). Further, an alpha coefficient of .89 was reported for 85 Finnish adolescents with disabilities (Lintunen, Heikinaro-Johansson, et al., 1995). Simplex reliability coefficients for Perceived Fitness (Lintunen, Leskinen, et al., 1995) among the boys ranged from .78 to .91 during the annual 4-year follow-up assessments. Among the girls, the estimates of the measurement error variances were close to zero and could thus be fixed at 1. Thus, the reliability of the Perceived Fitness sum index was very high. The simplex stability coefficients for Perceived Fitness among the boys were .86, .79, .97, and .87 between the annual measurements from the ages of 11 to 15. The corresponding Pearson product moment correlation coefficients were .70, .64, .83, and .79. The simplex stability coefficients (and also the correlation coefficients) among the girls were .67, .71, .80, and .82. According to these results, Perceived Fitness became more stable during adolescence.

*Validity: The discriminant validity of the Perceived Fitness subscale was supported: Exercise activity (i.e., sedentary, active, and very active participation in supervised exercise activities) (Lintunen, 1995), timing of biological maturation (Lintunen, Rahkila, Silvennoinen, & Osterback, 1988) and physical disability (Lintunen, Heikinaro-Johansson, et al., 1995) mediated participants' responses to the Perceived Fitness subscale.

Convergent validity was supported in that participants' responses on the Perceived Fitness subscale were significantly related to their responses to Rosenberg's Self-Esteem Scale among boys ($r=.40, .29., .47., .29$) but not among girls ($r=.07, 20. 28, .11$) during successive, annual measurements taken from the ages of 11 to 15 years (Lintunen, Leskinen, et al., 1995). It should be noted that boys valued fitness highly whereas the girls valued fitness only moderately.

Concurrent validity was supported in that actual estimates of physical fitness explained perceived physical fitness. Lisrel-analysis indicated that there was a regression relationship between the latent factor of Physical Fitness with four indicators and Perceived Fitness (Lintunen, 1995). The factor of Physical Fitness explained 31%, 43%, and 66% of the variance of Perceived Fitness among girls ($n=49$) and 31%, 16%, and 7% of the variance among the boys ($n=64$) at the ages of 11, 13, and 15, respectively.

**Norms: Not cited. Psychometric data were reported for physically sedentary, active, and very active Finnish boys (*n*=64; *M* age at beginning of study= 11.0 years; *SD*=1.10) and girls (*n*=49; *M* age at beginning of study= 10.7 years; *SD*= 0.9) at the age of 11, 12, 13, 14, and 15 years; for 51 female and 34 male adolescents (*M* age= 15.1 years; *SD*= 1.5) with disabilities; and for a sample of 116 female and 116 male adolescents (ages 13-16 years) from central Finland.

**Availability: Contact Taru Lintunen, Department of Physical Education, University of Jyvaskyla, P. O. Box 35, FIN-40351, Jyvaskyla, Finland. (Phone # 358-41-602113; FAX # 358-41-602101; E-mail: lintunen@pallo.jyu.fi)

References
*Lintunen, T. (1995). *Self-perceptions, fitness, and exercise in early adolescence: A four-year follow-up study.* (Studies in Sport, Physical Education and Health, No. 41). Jyvaskyla, Finland: Jyvaskyla University Printing House.
*Lintunen, T., Heikinaro-Johansson, P., & Sherrill, C. (1995). Use of the Perceived Physical Competence Scale with adolescents with disabilities. *Perceptual and Motor Skills, 80,* 571-577.
*Lintunen, T., Leskinen, E., Oinonen, M., Salinto, M., & Rahkila, P. (1995). Change, reliability, and stability in self-perceptions in early adolescence: A four-year follow-up study. *International Journal of Behavioral Development, 18,* 351-364.
Lintunen, T., Rahkila, P., Leskinen, E., & Salmela, T. (1989). Relationship between physical fitness, perceived physical competence and self-esteem in 11-year-old boys and girls. *Abstracts of the 7th World Congress of Sport Psychology* (p. 77). Singapore.
*Lintunen, T., Rahkila, P., Silvennoinen, M., & Osterback, L. (1988). Psychological and physical correlates of early and late biological maturation in 9- to 11-year-old girls and boys. In R. M. Malina (Ed.), *Young athletes: Biological, psychological, and educational perspectives* (pp. 85-91). Champaign, IL: Human Kinetics.

160 Perceived Physical Fitness Scale [PPFS]
Ben R. Abadie

Source: Abadie, B. R. (1988). Construction and validation of a perceived physical fitness scale. *Perceptual and Motor Skills, 67,* 887-892.

Purpose: To assess an individual's perceptions of his or her physical fitness.

Description: The PPFS contains 12 items that assess an individual's perceptions of his or her physical fitness in relation to cardiorespiratory endurance, muscular strength, muscular endurance, flexibility, and body composition. For example, participants are asked to respond to the item "I possess less muscular strength than most individuals my age." Participants respond to each item using a 5-point Likert scale.

Construction: A total of 15 items were developed to represent the five above components of physical fitness. Three experts (one physical educator and two exercise physiologists) established the content validity of the items. Based on an item analysis of the responses of 144 men and 166 women to the PPFS, 12 items were retained.

Reliability: An alpha reliability coefficient of .78 was reported (n=310). A test-retest reliability coefficient of .92 was indicated among 111 of these individuals across a 7- to 10-day interval.

Validity: A principal component factor analysis (n=310) resulted in the identification of four factors (representing 62.9 percent of the variance) that were labeled Physical Condition, Flexibility, Muscular Condition, and Body Composition. Discriminant validity was supported in that high physically fit older adults (n=19) scored higher on the PPFS than did low fit older adults (n=22). Furthermore, 49 young adults (M age < 50) who participated in exercise during the last 3 months scored higher on the PPFS than did young adults (n=41) who did not exercise during that time period. In addition, derived factor scores on the PPFS were correlated with actual measures of physical fitness among young (n=28, M age=27.8 years) and older (n=30, M age=68.3 years) adults, except for the muscular strength and flexibility measures obtained among the older adults.

Norms: Not cited. Psychometric data were reported for 144 men and 166 women.

**Availability: Contact Ben R. Abadie, Department of Physical Education, Health and Recreation, Box 6186, Mississippi State University, Mississippi State, MS 39762-6186. (Phone # 601-325-7235; FAX # 601-325-8784; E mail: bra1@ra.msstate.edu)

Reference
Abadie, B. R. (1988). Relating trait anxiety to perceived physical fitness. *Perceptual and Motor Skills, 67,* 539-543.

161 Physical Estimation and Attraction Scales (PEAS)

Robert J. Sonstroem

Source: Sonstroem, R. J. (1978). Physical Estimation and Attraction Scales: Rationale and research. *Medicine and Science in Sports, 10,* 97-102.

Purpose: To assess (a) self-perceptions of physical fitness and athletic ability, hypothesized to be a component of global self-esteem (estimation); and (b) interest in vigorous physical activity (attraction).

Description: The PEAS is an 89-item true-false test containing two subscales--Physical Estimation (EST) and Attraction (ATTR). The test has three versions for different age and sex groups: boys, men, and females.

Construction: Based on an item analysis of male high school students' (*n*=165) responses to an original pool of 51 EST and 39 ATTR items, a total of 76 items were retained. Borrowing from Kenyon's work on the Attitudes Toward Physical Activity inventory, 54 new items were developed. These items were combined with an enlarged pool of 55 EST items and 46 ATTR items, and the resulting 155-item pool was administered to 710 male students at three high schools. Principal component factor analyses of their responses led to the retention of 89 items representing a seven-factor solution (and accounting for 49.31% of the variance).

Reliability: Kuder-Richardson-20 internal consistency coefficients of .87 (EST) and .89 (ATTR) were reported. Test-retest reliability coefficients of .92 (EST) and .94 (ATTR) were reported for 40 high school males over a 2-week interval.

Validity: Using three independent samples of high school males (*n*=115; *n*=187; and *n*=109) and 112 boys in grades 7-8, statistically significant but low correlation coefficients (ranging from .21 to .51) were reported for their EST responses and various global measures of self-esteem and life adjustment (e.g., Tennessee Self Concept Scale), thus supporting the convergent validity of this subscale. EST responses also correlated positively with various measures of physical ability, whereas global self-esteem did not, thus supporting estimation as a mediating variable in a physical fitness and self-esteem relationship. Participants' responses on ATTR were related to self-report levels of participation in physical activity. Discriminant validity was evidenced by low correlation coefficients of EST scores with Lie Scale scores and Marlowe-Crowne Social Desirability scale scores, as well as low relationships between ATTR and social desirability.

Norms: Not cited.

Availability: Contact Robert J. Sonstroem, Department of Physical Education, 106 Tootell Center, University of Rhode Island, Kingston, RI 02881-0810. (Phone # 401-874-5434)

References
*Dishman, R. K. (1980). The influence of response distortion in assessing self-perceptions of physical ability and attitude toward physical activity. *Research Quarterly for Exercise and Sport, 51,* 286-298.

*Fox, K. R., Corbin, C. B., & Couldry, W. H. (1985). Female physical estimation and attraction to physical activity. *Journal of Sport Psychology, 7,* 125-136.

*Safrit, M. J., Wood, T. M., & Dishman, R. K. (1985). The factorial validity of the Physical Estimation and Attraction Scales for adults. *Journal of Sport Psychology, 7,* 166-190.

*Sonstroem, R. J. (1974). Attitude testing examining certain psychological correlates of physical activity. *Research Quarterly, 45,* 93-103.

*Sonstroem, R. J., & Morgan, W. P. (1989). Exercise and self-esteem: Rationale and model. *Medicine and Science in Sports and Exercise, 21,* 329-337.

 *[Physical Fitness Self-Efficacy Scale] [PFSES]
John E. Bezjak and Jerry W. Lee

Source: Bezjak, J. E., & Lee, J. W. (1990). Relationship of self-efficacy and locus of control constructs in predicting college students' physical fitness behaviors. *Perceptual and Motor Skills, 71,* 499-508.

Purpose: To assess "...participants' perceived competence and confidence in performing tasks involving components of health-related physical fitness" (p. 501).

Description: The PFSES contains 15 items such as "I have a lot of stamina" or "I have strong muscles." Participants respond to each item on a 6-point Likert scale with the anchorings 1 (*strongly disagree*) to 6 (*strongly agree*).

Construction: Not reported.

Reliability: A Cronbach alpha internal consistency coefficient of .84 (*N*=300 approximate) was reported.

Validity: Self-efficacy scores were related to participants' (*N*=211) frequency and duration of reported participation in health-related physical fitness activities.

Norms: Not cited. Psychometric data were reported for 300 undergraduate students (*n*=161 females; *n*= 139 males), and descriptive statistics and psychometric data were reported for 211 undergraduate students (*n*=114 females; *n*=93 males). The subjects were sampled from colleges and universities in the Riverside, California, area.

Availability: Last known address: John E. Bezjak, Department of Institutional Research, University of Phoenix, 4615 East Elwood Street, Phoenix, AZ 85040.

Reference

*Bezjak, J. E., & Langga-Sharifi, E. (1991). Validation of the Physical Fitness Opinion Questionnaire against marathon performance. *Perceptual and Motor Skills, 73*, 993-994.

*Physical Self-Concept Scale (PSCS)
Garry E. Richards

Source: Richards, G. E. (1987, January). *Outdoor education in Australia in relation to the Norman conquest, a Greek olive grove, and the external perspective of a horse's mouth.* Paper presented at the 5th National Outdoor Education Conference, Perth, Western Australia.

Purpose: To assess self-perceptions of the physical well-being.

Description: The PSCS contains 43 items within seven subscales: Body Build, Appearance, Health, Physical Competence, Strength, Action, and

Satisfaction. Participants respond to each item using an 8-point ordinal scale with the anchorings 1 (*definitely false*) to 8 (*definitely true*).

Construction: Items for the PSCS were developed from a review of the literature. Exploratory principal components factor analysis (oblique rotation) supported a seven-factor structure.

Reliability: Cronbach alpha internal consistency coefficients were reported for four independent samples of male or female children and adults. The coefficients ranged from .93 (Appearance and Physical Competence) among female adults, to .79 (Health) among male adults. These reported alpha coefficients per subscale represent the mean of two alpha coefficients computed for two administrations of the PSCS three weeks apart.

Test-retest reliability coefficients across a 3-week period for these samples ranged from .77 to .90.

Validity: Not discussed.

Norms: The author reports descriptive and psychometric data for 2,612 individuals across gender, age, educational and socioeconomic backgrounds.

Availability: Contact Garry E. Richards, Executive Director, Australian Outward Bound School, c/-P.O. Tharwa, A.C.T. 2620 Australia. (Phone # (06) 237-5158; FAX # (06) 237-5224)

 164

*Physical Self-Description Questionnaire (PSDQ)
Herbert W. Marsh, Garry E. Richards, Steven Johnson, Lawrence Roche, and Patsy Tremayne

Source: Marsh, H. W., Richards, G. E., Johnson, S., Roche, L., & Tremayne, P. (1994). Physical Self-Description Questionnaire: Psychometric properties and a multitrait-multimethod analysis of relations to existing instruments. *Journal of Sport & Exercise Psychology, 16*, 270-305.

Purpose: To assess participants' physical self-concept from a multidimensional, hierarchical perspective.

Description: The PSDQ contains 70 items and 11 scales: Strength, Body Fat, Activity, Endurance/Fitness, Sports Competence, Coordination, Health, Appearance, Flexibility, Global Physical Self-Concept, and Global Esteem. Participants respond to each item using a 6-point true/false response scale. The PSDQ was designed for adolescents 12 years of age or older, but the authors indicate that the PSDQ should also be appropriate for adults.

Construction: Marsh and Redmayne (1994) developed an initial version of the PSDQ containing six physical self-concept scales. This research was extended using a sample of 315 adolescents who were administered a longer version of the current PSDQ. Item analyses, reliability assessments, and factor analysis led to the retention of 11 scales and the 70 item PSDQ.

Reliability: Cronbach alpha coefficents ranged from .82 to .92 (median=.88) and from .87 to .96 (median=.91) for two independent samples (n=315; n=395) of adolescents. Marsh (in press-c) reported median test-retest stability coefficients of .83 (3-month period) and .69 (14-month period).

Validity: Confirmatory factor analysis supported the a priori 11-factor structure underlying the multidimensional physical self-concept. Although the factor solutions for males and females were similar, responses by females were somewhat more reliable, variable, and more differentiated than males. In addition, the use of multitrait-multimethod analyses to evaluate the relationships of participants' responses to the PSDQ with their responses to the Physical Self-Perception Profile and the Physical Self-Concept scale indicated good support for the convergent and discriminant validity of the PSDQ.

In a recent study (Marsh, in press-a), 23 external criteria (e.g., body composition, endurance, strength) were predicted a priori to be most highly correlated with one of the PSDQ scales. Every predicted correlation was statistically significant. In support of discriminant validity, most predicted correlations were higher than other correlations involving the same criterion (Marsh, in press-a).

260

Norms: Not reported. Psychometric data were reported for 315 adolescents (208 boys; 107 girls) participating in the Australian Outward Bound school programs, and for 396 adolescents (217 males; 178 females) attending a private, comprehensive high school in Sydney, Australia.

Availability: Contact Herbert W. Marsh, University of Western Sydney, Macarthur, P.O. Box 555, Campbelltown, New South Wales 2560, Australia. [Phone # (046) 20 3563; FAX (046) 28 5353; E-mail: h.marsh@uws.edu.au]

References

*Chi, L., & Lin, H-H. (1995). The prediction of physical self-concept among youth dancers [Abstract]. *Journal of Sport & Exercise Psychology, 17* (Suppl.), S40.

*Marsh, H. W. (1993) The multidimensional structure of physical fitness: Invariance over gender and age. *Research Quarterly for Exercise and Sport, 64,* 256-273.

*Marsh, H. W. (1994). The importance of being important: Theoretical models of relations between specific and global components of physical self-concept. *Journal of Sport & Exercise Psychology, 16,* 306-325.

*Marsh, H. W. (in press-a). Construct validity of Physical Self Description Questionnaire responses: Relations to external criteria. *Journal of Sport & Exercise Psychology.*

*Marsh, H. W. (in press-b). The measurement of physical self concept: A construct validation approach. In K. Fox (Ed.), *The physical self: From motivation to well-being.* Champaign, IL: Human Kinetics.

*Marsh, H. W. (in press-c). Physical Self Description Questionnaire: Stability and discriminant validity. *Research Quarterly for Exercise and Sport.*

Marsh, H. W., Perry, C., Horsely, C., & Roche, L. (1995). Multidimensional self-concepts of elite athletes: How do they differ from the general population? *Journal of Sport & Exercise Psychology, 17,* 70-83.

*Marsh, H. W., & Redmayne, R. S. (1994). A multidimensional physical self-concept and its relation to multiple components of physical fitness. *Journal of Sport & Exercise Psychology, 16,* 43-55.

*Marsh, H. W., & Roche, L. A. (in press). Predicting self esteem from perceptions of actual and ideal ratings of body fatness: Is there only one ideal "supermodel"? *Research Quarterly for Exercise and Sport.*

165	**Physical Self-Efficacy Scale (PSE)** Richard M. Ryckman, Michael A. Robbins, Billy Thornton, and Peggy Cantrell

Source: Ryckman, R. M., Robbins, M. A., Thornton, B., & Cantrell, P.

(1982). Development and validation of a Physical Self-Efficacy Scale. *Journal of Personality and Social Psychology, 42,* 891-900.

Purpose: To measure individual differences in perceived physical ability and confidence in physical self-presentation in social situations.

Description: The PSE contains a 10-item Perceived Physical Ability (PPA) subscale and a 12-item Physical Self-Presentation Confidence (PSPC) subscale. An example of an item from the PPA subscale is "I have excellent reflexes." An example of a PSPC subscale item is "People think negative things about me because of my posture." Participants respond to all items using a 6-point Likert format.

Construction: A pool of 90 items was developed focusing on individuals' generalized expectancies concerning perceived physical skills, and their level of confidence in displaying and being evaluated by others on physical skills. Principal component factor analysis of the responses of 363 undergraduate students resulted in the retention of three factors, one of which was eliminated because it was contaminated by social desirability response distortions. A total of 22 items were retained forming the two subscales noted above.

Reliability: Alpha reliability coefficients (n=363) for the PSE and the PPA and PSPC subscales were .81, .84, and .74, respectively. Test-retest reliability coefficients (n=83 undergraduate students) across a 6-week interval were .80 (PSE), .85 (PPA), and .69 (PSPC).

Validity: Convergent validity (n=90 undergraduate students) was reported with the Tennessee Physical Self-Concept subscale (r=.58). Among a sample of 207 undergraduate students, concurrent validity was also demonstrated using locus of control, sensation seeking, and trait anxiety measures. Discriminant validity was evident because the PPA was less related to global self-consciousness than was the PSPC subscale. Predictive validity was also supported among two additional samples of undergraduate students in that individuals with positive perceptions of physical skills outperformed individuals with poorer self-regard on three motor skill tasks.

Norms: Psychometric data were reported for various samples of undergraduate students (above) who were enrolled in introductory classes.

262

(See also studies by Ryckman and his colleagues listed in the reference list.)

**Availability: Contact Richard M. Ryckman, Department of Psychology, 5742 Clarence Cook Little Hall, University of Maine, Orono, ME 04469-5742. (Phone # 207-581-2046; FAX # 207-581-6128; E-mail: ryckman@maine.maine.edu)

References

*Bosscher, R. J., Laurijssen, L., & De Boer, E. (1993). Measuring physical self-efficacy in old age. *Perceptual and Motor Skills, 77,* 470.

Cogan, K. D., Highlen, P. S., Petrie, T. A., Sherman, W. M., & Simonsen, J. (1991). Psychological and physiological effects of controlled intensive training and diet on collegiate rowers. *International Journal of Sport Psychology, 22,* 165-180.

*Cusumano, J. A., & Robinson, S. E., & Morooka, F. (1989). Physical self-efficacy levels in Japanese and American university students. *Perceptual and Motor Skills, 69,* 912-914.

*Duda, J. L., Smart, A. E., & Tappe, M. K. (1989). Predictors of adherence in the rehabilitation of athletic injuries: An application of personal investment theory. *Journal of Sport & Exercise Psychology, 11,* 367-381.

*Duda, J. L., & Tappe, M. K. (1988). Predictors of personal investment in physical activity among middle-aged and older adults. *Perceptual and Motor Skills, 66,* 543-549.

Duncan, T., & McAuley, E. (1987). Efficacy expectations and perceptions of causality in motor performance. *Journal of Sport Psychology, 9,* 385-393.

Escarti, A., Garcia-Ferriol, A, & Cervello, E. (1993). Relationship between the perception of the coaches competence with physical self-efficacy and motivation level. *Proceedings of the Eighth World Congress of Sport Psychology* (pp. 211-217). Lisbon, Portugal.

*Gayton, W. F., Matthews, G. R., & Burchstead, G. N. (1986). An investigation of the validity of the Physical Self-efficacy Scale in predicting marathon performance. *Perceptual and Motor Skills, 63,* 752-754.

*Godin, G., & Shepard, R. J. (1985). Gender differences in perceived physical self-efficacy among older individuals. *Perceptual and Motor Skills, 60,* 599-602.

*Holloway, J. B., Beuter, A., & Duda, J. L. (1988). Self-efficacy and training for strength in adolescent girls. *Journal of Applied Social Psychology, 18,* 699-719.

*Kavussanu, M., & McAuley, E. (1995). Exercise and optimism: Are highly active individuals more optimistic? *Journal of Sport & Exercise Psychology, 17,* 246-258

*LaGuardia, R., & Labbe, E. E. (1993). Self-efficacy and anxiety and their relationship to training and race performance. *Perceptual and Motor Skills, 77,* 27-34.

*Lox. C. L., McAuley, E., & Tucker, R. S. (1995). Exercise as an intervention for enhancing subjective well-being in an HIV-1 population. *Journal of Sport & Exercise Psychology, 17,* 345-362.

Martin, K. A., & Hall, C. R. (1995). Using mental imagery to enhance intrinsic motivation. *Journal of Sport & Exercise Psychology, 17,* 54-69.

*McAuley, E., & Gill, D. (1983). Reliability and validity of the Physical Self-Efficacy Scale in a competitive sport setting. *Journal of Sport Psychology, 5,* 410-418.

McCullagh, P., Matzkanin, K. T., & Figge, Jr., J. K. (1990). Personal investments in exercise: An examination of adult swimmers [Abstract]. *Proceedings of the Association for the Advancement of Applied Sport Psychology annual convention* (p. 77). San Antonio, TX.

Mueller, L. M. (1992). The effect of general and task-specific self-efficacy on the performance of a fine motor task. *Journal of Sport Behavior, 15,* 130-140.

Robertson, K. S., Mellors, S., Hughes, M., Sanderson, F. H., & Reilly, T. (1990). Psychological health status of squash players of differing standards [Abstract]. *Journal of Sports Sciences, 8,* 71-72.

*Ryckman, R. M., & Hamel, J. (1993). Perceived physical ability differences in the sport participation motives of young athletes. *International Journal of Sport Psychology, 24,* 270-283.

*Ryckman, R. M., Robbins, M. A., & Thorton, B. (1982). *Personality correlates of perceived physical self-efficacy in university men and women.* Paper presented at the Multi-Ethnic Conference on Assessment, Tampa, FL.

*Ryckman, R. M., Robbins, M. A., Thorton, B., & Kaczor, L. (1983). *Physical self-efficacy, exercise routines, and sports participation in university men and women.* Paper presented at the Southeastern Psychological Association Convention, Atlanta, GA.

*Salmoni, A. W., & Sidney, K. H. (1989). The effect of exercise on physical self-efficacy in the elderly [Abstract]. *Psychology of motor behavior and sport* (p 151). Kent, OH: Proceedings of the North American Society for the Psychology of Sport and Physical Activity annual convention.

*Thorton, B., & Ryckman, R. M. (1991). Physical attractiveness, physical effectiveness, and self-esteem in adolescence: A cross-sectional analysis. *Journal of Adolescence, 14,* 85-98.

*Thornton. B., Ryckman, R. M., Robbins, M. A., Donolli, J., & Biser, G. (1987). Relationship between perceived physical ability and indices of actual physical fitness. *Journal of Sport Psychology, 9,* 295-300.

*Wells, C. M., Collins, D., & Hale, B. D. (1993). The self-efficacy-performance link in maximum strength performance. *Journal of Sports Sciences, 11,* 167-175.

Wong, E. H., & Lox, C. L. (1993). Relationship between sports context, competitive trait anxiety, perceived ability, and self presentation confidence. *Perceptual and Motor Skills, 76,* 847-850.

166 Physical Self-Perception Profile (PSPP)
Kenneth R. Fox and Charles B. Corbin

Source: Fox, K. R., & Corbin, C. B. (1989). The Physical Self-Perception Profile: Development and preliminary validation. *Journal of Sport & Exercise Psychology, 11,* 408-430.

Purpose: To examine perceptions of the physical self from a multidimensional perspective.

Description: The PSPP consists of five 6-item subscales: Perceived sports competence (Sport), perceived bodily attractiveness (Body), perceived physical strength and muscular development (Strength), perceived level of physical conditioning and exercise (Condition), and physical self-worth (PSW). Participants respond to each item using a four-choice structured alternative format; scores range from 6 to 24 on each subscale.

Construction: During Phase I (subdomain identification), a literature review of existing related instrumentation was conducted, participants' responses (from a previous research study) to two of these instruments were subjected to factor analysis, and the open-ended responses given by 63 college males and 80 college females as to why they felt good about their physical self were evaluated. Based on these criteria, four subdomains were identified: perceived body attractiveness, sports competence, physical strength, and fitness and exercise.

During Phase II (instrument construction), six-item subscales were constructed for each of the subdomains using a four-choice structured alternative format. In addition, a six-item subscale was developed to assess physical self-worth at the domain level. Based on the responses of 24 female and 28 male students, some items were subsequently revised.

During Phase III, further analyses among 71 male and 80 female college students were made of item characteristics, as well as subscale internal consistency, stability, factor structure, and social desirability response distortions. Exploratory factor analysis with oblique rotation supported a four-factor structure; however, the physical conditioning subscale appeared to have ambiguous items leading to a revision of this subscale.

Upon confirmation of the factorial validity and internal reliability of the revised subscales (n=128 males; n=106 females), the subscale responses of 49 males and 41 college females were evaluated for test-retest stability across 16 or 23 days. In addition, these individuals were administered the Marlowe-Crowne Social Desirability Scale (1982) to examine the extent to which item responses were susceptible to social desirability.

During Phase IV, the responses of 180 male and 175 female undergraduate students were analyzed using LISREL to confirm the factor structure of the perception profile. In addition, the relationships of subscale responses to measures of global self-esteem and physical activity behavior were examined to establish the preliminary construct validity of the PSPP. Based on these analyses, a 30-item five-scale PSPP emerged.

Reliability: Cronbach alpha reliability coefficients ranged from .81 to .92 among 128 male and 106 female undergraduates. Test-retest reliability coefficients ranged between .74 and .92 for a 16-day period, and between .81 and .88 across 23 days.

Validity: Exploratory factor analyses supported a four-factor structure explaining 66.2% of the variance. Confirmatory factor analysis ($n=375$) indicated that participants' responses to the PSPP were adequately described by four factors. In addition, the PSPP was successful in discriminating between physically active and nonactive undergraduate students, and was predictive of the type of physical activity engaged in by these students.

Norms: Psychometric data for the final version were based on the responses of 589 undergraduate students enrolled at a midwestern university.

**Availability: Contact Kenneth R. Fox, Exercise and Sport Sciences, School of Education, University of Exeter, St. Luke's. Heavitree Road, Exeter EX1 2LU, England. (Phone # +44 01392 264890; FAX # +44 01392 264792; E-mail: krfox@exeter.ac.uk). Copies of the PSPP manual are available either from the first author or from the Office for Health Promotion, Northern Illinois University, DeKalb, IL 60115 (Phone # 815-753-0112). The first author noted (K. R. Fox, personal communication, April 5, 1996) that children's (e.g., Whitehouse, 1995) and adult (e.g., Chase, Corbin, & Fox, in review) versions of the PSPP are now available; also, the first author has prepared a shortened version of the PSPP for use, particularly in health settings. The first author also has information available concerning Spanish, Portuguese, French, and Greek translations of the PSPP.

References

*Brewer, B. W. Self-identity and specific vulnerability to depressed mood. *Journal of Personality, 61,* 343-364.

*Brewer, B. W., van Raalte, J. L., & Linder, D. E. (1993). Athletic identity: Hercules muscles or Achilles heel? *International Journal of Sport Psychology, 24,* 237-254.

Buxton, K. E., & Ashford, B. (1994). Participation motives and physical self-perceptions in high- and low-frequency female aerobic dance participants. *Journal of Sports Sciences, 12,* 184.

*Caruso, C. M., & Gill, D. L. (1992). Strengthening physical self-perceptions through exercise. *Journal of Sports Medicine and Physical Fitness, 32,* 416-427.

*Chase, L. A., & Corbin, C. B. (1993). Activity involvement and physical self-perceptions in the older population [Abstract]. *Research Quarterly for Exercise and Sport, 64* (Suppl.). A-99-100.

*Chase, L. A., Corbin, C. B., & Fox, K. R. (in review). Physical self-perceptions of older adults. *Journal of Aging and Physical Activity.*

*Crocker, P., Chad, K., Humbert, L., & Graham, T. (1994). The effects of a 10-week jump-rope program on physical self-perceptions in grade nine students [Abstract]. *Journal of Sport & Exercise Psychology, 16* (Suppl.), S44.

*Daly, A. J., & Parfitt, G. (1995). The effects of exercise withdrawal on physical self-perceptions [Abstract]. *Journal of Applied Sport Psychology, 7* (Suppl.), S54.

*Damm, S. G., & Ashford, B. (1994). Physical self-perceptions and goal orientations in British schoolchildren aged 13-14 years; Gender and ability differences [Abstract]. *Journal of Sports Sciences, 12,* 188.

*Ebbeck, V. (1992). The mediating role of perceived importance, certainty, and ideal comparison variables in the perceived competence/physical self-worth relationship [Abstract]. *Proceedings of the Association for the Advancement of Applied Sport Psychology annual convention* (p. 24). Colorado Springs, CO.

*Ebbeck, V. (1993). Sources of information used to judge physical self-worth: A comparison of high and low self-esteem groups [Abstract]. *Journal of Sport & Exercise Psychology, 15* (Suppl.), S25.

*Eklund, R. (1995). Self-esteem and social physique anxiety [Abstract]. *Journal of Sport & Exercise Psychology, 17* (Suppl.), S49.

*Fox, K. R., & Dirkin, G. R. (1992). Psychosocial predictors and outcomes of exercise in patients attending multidisciplinary obesity treatment. *International Journal of Obesity, 16,* 84.

Fox, K. R., Mucci, W. H., & Dirkin, G. R. (1990). Exercise psychology of obese adults attending clinical treatment: A longitudinal study [Abstract]. *Journal of Sports Sciences, 8,* 70

Fox, K. R., & Vehnekamp, T. J. (1990). Gender comparisons of self-perceptions, physical fitness, exercise and dietary habits in college students [Abstract]. *Journal of Sports Sciences, 8,* 282-283.

*Green, L., Walker, D., & Nelson, K. (1993). Cognitions and causal attributions of low and high self-perception collegiate students during success and failure learning situations in aerobic dance [Abstract]. *Research Quarterly for Exercise and Sport, 64* (Suppl.), A-87-88.

Helmcamp, A., & Petrie, T. A. (1993). The relationship of exercise duration to disordered eating, physical self-esteem, and beliefs about attractiveness [Abstract]. *Proceedings of the Association for the Advancement of Applied Sport Psychology annual convention* (p. 67). Montreal, Canada.

*Leveillee, C. M., Sonstroem, R. J., & Reibe, D. (1994). Self perceptions and eating disorder differences in routine and ultra adult female exercisers [Abstract]. *Medicine and Science in Sport and Exercise, 26* (Suppl.), S155

*Linford, J., & Fazey, D. (1994). Goal orientation of physical education lessons and the perceived physical competence levels of young adolescents [Abstract]. *Journal of Sports Sciences, 12,* 199-200.

*Marsh, H. W., Richards, G. E., Johnson. S., Roche, L., & Tremayne, P. (1994). Physical Self-Description Questionnaire: Psychometric properties and a multitrait-multitimethod analyses of relations to existing instruments. *Journal of Sport & Exercise Psychology, 16,* 270-305.

*Marsh, H. W., & Sonstroem, R. J. (1995). Importance ratings and specific components of physical self-concept: Relevance to predicting global components of self-concept and exercise. *Journal of Sport & Exercise Psychology, 17,* 84-104.

*Mutrie, N., & Davison, R. (1994). Physical self-perception in exercising older adults [Abstract]. *Journal of Sports Sciences, 12,* 203.

*Page, A., Ashford, B., Fox, K. R., & Biddle, S. J. H. (1993). Evidence of cross-cultural validity for the Physical Self-Perception Profile. *Personality and Individual Differences, 14,* 585-590.

*Page, A., Fox, K., & Biddle, S. (1992). Physical self-perception in British subjects: Relationships with self-esteem and exercise involvement [Abstract]. *Journal of Sports Sciences, 10,* 603-604.

*Page, A., Fox, K. R., McManus, A., & Armstrong, N. (1994). Profiles of self-perception change following an 8 week aerobic training programme [Abstract]. *Journal of Sports Sciences, 12,* 204.

Petrie, T. A., Diehl, N. S., Rogers, R., & Johnson, C. L. (1995). The Social Physique Anxiety Scale: Reliability and construct validity [Abstract]. *Journal of Applied Sport Psychology, 7* (Suppl.), S99.

*Sonstroem, R. J., Harlow, L. L., & Josephs, L. (1994). Exercise and self-esteem: Validity of model expansion and exercise associations. *Journal of Sport & Exercise Psychology, 16,* 29-42.

*Sonstroem, R. J., Speliotis, E. D., & Fava, J. L. (1992).Perceived physical competence in adults: An examination of the Physical Self-Perception Profile. *Journal of Sport & Exercise Psychology, 14,* 207-221.

*Welk, G. J., & Corbin, C. B. (1995). Physical self-perceptions of high school athletes. *Pediatric Exercise Science, 7,* 152-161.

*Whalen, J. P., & Brewer, B. W. (1992). Competence/importance discrepancies within the subdomains of global physical self-worth [Abstract]. *Proceedings of the Association for the Advancement of Applied Sport Psychology annual convention* (p. 131). Colorado Springs, CO.

*Whitehead, J. R. (1991). Preliminary validation of the Physical Self-Perception Profile questionnaire for seventh and eight grade students [Abstract]. *Proceedings of the North American Society for the Psychology of Sport and Physical Activity annual convention* (p. 205). Pacific Grove, CA.

*Whitehead, J. R. (1995). A study of children's physical self perceptions using an adapted physical self-perception profile questionnaire. *Pediatric Exercise Science, 7,* 132-151.

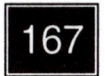

*Pictorial Scale of Perceived Physical Competence [PSPPC]

Dale A. Ulrich and Douglas H. Collier

Source: Ulrich, D. A., & Collier, D. H. (1990). Perceived physical competence in children with mental retardation: Modification of a pictorial scale. *Adapted Physical Activity Quarterly, 7,* 338-354.

Purpose: To assess self-perceptions of motor skill competence among elementary-school-aged children.

Description: Children are shown two pictures of 10 motor skills (e.g., dribbling a ball, kicking a ball). One picture depicts a child who is "pretty good" at the skill, and the other picture depicts a child who is "not very good" at the skill. Participants are asked to select the picture that they feel most like. They are also asked to indicate if they feel the child in the picture they selected was either "a lot" like them or "a little" like them. Scores of 1 to 4 are assigned on the PSPPC. A score of 1 designates a child who selects the pictures of a not a very good performer and who feels like that; a score of 4 is assigned to the child who selects the picture of a pretty good performer and feels like that person.

Construction: The PSPPC represents a modification of Harter's (Harter & Pike, 1984) Pictorial Scale of Perceived Competence and Social Acceptance for young children. Three items were deleted from this scale because the investigators did not feel they represented fundamental gross motor skills as commonly taught in elementary school motor-development programs. Also, a hopping item was eliminated because 10- to 12-year-olds do not enjoy this locomotor skill. Additional items were added based on the recommendations of elementary and adapted physical education instructors. Exploratory factor analysis (maximum likelihood factor analysis with oblique rotation) produced two factors, with the first factor accounting for 79% of the variance and the second factor accounting for 14% of the variance. Seven items loaded on Factor 1.

Reliability: Cronbach alpha reliability coefficients of .82 (total scale), .85 (Factor 1), and .72 (Factor 2) were reported (N=87). Test-retest reliability coefficients (N=87) across 3 to 5 days ranged from .26 (skip) to .63 (dribble), with a test-retest reliability coefficient of .77 reported for the overall mean score.

Validity: Not discussed.

Norms: Not cited. Descriptive and psychometric data were reported for 7- to 12-year-old children (42 boys and 45 girls) who were mildly mentally retarded.

Availability: Contact Dale A. Ulrich, Department of Kinesiology, Indiana University, Bloomington, IN 47405. (Phone # 812-855-5538; FAX # 812-855-6778; E-mail: ulrich@indiana.edu)

Reference

Harter, S., & Pike, R. (1984). The Pictorial Scale of Perceived Competence and Social Acceptance for young children. *Child Development, 55,* 1969-1982.

Playground Movement Confidence Inventory [PMCI]

Michael E. Crawford and Norma Sue Griffin

Source: Crawford, M. E., & Griffin, N. S. (1986). Testing the validity of the Griffin/Keogh Model for Movement Confidence by analyzing the self-report playground involvement decisions of elementary school children. *Research Quarterly for Exercise and Sport, 57,* 1, 8-15.

Purpose: To assess a children's sense of adequacy in a movement situation based on the interaction of personal perceptions of competence in performance, the potential for harm, and the potential for enjoyment.

Description: Six playground tasks are pictorially presented to children. The three subscales (Competence, Harm, and Enjoyment) center on questions about the confidence and performance decisions of the children in relation to each playground task shown. Items are assessed using a 4-point ordinal scale.

Construction: A large pool of movement tasks commonly performed on a playground was evaluated by experts and was subjected to a series of field trials. The six tasks selected were judged to be age appropriate and most representative of the range of playground movement choices/behavior for these children.

Reliability: Alpha reliability coefficients (*n*=250 fifth-grade students), computed by subscale, were .86 (Competence), .87 (Harm), and .84 (Enjoyment). Test-retest reliability coefficients for this sample were .79 (Competence), .75 (Harm), .78 (Enjoyment), and .78 for the combined inventory score.

Validity: The PMCI successfully discriminated between high versus low confidence and high versus low experience children. The index of discriminatory power was 84.65% correct classification accuracy, and the validity coefficient for scale classification power was .98. Construct validity was supported through principal component factor analysis. The three hypothesized factors emerged (competence, harm, enjoyment) accounting for 54% of the total variance (with 90% of this variance explained by the competence factor).

Norms: Not reported. Psychometric data are cited for 250 fifth-grade students in the Omaha Public Schools who were selected through cluster sampling; geographical stratification of the school district was utilized to ensure socioeconomic representativeness of the sample. Fifty-one percent of the sample was male, and 49% was female.

Availability: Contact Norma Sue Griffin, Department of Speech Education, 301 Barkley Center, University of Nebraska-Lincoln, Lincoln NE 68588-0732. (Phone # 402-472-5486; E-mail: ngriffin@unlinfo.unl.edu)

*[Running Self-Efficacy Scale] [RSES]
Rick LaGuardia and Elise E. Labbe

Source: LaGuardia, R., & Labbe, E. E. (1993). Self-efficacy and anxiety and their relationship to training and race performance. *Perceptual and Motor Skills, 77,* 27-34.

Purpose: To assess self-efficacy of running performance and confidence of self-presentation in running performance.

Description: The RSES contains 14 items and two subscales: Perceived Running Ability (8 items) and Self-Presentation Confidence (6 items). Runners respond to each item using a 7-point Likert scale.

Construction: Items were developed to reflect expected outcomes of running events that high school and college cross-country and track and field runners compete in. Also included were road race distances. (E. Labbe, personal communication, April 16, 1996).

Reliability: Not indicated.

Validity: Runners' (*N*=63) scores on the RSES were negatively correlated (*r*'s ranged from -.38 to -.42) with their pace times for three races. Also, their state anxiety scores and scores on the Self-Presentation Confidence subscale were negatively correlated.

Norms: Not cited. Psychometric data were presented for 33 men and 14 women who were members of two local running clubs and for 10 men and 6 women who were members of a local university track team.

**Availability: Contact Elise E. Labbe, Department of Psychology, University of South Alabama, Mobile, AL 36688-0002. (Phone # 334-460-7149; FAX # 334-460-7267)

170	***[Self-Efficacy for Exercise Behavior Scale] [SEEBS]**

Bess H. Marcus, Vanessa C. Selby, Raymond S. Niaura, and Joseph S. Rossi

Source: Marcus, B. H., Selby, V. C., Niaura, R. S., & Rossi, J. S. (1992). Self efficacy and the stages of exercise behavior change. *Research Quarterly for Exercise and Sport, 63,* 60-66.

Purpose: To measure participants' confidence in their ability to persist with regular exercise under various impediments.

Description: Participants are asked if they are confident they can persist in regular exercise when they are tired, in a bad mood, on vacation, and so forth. Participants respond to each of five items using a 5-point ordinal scale with the anchorings 1 (*not at all confident*) to 5 (*very confident*).

Construction: Items were selected to represent the categories negative affect, resisting relapse, and making time for exercise. These categories (or factors) were derived from previous factor analytic research on exercise and smoking behavior.

Reliability: A Pearson product-moment test-retest reliability coefficient of .90 (*N*=20) was reported across a 2-week period.

272

Validity: Not discussed.

Norms: Not cited. Descriptive statistics are presented for 1,063 employees (70% were male; M age=41.1 years, SD= 10.8) at a Rhode Island division of a government agency and for 429 employees of a Rhode Island medical center, 85% of whom were women (M age=40.5 years; SD=11.0). A third sample (N=20) of employees of a Rhode Island medical center was used to establish reliability estimates.

**Availability: Contact Bess H. Marcus, Division of Behavioral Medicine, The Miriam Hospital and Brown University School of Medicine, RISE Building, 164 Summit Ave., Providence, RI 02906 (Phone # 401-331-8500, ext. 3707; FAX # 401-331-2453)

References
*Gorely, T., & Gordon, S. (1995). An examination of the transtheoretical model and exercise behavior in older adults. *Journal of Sport & Exercise Psychology, 17*, 312-324.

*Marcus, B. H., Eaton, C. A., Rossi, J. S., & Harlow, L. L. (1994). Self-efficacy, decision-making, and stages of change: An integrative model of physical exercise. *Journal of Applied Social Psychology, 24*, 489-508.

*Marcus, B. H., & Owen, N. (1992). Motivational readiness, self-efficacy and decision-making for exercise. *Journal of Applied Social Psychology, 22*, 3-16.

*Marcus, B. H., Pinto, B. M., Simkin, L. R., Audrain, J. E., & Taylor, E. R. (1994). Application of theoretical models to exercise behavior among employed women. *American Journal of Health Promotion, 9*, 49-55.

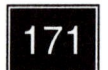

Stunt Movement Confidence Inventory (SMCI)
Norma S. Griffin and Michael E. Crawford

Source: Griffin, N. S., & Crawford, M. E. (1989). Measurement of movement confidence with a stunt movement confidence inventory. *Journal of Sport & Exercise Psychology, 11*, 26-40.

Purpose: To measure self-perceptions of movement confidence among children.

Description: The SMCI contains pictorial representations of six movement tasks such as performing a stunt on a skateboard and jumping while roller-skating. The six tasks were selected and designed to present performance demands involving height, speed, strength, balance and/or coordination; stunting was presented as a means of introducing movement challenge. Initial items of the SMCI focus on subject self-ratings of confidence and experience (using a 4-point ordinal scale) in relation to each task. Children are then asked to respond to nine items per task (on a 4-point rating scale) based on performance perceptions. These nine items represent the three factors of personal perceptions of competence, perceived potential for enjoying movement, and perceptions of the potential for physical harm.

Construction: The movement confidence model was selected as a theoretical focus for evaluating children's movement perceptions and decisions. This model guided construction of the two dependent variables measuring perceptions of movement confidence and experience, the six pictorially represented movement tasks, and the three movement confidence factor subscales.

Reliability: Alpha reliability coefficients (n=356 elementary school children) were .90, .93, and .91 for the subscales of competence, enjoyment, and harm, respectively. Test-retest reliability coefficients across a 2-week interval among these subjects were .82 (experience with task), .80 (movement confidence), .88 (competence), .79 (enjoyment), and .85 (harm).

Validity: Multiple discriminant analysis indicated that the SMCI was sufficiently stable to discriminate among high and low confidence/experience groups. This was confirmed by analytical validation of the SMCI indicating minimal R shrinkage. Construct validity was examined through factor analysis that supported the importance of the three model factors of enjoyment, competence, and harm in providing a meaningful analysis of performance decisions.

Norms: Psychometric data are based on a representative sample (n=356), using cluster sampling procedures, of all children in the fourth and fifth grades of the Omaha, Nebraska, public school system. No differences were found on the total score of the SMCI when the data were examined as a function of subject gender and ethnic group.

Availability: Contact Norma S. Griffin, Department of Speech Education, 301 Barkley Center, University of Nebraska-Lincoln, Lincoln, NE 68588-0732. (Phone # 402-472-5486)

Chapter 12

Confidence (Sport)

Tests in this chapter assess perceptions of sport performance competence and perceptions of competence in the coaching role. The strength of perceived self-efficacy in relation to sport performance, and perceptions of self-acceptance within the sport domain are also evaluated.

172 *Chemical Health Intervention Confidence Scale [CHICS]

James P. Corcoran and Deborah L. Feltz

Source: Corcoran, J. P. & Feltz, D. L. (1993). Evaluation of chemical health education for high school athletic coaches. *The Sport Psychologist, 7,* 298-308.

Purpose: To assess coaches' self-efficacy/confidence beliefs to employ chemical information and intervention skills with their athletes.

Description: The CHICS contains nine items. For example, coaches are asked how confident they are in their "knowledge of chemicals used by athletes today," and how confident they are in their "ability to confront unacceptable behavior that is exhibited on your team." Coaches respond on a 10-point Likert scale with the anchorings 0 (*not at all confident*) to 9 (*extremely confident*).

Construction: Not discussed.

Reliability: A Cronbach alpha reliability coefficient ($N=218$) of .92 and a test-retest reliability coefficient ($N=17$) of .83 were reported.

Validity: Construct validity was supported in that participants ($n=113$) exposed to a chemical health education and coaching program over 4 months exhibited greater confidence than did control subjects ($n=105$) in terms of their knowledge and use of critical chemical information and chemical health intervention skills. However, there was little evidence to support a relationship between knowledge versus confidence about critical chemical information and chemical health intervention skills.

Norms: Not cited. Psychometric data were reported for 218 high school coaches from the Midwest representing 21 sports. These coaches were predominantly Caucasian males (60%) with a mean age of 34.8 years ($SD=9.50$).

**Availability: Contact Deborah L. Feltz, Youth Sport Institute, Michigan State University, I. M. Sports Circle, East Lansing, MI 48824. (Phone # 517-355-4732; FAX # 517-353-2944; E-mail: dfeltz@msu.edu)

173 *Coaching Competence Questionnaire (CCQ)

Elizabeth L. Zimney and Heather Barber

Source: Zimney, E. L., & Barber, H. (1995, September). *An examination of athlete behaviors as a source of competence information for intercollegiate coaches.* Paper presented at the annual conference of the Association for the Advancement of Applied Sport Psychology, New Orleans, LA.

Purpose: To assess coaches' perceived competence in specific and general areas of coaching.

Description: The CCQ contains eight subscales: Practice and Seasonal Planning, Communication Skills, Ability to Motivate Athletes, Teaching Sport Skills, General Coaching Competence, Training and Conditioning, Coaching During Competition, and Sport-Specific Knowledge of Strategies and Tactics.

Construction: Items for the CCQ were derived from a review of the literature and pilot research. Ten independent coaches and researchers were used to establish the content validity of the CCQ.

Reliability: Cronbach alpha internal consistency coefficients ($N=104$) ranged from .83 to .94.

Validity: Not reported.

Norms: Not cited. Descriptive and psychometric data were reported for 36 female and 68 male coaches (M age=40.37 years) of eight sports at the Division I, II, or III levels.

Availability: Contact Heather Barber, Department of Kinesiology, University of New Hampshire, 209 Hampshire Hall, Durham, NH 03824. (Phone # 603-862-2058; FAX # 603-862-0154; E-mail: hb@christa.unh.edu)

Reference

*Barber, H., & Weiss. M. R. (1992). An examination of sources and levels of perceived competence in male and female interscholastic coaches [Abstract]. *Proceedings of the North American Society for the Psychology of Sport and Physical Activity annual convention* (p. 133). Pittsburgh, PA.

*Collective Efficacy Scales (CE)
Kim D. Dorsch, W. Neil Widmeyer, David M. Paskevich, and Lawrence R. Brawley

Source: Dorsh, K. D., Widmeyer, W. N., Paskevich, D. M., & Brawley, L. R. (1995). Collective efficacy: Its measurement and relationship to cohesion in ice hockey [Abstract]. *Journal of Applied Sport Psychology, 7* (Suppl.), S56.

Purpose: To assess "...a member's view of the group's beliefs regarding their team's collective capabilities" within a designated sport (S56).

Description: Eight scales assess different aspects of collective efficacy using 0-100% confidence scales.

Construction: Not indicated.

Reliability: Cronbach alpha coefficients (N=308) ranged from .86 to .95.

Validity: Using discriminant function analysis, it was found that participants' (N=308) scores on the CE scales effectively discriminated their categorizations as extreme task cohesion groups.

Norms: Not cited. Psychometric data were reported for 308 male ice hockey players representing 19 teams at the university and junior levels.

Availability: Contact W. Neil Widmeyer, Department of Kinesiology, University of Waterloo, Waterloo, Ontario, Canada N2L 3G1. (Phone # 519-885-1211, ext. 3955; FAX # 519-746-6776; E-mail: widmeyer@healthy.uwaterloo.ca)

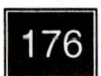 **Diving Efficacy Scale** (DES)
Deborah L. Feltz, Daniel M. Landers, and Ursula
Raeder

Source: Feltz, D. L., Landers, D. M., & Raeder, U. (1979). Enhancing self-efficacy in high-avoidance motor tasks: A comparison of modeling techniques. *Journal of Sport Psychology, 1,* 112-122.

Purpose: To assess the strength of self-efficacy among novice divers.

Description: The DES contains eight diving-related items that are presented in increasing order of difficulty. Divers rate the strength of their expectations for each diving task on a 100-point probability scale, ranging in 10-unit intervals from *great uncertainty* to *complete certainty.*

Construction: The design of the scale was modified from Bandura's efficacy scale.

Reliability: Test-retest reliability of the DES was .98 across a one-week interval among seven college students.

Validity: Not discussed.

Norms: Not cited

**Availability: Contact Deborah L. Feltz, Department of Physical Education, 138 IM Sports Circle, Michigan State University, East Lansing, MI 48824. (Phone # 517-355-4732; FAX # 517-353-2944; E-mail: dfeltz@msu.edu)

176 ***Elite Athlete Self Description Questionnaire** (EASDQ)
Herbert W. Marsh, John Hey, Steven Johnson, and
Clark Perry

Source: Marsh, H. W., Hey, J., Johnson, S., & Perry, C. (in press). Elite Athlete Self Description Questionnaire: Hierarchical confirmatory factor analysis of responses by two distinct groups of elite athletes. *International Journal of Sport Psychology.*

Purpose: To assess various components of the elite athlete self-concept.

Description: The EASDQ contains 28 items and six scales: Skill (e.g.,"I recognize myself as very skillful in my best sport/event"); Body (e.g., "I excel in my best sport/event because of the suitability of my body shape"); Aerobic (e.g., "Compared to my team mates/competitors I am aerobically superior in my best sport/event"); Anaerobic (e.g., "My capacity for short bursts of high intensity activity makes me a good performer in my best sport/event"); Mental (e.g., "I am mentally able to motivate myself appropriate to the situation when appropriate"); and Performance (e.g., "I excel at my best sport/event because I am able to give a peak performance when necessary"). Participants respond to each item using a six-category true-false ordinal response scale.

Construction: The EASDQ was developed, based on an intuitive model, in which it was..."hypothesized that overall performance by elite athletes was a function of skill levels, body suitability, physiological (aerobic and anaerobic) competence, and mental competence" (p. 4). Six scales, postulated as components of the elite athlete self-concept were developed. A pool of items was developed for each scale to reflect "... aspects such as self-perceptions of competence in relation to relative and absolute standards and the inferred perceptions of others (coaches and other elite athletes)" (p. 5). The pool of items was evaluated by sport psychology experts for their suitability with elite athletes. An initial draft of the EASDQ was then administered to small groups of elite athletes who commented on item clarity and wording.

Reliability: Cronbach alpha internal consistency coefficients for two samples (Australian Institute of Sport athletes, $n=151$; elite high school athletes, $n=349$) combined ranged from .83 (Performance) to .89 (Body) with a mean alpha coefficient of .85. Separate sample mean alpha coefficients of .86 (AIS athletes) and .84 (high school athletes) were also reported.

Validity: Confirmatory factor analysis of the responses of both groups combined and of each separate sample supported the six a priori factor structure; there was also support for the factorial invariance (and, therefore, the generalizability) of participants' responses across the two samples. Hierarchical confirmatory factor analysis indicated a single higher order factor and the invariance of the hierarchical structure across the two samples.

Norms: Not indicated. Psychometric data were reported for 151 elite athletes (62% male, 38% female; M age= 21 years) in residence at the Australian Institute of Sport and 349 elite athletes (63% male, 37% female) enrolled in Year 7 to Year 10 of a prestigious Australian high school.

Availability: Contact Herbert W. Marsh, University of Western Sydney, Macarthur, P. O. Box 555, Campbelltown, New South Wales 2560, Australia. [Phone # (046) 20 3563; FAX # (046) 28 5353; E-mail: h.marsh@uws.edu.au].

Reference
*Marsh, H. W., Perry, C., Horsely, C., & Roche, L. A. (1995). Multidimensional self-concepts of elite athletes: How do they differ from the general population? *Journal of Sport & Exercise Psychology, 17,* 70-73.

*Free-Throw Self-Efficacy Scale [FTSES]
Jeffrey M. Shaw, David A. Dzewaltowski, and Mary McElroy

Source: Shaw, J. M., Dzewaltowski, D. A., & McElroy, M. (1992). Self efficacy and causal attributions as mediators of perceptions of psychological momentum. *Journal of Sport & Exercise Psychology, 14,* 134-147.

Purpose: To assess self-efficacy toward competitive basketball free-throw shooting.

Description: The FTSES contains eight items such as "How confident are you that you can beat your opponent?" Participants rate their self confidence in 10% increments ranging from 0% perceived confidence to 100% perceived confidence.

Construction: Not discussed.

Reliability: Reliability coefficients (N=60) ranged from .80 to .87.

Validity: Not discussed.

Norms: Not cited. Psychometric data were reported for 60 male undergraduate students enrolled in physical education classes.

**Availability: Contact David A. Dzewaltowski, Department of Kinesiology, 8 Natatorium, Kansas State University, Manhattan, KS 66506-0302. (Phone # 913-532-0708; FAX # 913-532-6486; E-mail: dadx@ksu.ksu.edu)

178 Gymnastic Efficacy Measure (GEM)
Edward McAuley

Source: McAuley, E. (1985). Modeling and self-efficacy: A test of Bandura's model. *Journal of Sport Psychology, 7, 283-295.*

Purpose: To assess an individual's belief that he or she can execute successfully a balance beam skill in gymnastics.

Description: Six gymnastic activity items for the balance beam are arranged in hierarchical order of difficulty, with the target task (a dive forward roll mount onto a gymnastic balance beam from a springboard) listed as the final item. For items (tasks) that participants feel they can perform, they rate on a 100-point probability scale how certain they are about performing them. A rating of 100 points indicates absolute certainty; a rating of 10 points indicates that the individual is highly uncertain about performing the task. Self-efficacy cognitions are assessed by totaling these certainty ratings across across the six items and then dividing by the total number of items.

Construction: Not discussed.

Reliability: Not discussed.

Validity: Path analytic techniques were used to demonstrate that participants' (N=39) self-efficacy cognitions were a significant predictor of their performance of three forward roll mounts onto the balance beam.

Norms: Not indicated. Psychometric data were presented for 39 undergraduate students enrolled in physical education skills classes.

Availability: Contact Edward McAuley, Department of Kinesiology, 215 Freer Hall, University of Illinois, 906 South Goodwin Avenue, Urbana, IL 61801. (Phone # 217-333-6487; FAX # 217-244-7322; E-mail: a-mc3@staff.uiuc.edu)

179 *Influential Athlete Behavior Questionnaire (IABQ)
Elizabeth L. Zimney and Heather Barber

Source: Zimney, E. L., & Barber, H. (1995, September). *An examination of athlete behaviors as a source of competence information for intercollegiate coaches.* Paper presented at the annual conference of the Association for the Advancement for Applied Sport Psychology, New Orleans, LA.

Purpose: To assess coaches' perceptions of competence based on 10 sources of competence information provided by their athletes' behaviors.

Description: The IABQ contains 10 subscales: Performance Outcome, Performance Improvement, Performance Decline, Positive Verbal Feedback, Positive Nonverbal Feedback, Negative Verbal Feedback, Negative Nonverbal Feedback, Athlete Effort, Athlete Enjoyment, and Athlete Attitude.

Construction: Items for the IABQ were derived from a review of literature and pilot testing. The items were reviewed by 10 coaches and researchers for content validity.

Reliability: Cronbach alpha internal consistency coefficients ($N=104$) ranged from .65 (Positive Nonverbal Feedback) to .87.

Validity: Not discussed.

Norms: Not reported. Descriptive and psychometric data were reported for 36 female coaches and 68 male coaches (M age=40.37 years). These individuals coached women's cross-country, field hockey, women's soccer, women's tennis, men's cross-country, football, men's soccer, or men's tennis at the NCAA Division I, II, or III level.

Availability: Contact Heather Barber, Department of Kinesiology, University of New Hampshire, 209 Hampshire Hall, Durham, NH 03824. (Phone # 603-862-2058; FAX # 603-862-0154; E-mail: hb@christa.unh.edu)

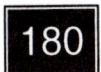

*Multi-Dimensional Coaching Efficacy Scale (MCES)
Deborah L. Feltz, M. A. Chase, S. G. Simensky, C. N. Hodge, J. Shi, and I. Lee

Source: Feltz, D. L., Chase, M. A., Simensky, S. G., Hodge, C. N., Shi, J., & Lee, I. (1994). Development of the multi-dimensional Coaching Efficacy Scale [Abstract]. *Journal of Sport & Exercise Psychology, 16* (Suppl.), S51.

Purpose: To assess "... the extent to which coaches believe they can affect the learning and performance of their athletes" (p. S51).

Description: The MCES contains 24 items and four subscales: (a) Competition, (b) Interpersonal, (c) Technique, and (d) Character Building.

Construction: An initial pool of 41 items was administered to 400 high school coaches (48% return rate). Exploratory factor analysis of their responses to the MCES led to a four-factor solution accounting for 64% of the variance, and the retention of 24 items. The largest factor, labeled Competition, accounted for 43% of the variance.

Reliability: Not discussed.

Validity: Concurrent validity of the MCES was supported in that coaches' responses to the MCES were correlated to their responses to measures of self-esteem ($r=.43$), expectancy for success ($r=.53$), and internal locus of control ($r=.37$).

288

Norms: Not cited. Psychometric data were reported for 192 high school coaches.

**Availability: Contact Deborah Feltz, Michigan State University, East Lansing, MI 48824. (Phone # 517-355-4732; FAX # 517-353-2944; E-mail: dfeltz@msu.edu)

 **Perceived Physical Competence Subscale for Children [PPCSC]**
Susan Harter

Source: Harter, S. (1982). The Perceived Competence Scale for Children. *Child Development, 53,* 87-97.

Purpose: To assess a child's perceptions of his or her physical competence in sports and outdoor games.

Description: The PPCSC is one of four subscales of Harter's Perceived Competence Scale for Children (PCSC). The PCSC assesses a child's sense of competence across the cognitive, social, and physical domains. A fourth subscale is labeled General Self-Worth. The PPCSC contains seven items. A structured alternative format is used. The child is first asked to indicate which kind of kid he or she is most like, based on two alternatives per item. The child is then asked whether the corresponding description selected is "sort of true" or "really true" of him or her. Each item is scored from 1 (low perceived physical competence) to 4 (high perceived physical competence).

Construction: A 40-item version of the PCSC was initially constructed. Items were selected based on interviews with children or were adapted from existing scales. Factor analysis of the responses of 215 third-through sixth-grade children led to the revision of at least one item per subscale. Subsequent factor analysis of the responses of a new sample of 133 children to the PCSC led to the final 28-item version.

Reliability: A Cronback alpha internal consistency coefficient of .83 was reported for the PPCSC among 341 children, grades 3-6. Across four additional samples, alpha reliabilities ranged from .77 to .86 for this subscale. Test-retest reliability coefficients (corrected for attenuation) across 3 months (n=208) and 9 months (n=810) were .87 and .80, respectively.

Validity: Construct validity of the PCSC was supported through factor analysis. Across four independent samples, the hypothesized four-factor model of perceived competence emerged. Concurrent validity of the PPCSC was supported, in that teacher ratings of childrens' actual physical competence in the gymnasium correlated positively with these childrens' corresponding scores on the PPSCS. Discriminant validity was evident in that children (n=23) selected for sport teams scored higher on the PPCSC than did their classmates (n=57).

Norms: Descriptive and psychometric data were presented for (a) 341 third- through sixth-graders from California and Connecticut, (b) 714 third- through sixth-graders from New York, (c) three independent samples of children (n=470) from Colorado representing the same age range, (d) an additional California sample of 746 children in grades 3-9. Each sample contained an approximately equal number of boys and girls. Samples were drawn from middle- and upper-middle-class populations.

Availability: Contact Susan Harter, Department of Psychology, FRH 147, University of Denver, University Park, Denver, CO 80208. (Phone # 303-871-3790; E-mail: sharter@du.edu)

References

*Feltz, D. L., & Brown, E. W. (1984). Perceived competence in soccer skills among young soccer players. *Journal of Sport Psychology, 6,* 385-394.

Feltz, D. L., & Petlichkoff, L. (1983). Perceived competence among interscholastic sport participants and dropouts. *Canadian Journal of Applied Sport Sciences, 8,* 231-235.

Roberts, G. C., Kleiber, D. A., & Duda, J. L. (1981). An analysis of motivation in children's sport: The role of perceived competence in participation. *Journal of Sport Psychology, 3,* 206-216.

*Weiss, M. R., & Duncan, S. C. (1992). The relationship between physical competence and peer acceptance in the context of children's sport participation. *Journal of Sport & Exercise Psychology, 14,* 177-191.

*Weiss, M. R., McAuley, E., Ebbeck, V., & Wiese, D. M. (1990). Self-esteem and causal attributions for children's physical and social competence in sport. *Journal of Sport & Exercise Psychology, 12,* 21-36.

*Williams, L., & Gill, D. L. (1995). The role of perceived competence in the motivation of physical activity. *Journal of Sport & Exercise Psychology, 17,* 363-378.

182 Perceived Soccer Competence Subscale [PSCS]

Deborah L. Feltz and Eugene W. Brown

Source: Feltz, D. L., & Brown, E. W. (1984). Perceived competence in soccer skills among young soccer players. *Journal of Sport Psychology,* 6, 385-394.

Purpose: To assess children's perceptions of their competence in soccer.

Description: The PSCS contains seven items. A structured alternative format is used in which children must first decide which kind of person they are most like. Then they decide if the description is "sort of true" or "really true" of themselves. For example, participants are asked to select between "Some kids do very well at soccer" and "Others don't feel that they are very good when it comes to soccer." Item responses are scored on a 4-point ordinal scale, where a score of 1 is indicative of low perceived soccer competence and a score of 4 is indicative of high perceived soccer competence.

Construction: The PSCS was modified from Harter's (1982) Physical subscale of the Perceived Competence Scale for Children. The word "soccer" was substituted for the word "sport" in the original subscale; plus, a few minor changes were made in the wording of items to fit the context of soccer.

Reliability: A Cronbach alpha internal reliability coefficient of .75 was reported among 217 youth soccer participants.

Validity: Concurrent validity was supported in that children's (n=217) responses to the PSCS were correlated (r=.45) with General Self-Esteem and also with the Physical subscale (r=.66) of Harter's Perceived Competence Scale for Children. Multiple regression analyses indicated that these children's responses to the PSCS were more predictive of their soccer abilities than either the Physical Perceived Competence subscale or the General Self-Esteem scale.

Norms: Descriptive and psychometric data were presented for 205 male and 12 female youth soccer participants ranging in age from 8 to 13 years.

**Availability: Contact Deborah L. Feltz, Department of Physical Education, IM Sports Circle, Room 138, Michigan State University, East Lansing, MI 48824. (Phone # 517-355-4732; FAX # 517-353-2944; E-mail: dfeltz@msu.edu)

References

Glenn, S. D., & Horn, T. S. (1993). Psychological and personal predictors of leadership behavior in female soccer athletes. *Journal of Applied Sport Psychology, 5,* 17-34.

Harter, S. (1982. The Perceived Competence Scale for Children. *Child Development, 53,* 87-97.

*Hopper. C., Gutherie, G. D., & Kelly, T. (1991). Self-concept and skill development in youth soccer players. *Perceptual and Motor Skills, 71,* 275-285.

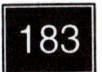

*Self-Acceptance Scale for Athletes (SASA)
Barbara Teetor Waite, Bruce Gansneder, and Robert J. Rotella

Source: Waite, B. T., Gansneder, B., & Rotella, R. J. (1990). A sport-specific measure of self-acceptance. *Journal of Sport & Exercise Psychology, 12,* 264-279.

Purpose: To assess individual differences in perceived self-acceptance within the sport domain, defined as the "...valuing and feeling good about oneself regardless of one's shortcomings or failures as an athlete" (p. 266).

Description: Two dimensions of sport-specific self-acceptance are assessed: self-accepting self-regard (SASR) and independence of self regard (IOS). The SASR subscale contains five items; participants are asked to respond on a 4-point Likert scale to items such as "I consider myself to be of greater worth than others." The IOS subscale contains eight items in which participants are asked to indicate on a 4-point ordinal scale the degree to which winning, staying in shape, and other sport-specific domains are important to their self-regard.

Construction: The SASA was developed by (a) incorporating relevant theoretical and empirical literature and (b) establishing a list of sport specific domains to provide the content of specific items. Graduate students (*N*=22) who were or who had been competitive athletes and/or coaches rated the importance of 14 sport-related domains, of which 8 were selected as most important for item development. A university doctoral committee reviewed the SASA for face and content validity, and a university instrument review panel provided input on face validity, format, word choice, and instrument design. Subsequently, the SASA was pilot tested (N=20 sport psychology graduate students; N=52 Division I collegiate athletes) to further enhance item clarity and relevance.

Reliability: Cronbach alpha reliability coefficients (N=131 college athletes) for the SASR and IOS subscales and the entire SASA were .58, .79, and .80, respectively. Test-retest reliability coefficients (7- to 14-day intervals) among approximately 60 of these athletes were .75, .62, and .71 for the SASR, IOS, and total SASA scores, respectively.

Validity: Construct validity was supported through the factor analysis (varimax rotation) of these athletes' (N=131) responses to the SASA. Two factors emerged (SASA and IOS) that accounted for 42% of the variance. Convergent validity was supported by the positive correlation of these athletes' responses to the SASA and global measures of self-esteem, general self-acceptance, and stability of self-concept. Discriminant validity was supported by demonstrating that the correlation coefficient between self-acceptance and perceived competence was significantly lower than the correlation coefficient representing the relationship between self-esteem and perceived competence. Further, athletes categorized as high or low on self-acceptance and self-esteem differed with regard to stability of self-concept; the high self-acceptance/high self-esteem group evidenced higher stability of self-concept than those of all other groups.

Norms: Not cited. Psychometric data were reported for 131 athletes randomly selected (and stratified by sport) from a Division I state university.

**Availability: Contact Barbara Teetor Waite, P. O. Box 5072, Coralville, IA 52241-5072 (Phone # 319-354-4000; FAX # same; E-mail: sprtdoc@aol.com)

184 [Self-Confidence of Ability Questionnaire] [SCAQ]
Klaus Willimczik, S. Rethorst, and H. J. Riebel

Source: Willimczik, K., Rethorst, S., & Riebel, H. J. (1986). Cognitions and emotions in sports games--a cross-cultural comparative analysis. *International Journal of Physical Education, 23*(1), 10-16.

Purpose: To measure self-confidence in one's ability in sport.

Description: The SCAQ contains five items that include both volleyball-specific items and items relating to the sport-specific concept of ability. For example, "before the start of the game, I am confident of giving a good performance." Participants respond based on a scale of 0 (*not at all true*) to 6 (*completely true*).

Construction: Not discussed.

Reliability: Internal consistency coefficients of .66 (n=137 male and female German volleyball players) and .63 (n=150 male and female Indonesian volleyball players) were reported.

Validity: Not discussed.

Norms: Not cited. Psychometric data were based on the responses of 68 male German volleyball players, 69 female German volleyball players, 90 male Indonesian volleyball players, and 60 female Indonesian volleyball players to the SCAQ.

Availability: Contact Klaus Willimczik, Abteilung Sportwissenschaft, Universitat Bielefeld, Universitatsstr., D-4800 Bielefeld 1, Germany. (Phone # +521/106-5127)

185 Sport Competence Information Scale (SCIS)
Thelma S. Horn

Source: Horn, T. S., Glenn, S. D., & Wentzell, A. B. (1993). Sources of information underlying personal ability judgments in high school athletes. *Pediatric Exercise Science, 5,* 263-274.**

Purpose: To measure children's and adolescents' preferences for particular sources of competence information in a sport setting.

Description: The SCIS is a 39-item self-report inventory that represents 13 sources of competence information. These sources include Parental Feedback, Coach Feedback, Peer Feedback, Peer Comparison, Speed or Ease of Learning, Amount of Effort Exerted, Attraction Toward Sport, Game Performance Statistics, Game Outcome, Internal Information, Skill Improvement, Spectator Feedback, and Achievement of Self-Set Goals. The scale format consists of three scenarios, each of which describes competence judgments that athletes might make in regard to their performance in that sport context. The three competence scenarios correspond with three of the items constituting Harter's Perceived Competence Scale (Harter, 1982).

For each scenario, the competence judgment situation or context is briefly described. Then the individual respondent is asked to indicate, on a specified scale, how important each of the 13 sources of information is in helping her or him make that competence judgment. A 5-point Likert-type response format is used with verbal anchors ranging from *extremely important* to *not at all important.* As noted before, the SCIS contains three of the scenarios. Thus, the respondent rates the importance of each of the 13 sources of information in three different competence judgment contexts.

Although the current version of the SCIS is designed for use with athletes from a variety of sports (i.e., it is not specific to one sport), other researchers have modified the SCIS for use with athletes or individuals from a particular sport or physical activity (e.g., Ebbeck, 1990). Responses obtained via the use of the SCIS can be scored either by summing up the scores for the individual sources (n=13) or by conducting a factor analysis to determine the underlying structure of the instrument for each sample of subjects (see Horn & Amorose, in press).

Construction: The individual items composing the SCIS were identified and/or selected based on a series of steps. First, a content review of the theoretical and empirical literature on competence judgments was conducted. In addition, the Competence Information Scale, which was developed by Minton (1979) based on interviews with children in grades

---

**Note: This test summary was prepared by the author (T. Horn, personal communication, May 1, 1996).

four to six, was modified by Horn and Hasbrook (1986) to develop the original version of the SCIS. This version was subsequently administered to two samples of children (ages 8-12) and adolescents (ages 13 to 19). In both cases, study participants were asked to respond to sources of information contained in the early version of the SCIS but were also asked, via an open-ended question, to identify any additional information sources they might use in a competitive sport setting. Based on these pilot results, the initial version of the SCIS was revised. Subsequent use of the SCIS in a series of data collection projects (Horn et al., 1993; Phelps & Horn, 1992) has resulted in the continuous refinement of the scale in order to increase its readability and reliability.

Reliability: The internal consistency of the items composing each of the individual source subscales and/or identified factor subscales has been evaluated in several studies (e.g., Ebbeck, 1990; Horn & Weiss, 1991; Horn et al., 1993; Weiss, Ebbeck, & Horn, in press; Williams, 1990). Generally, obtained Cronbach alpha coefficients have been found to meet or exceed .70.

Validity: The content validity of the SCIS is based on an extensive review of the literature in the self-perceptions area of study. In addition, some evidence for the construct validity of selected subscales has been demonstrated through correlation of individuals' preferences for particular sources of information with certain of their psychological characteristics. Based on the theoretical and empirical literature on locus of control, for example, Horn and Hasbrook (1987) hypothesized that children who score high on the external perceptions of control subscales would be more apt to use external sources of information (e.g., game outcome, feedback from significant others) to evaluate or judge their sport competence, whereas children with higher scores on the internal locus of control subscale would be more apt to use internally-based competence information sources (e.g., self-comparison, achievement of self-set goals). Support was found for these hypotheses. Furthermore, consistent with developmental theory, these associations were strongest for the older children in the sample. In a follow-up study, Horn and Weiss (1991) found support for their hypothesis that children who differ in accuracy of personal competence judgments (i.e., as measured by the amount of discrepancy between actual and perceived estimates of sport competence) would also differ in the particular sources of information they choose to use to evaluate their competence. In a more recent study,

Weiss et al. (in press) again found support for an anticipated theoretical association between selected psychological characteristics (e.g., competitive trait anxiety, self-esteem, perceived competence) and children's preferences for particular competence information sources. Finally, Williams (1994) also provided some support for the construct validity of the SCIS in her study showing that high school athletes' scores on the Task and Ego Orientation in Sport Questionnaire (TEOSQ) were significantly related to the sources of information they use to judge their sport competence.

Norms: Not cited.

**Availability: Contact Thelma Horn, Department of PHS, Phillips Hall, Miami University, Oxford, OH 45056. (Phone # 513-529-2723; FAX # 513-529-5006; E-mail: tshorn@miamiu.acs.muohio.edu)

References

*Ebbeck, V. (1990). Sources of performance information in the exercise setting. *Journal of Sport & Exercise Psychology, 12*, 56-65.

Harter, S. (1982). The Perceived Competence Scale for Children. *Child Development, 53*, 87-97.

*Horn, T. S., & Amorose, A. (in press). Sources of competence information. In J. Duda (Ed.), *Advances in sport and exercise psychology measurement*. Morgantown, WV: Fitness Information Technology.

*Horn, T. S., Glenn, S. D., & Wentzell, A. B. (1993). Sources of information underlying personal ability judgments in high school athletes. *Pediatric Exercise Science, 5*, 263-274.

*Horn, T. S., & Harris, A. (1996). Perceived competence in young athletes: Research findings and recommendations for coaches and parents. In F. L. Smoll & R. E. Smith (Eds.), *Children and youth in sport: A biopsychosocial perspective* (pp. 309-329). Dubuque, IA: Brown & Benchmark.

*Horn, T. S., & Hasbrook, C. A. (1986). Information components influencing children's perceptions of their physical competence. In M. Weiss & D. Gould (Eds.), *Sport for children and youths: The 1984 Olympic Scientific Congress proceedings* (Vol. 10) (pp. 81-88). Champaign, IL: Human Kinetics Publishers.

*Horn, T. S., & Hasbrook, C. A. (1987). Psychological characteristics and the criteria children use for self-evaluation. *Journal of Sport Psychology, 9*, 208-221.

*Horn, T. S., & Weiss, M. R. (1991). A developmental analysis of children's self-ability judgments in the physical domain. *Pediatric Exercise Science, 3*, 310-326.

Minton, B. (1979). *Dimensions of information underlying children's judgments of their competence*. Paper presented at the Society for Research in Child Development, San Francisco, CA.

*Phelps, D., & Horn, T. S. (1992). [Sex and sport type as factors affecting college athletes' preferences for particular sources of competence information]. Unpublished data.

*Weiss, M. R., Ebbeck, V., & Horn, T. S. (in press). Children's self-perceptions and sources of physical competence information: A cluster analysis. *Journal of Sport & Exercise Psychology.*

*Williams, L. (1994). Goal orientations and athletes' preferences for competence information sources. *Journal of Sport & Exercise Psychology, 16,* 416-430.

186 State Sport-Confidence Inventory (SSCI)
Robin S. Vealey

Source: Vealey, R. S. (1986). Conceptualization of sport-confidence and competitive orientation: Preliminary investigation and instrument development. *Journal of Sport Psychology, 8,* 221-246.

Purpose: To assess the belief or degree of certainty individuals possess at one particular moment about their ability to be successful in sport.

Description: The SSCI contains 13 items measured using a 9-point Likert scale. Participants are asked to indicate how confident they feel *right now* about competing in an upcoming contest. When responding, participants are asked to compare their confidence to the most self-confident athlete they know.

Construction: An initial battery of 19 items was evaluated by four experts with extensive background in sport psychology to establish item clarity and face and content validity. Fifteen items were retained and placed in a 5-point Likert scale format. Factor analyses of high school (n=99) and college (n=101) students' responses to the SSCI confirmed the unidimensionality of scale items. However, the obtained correlation coefficient (r=.21) between participants' responses to the SSCI and the Crowne-Marlowe Social Desirability Scale indicated that the SSCI was somewhat contaminated by social desirability response bias.

The SSCI was subsequently modified including conversion of the items to a 9-point Likert scale format. Additional testing utilizing samples of high school (n=103) and college (n=96) varsity athletes led to the retention of 13 items that demonstrated adequate variability, internal consistency, item-total score correlation coefficients greater than .50, and acceptable item discrimination coefficients. There was no evidence of social desirability contamination.

Reliability: An alpha reliability coefficient of .95 was obtained (n=199 high school and college athletes). Test-retest reliability was not evaluated because the SSCI was conceptualized as a state measure.

Validity: Concurrent validity was evident by the positive correlation (.69) of the SSCI with the state self-confidence scale of the CSAI-2. Also, participants' ($n=199$ high school and college athletes) responses to the SSCI were inversely related to both their competitive A-trait scores on the SCAT and their responses to the cognitive and somatic state anxiety scales of the CSAI-2. Construct validity of the SSCI was evident by demonstrating that pre- and postcompetitive state sport-confidence was positively correlated to participants' ($n=48$ elite gymnasts) initial trait sport-confidence and competitive orientation scores. However, participants' precompetitive state sport-confidence scores were not correlated with their subsequent gymnastic performance scores.

Norms: Not available. Psychometric data were reported for 212 high school athletes ($n=141$ females; $n=71$ males) and 206 college athletes ($n=103$ females; $n=103$ males), and for 48 elite gymnasts.

**Availability: Contact Robin S. Vealey, Department of Physical Education, Health, and Sport Studies, Phillips Hall, Miami University, Oxford, OH 45056. (Phone # 513-529-2720; FAX # 513-529-5006; E-mail: rsvealey@miamiu.muohio.edu)

References

Daw, J., & Burton, D. (1994). Evaluation of a comprehensive psychological skills training program for collegiate tennis players. *The Sport Psychologist. 8,* 37-57.

Feltz, D. L., Corcoran, J. P., & Lirgg, C. D. (1989).Relationship among team confidence, sport confidence and hockey performance [Abstract]. *Psychology of motor behavior and sport* (p. 102). Kent, OH: Proceedings of the North American Society for the Psychology of Sport and Physical Activity annual convention.

Gayton, W. F., & Nickless, C. J. (1987). An investigation of the validity of the Trait and State Sport-Confidence inventories in predicting marathon performance. *Perceptual and Motor Skills, 65,* 481-482.

Grieve, F., Whelan, J. P., Kottke, R., & Meyers, A. W. (1992). The effects of goal orientation on mood, perceived competence, task difficulty and task persistence in a basketball contest [Abstract]. *Proceedings of the Association for the Advancement of Applied Sport Psychology annual convention.* (p. 37). Colorado Springs, CO.

*Martin, J. J., & Gill, D. L. (1991). The relationships among competitive orientation, sport-confidence, self-efficacy, anxiety, and performance. *Journal of Sport & Exercise Psychology, 13,* 149-159.

Pease, D., Kozub, S. A., & Burgress, B. (1993). Gender comparisons of self-efficacy cognitions while performing a motor task [Abstract]. *Proceedings of the Association for the Advancement of Applied Sport Psychology annual convention* (p. 109). Montreal, Canada.

*Vealey, R. S., & Campbell, J. L. (1988). Achievement goals of adolescent figure skaters: Impact on self-confidence, anxiety, and performance. *Journal of Adolescent Research, 3,* 227-243.

*Yang, G., & Pargman, D. (1993). An investigation of relationships among sport-confidence, self-efficacy, and competitive anxiety and their ability to predict performance on a karate skill test. *Proceedings of the Eighth World Congress of Sport Psychology* (pp. 968-972). Lisbon, Portugal.

*Yang, G., & Pargman, D. (1995). The investigation of relationships among self-confidence, self-efficacy, competitive anxiety, and sport performance [Abstract]. *Journal of Applied Sport Psychology, 7* (Suppl.), S126.

Swim Skills Efficacy Scale (SSES)
Patricia I. Hogan and James P. Santomier

Source: Hogan, P. I., & Santomier, J. P. (1984). Effect of mastering swimskills on older adults' self-efficacy. *Research Quarterly for Exercise and Sport, 55,* 294-296.

Purpose: To measure the conviction that one can successfully execute the aquatic behavior required to produce certain outcomes.

Description: The SSES presents 11 swim-skill related items in order of increasing difficulty. The SSES considers the level, confidence, and strength of efficacy expectations.

Construction: Modified from Bandura's efficacy scales.

Reliability: A test-retest reliability coefficient of .99 was obtained across a one-week interval among 15 elderly participants.

Validity: Not discussed.

Norms: Not cited.

Availability: Last known address: James P. Santomier, Program in Physical Education and Sport, New York University, 635 E. Building, New York, NY 10003. (Phone # 212-598-2386)

188 | *Tennis Self-Efficacy Scale [TSES]
C. Michael Greenwood, David D. Dzewaltowski, and Ron French

Source: Greenwood, C. M., Dzewaltowski, D. D., & French, R. (1990). Self efficacy and psychological well-being of wheelchair tennis participants and wheelchair nontennis participants. *Adapted Physical Activity Quarterly, 7,* 12-21.

Purpose: To assess "...subjects' self-efficacy expectations toward playing tennis" (p. 15).

Description: Participants' strength of self-efficacy toward completing 10 tennis tasks (e.g., returning a tennis serve, serving a tennis ball) is measured by having them indicate from 0 to 100, in increments of 10, their perceived confidence in completing each tennis task. Total scores range from 0 (no confidence) to 100 (high confidence).

Construction: Not discussed

Reliability: A Cronbach alpha internal reliability coefficient of .92 was reported (N=127).

Validity: Discriminant validity was supported in that wheelchair tennis participants (N=87) were more confident about their performance on the tennis court than were wheelchair tennis nonparticipants (N=40). Concurrent validity was supported in that a positive correlation coefficient of .73 was obtained when examining the relationship of wheelchair tennis participants' confidence in playing tennis and their confidence for general wheelchair mobility tasks.

Norms: Not cited. Psychometric data were reported for 87 participants (n=77 males, n=10 females; M age=32.60 years, SD=8.20) in the 1987 Southwest National Wheelchair Tennis Championships and 40 wheelchair mobile individuals (n=32 males, n=8 females; M age=35.40 years, SD=10.54).

Availability: Contact David A. Dzewaltowski, Department of Kinesiology, 8 Natatorium, Kansas State University, Manhattan, KS

66506-0302. (Phone # 913-532-0708; FAX # 913-532-6486; E-mail: dadx@ksu.ksu.edu)

189 Trait Sport-Confidence Inventory (TSCI)
Robin S. Vealey

Source: Vealey, R. S. (1986). Conceptualization of sport-confidence and competitive orientation: Preliminary investigation and instrument development. *Journal of Sport Psychology, 8*, 221-246.

Purpose: To assess individual differences in the belief or degree of certainty individuals usually possess about their ability to be successful in sport.

Description: The TSCI contains 13 items that were placed in inventory format using a 9-point Likert scale. Participants are asked to indicate how confident they *generally feel* when competing in sport. When responding, participants are asked to compare their confidence to the most confident athlete they know. For example, participants are asked to "compare your confidence in YOUR ABILITY TO ACHIEVE YOUR COMPETITIVE GOALS to the most confident athlete you know."

Construction: An initial battery of 20 items were evaluated by four experts to establish item clarity and face and content validity. Sixteen items were retained and placed in a 5-point Likert scale format. Factor analyses of high school ($n=99$) and college ($n=101$) students' responses to the TSCI confirmed the unidimensionality of scale items. However, the obtained correlation coefficient ($r=.23$) between participants' responses to the TSCI and the Crowne-Marlowe Social Desirability Scale indicated that the TSCI was somewhat contaminated by social desirability response bias.

The TSCI was subsequently modified including conversion of the items to a 9-point Likert scale format. Additional testing utilizing samples of high school ($n=103$) and college ($n=96$) varsity athletes led to the retention of 13 items that demonstrated adequate variability, internal consistency ($r=.93$), item-total score correlation coefficients greater than .50, and acceptable item discrimination coefficients. There was no evidence of social desirability contamination.

Reliability: Alpha reliability was reported as .93. Test-retest reliability coefficients among a sample of high school (n=109) and college (n=110) athletes were .86 (1-day interval), .89 (1-week interval), and .83 (1-month interval).

Validity: Concurrent validity coefficients are reported with the Sport Competition Anxiety Test, the Physical Self-Efficacy Scale, Rotter's Internal-External Control Scale, and Rosenberg's Self-Esteem Scale utilizing high and college athletes (n=199). Construct validity was established by demonstrating among elite gymnasts (n=48) that the TSCI was a significant predictor of pre- and postcompetitive state sport-confidence and several subjective outcomes of performance.

Norms: Not available. Psychometric data were reported for 212 high school athletes (n= 141 females; n=71 males) and 206 college athletes (n=103 females; n=103 males) and for 48 elite gymnasts.

**Availability: Contact Robin S. Vealey, Department of Physical Education, Health, and Sport Studies, Phillips Hall, Miami University, Oxford, OH 45056. (Phone # 513-529-2720; FAX # 513-529-5006; E-mail: rsvealey@miamiu.muohio.edu)

References

Acevedo, E. O., Dzewaltowski, D. A., Gill, D. L., & Noble, J. M. (1992). Cognitive orientations of ultramarathoners. *The Sport Psychologist,6,* 242-252.

Bull, S. J. (1991). Personal and situational influences on adherence to mental skills training. *Journal of Sport & Exercise Psychology, 13,* 121-132.

Daw, J., & Burton, D. (1994). Evaluation of a comprehensive psychological skills training program for collegiate tennis players. *The Sport Psychologist, 8,* 37-57.

Deeter, T. E. (1989). Development of a model of achievement behavior for physical activity. *Journal of Sport & Exercise Psychology, 11,* 13-25.

Deeter, T. E. (1990). Re-modeling expectancy and value in physical activity. *Journal of Sport & Exercise Psychology, 12,* 86-91.

Dexter, E. K., & Duda, J. L. (1989). Predictors of competitive stress among female dancers [Abstract]. *Psychology of motor behavior and sport* (p.117). Kent, OH: Proceedings of the North American Society for the Psychology of Sport and Physical Activity annual convention.

Frost, R. O., & Henderson, K. J. (1991). Perfectionism and reactions to athletic competition. *Journal of Sport & Exercise Pychology, 13,* 323-335.

*Gayton, W. F., & Nickless, C. J. (1987). An investigation of the validity of the Trait and State Sport-Confidence inventories in predicting marathon performance. *Perceptual and Motor Skills, 65,* 481-482.

*Kakkos, V., & Zervas, Y. (1993). Competitive worries and self confidence as predictors of the precompetitive cognitive-emotional state. *Proceedings of the Eighth World*

Congress of Sport Psychology (pp. 855-859). Lisbon, Portugal.

*Martin, J. J., & Gill, D. L. (1991). The relationships among competitive orientation, sport-confidence, self-efficacy, anxiety, and performance. *Journal of Sport & Exercise Psychology, 13,* 149-159.

*Mills, B. D. (1995). Examining the relationship between trait sport confidence, goal orientation and competitive experience in female collegiate volleyball players [Abstract]. *Journal of Sport & Exercise Psychology, 17* (Suppl.), S81.

Prapavessis, H., & Grove, J. R. (1994). Personality variables as antecedents of precompetitive mood state temporal patterning. *International Journal of Sport Psychology, 25,* 347-365.

*Thompson, L. P., & Hoo, S. (1995). Relationships between coach expectations and observed feedback, athlete perceptions of feedback, and sport-confidence: A case study [Abstract]. *Research Quarterly for Exercise and Sport, 66* (Suppl.), A-77-78.

*Vealey, R. S. (1988). Sport-confidence and competitive orientation: An addendum on scoring procedures and gender differences. *Journal of Sport & Exercise Psychology, 10,* 471-478.

*Vealey, R. S., & Campbell, J. L. (1988). Achievement goals of adolescent figure skaters: Impact on self-confidence, anxiety, and performance. *Journal of Adolescent Research, 3,* 227-243.

*Yang, G., & Pargman, D. (1993). An investigation of relationships among sport-confidence, self-efficacy, and competitive anxiety and their ability to predict performance on a karate skill test. *Proceedings of the Eighth World Congress of Sport Psychology* (pp. 968-972). Lisbon, Portugal.

190 *Trampoline Routine Questionnaire [TRQ]
Jean Whitehead

Source: Whitehead, J. (1978). The construction of a questionnaire on confidence in trampolining. *British Journal of Physical Education, 9* (5), 136-137.

Purpose: To assess children's confidence for performing a set trampoline routine, where confidence was defined as "... an assured expectation of satisfactory performance" (p. 136).

Description: The TRQ contains 24 items. Ten items form a Practical subscale (e.g., "This routine is too complicated for me to attempt"). Ten items form an Emotional subscale (e.g., "I feel sick at the thought of trying this routine"). Four "blind" items are also included to disguise the focus of the test and to detect response inconsistencies. Children respond to each item using a 5-point Likert scale.

Construction: Statements were obtained from questions to children (N=51) regarding their thoughts when trampolining and from the feelings of the Cheshire Schools trampoline team before and after important competitions. A total of 110 items were retained for further scaling and were evaluated by 20 judges using the Thurstone scaling technique. Items with equivalent scores were retained for the Practical and Emotional subscales.

Reliability: A corrected split-half reliability coefficient of .91 was reported (N=50).

Validity: Teachers' anxiety ratings and children's trampoline performance expectations correlated -.53 and .47, respectively, with their scores on the TRQ.

Norms: Not cited. Psychometric data were reported for a random sample of 50 children, ages 11-12 years old, in their second year of secondary school.

**Availability: Contact Jean Whitehead, Chelsea School Research Centre, University of Brighton, Gaudick Road, Eastbourne, East Sussex, England BN20 7SP. (Phone # 01273-600900; FAX # 01273-643704; E-mail: jw73@bton.ac.uk)

Chapter 13

Imagery

Tests in this chapter assess individual differences in visual imagery of movement, the imagery of kinesthetic sensations, and in imagery utilization.

Chapter 13. Imagery 305

191 Imagery Use Questionnaire (IUQ)
Craig R. Hall, Kathryn A. Barr, and Wendy M. Rodgers

Source: Hall, C. R., Rodgers, W. M., & Barr, K. A. (1990). The use of imagery by athletes in selected sports. *The Sport Psychologist, 4,* 1-10.

Purpose: To examine factors related to imagery utilization in sport.

Description: The IUQ contains 37 items. For example, participants are asked to indicate the extent to which they use imagery before or during practice, or before or during a sport event. Participants respond to each item using a 7-point Likert scale except for two items that require yes/no responses. The scale anchor points are 1 (*never or very difficult*) to 7 (*always or very easy*).

Construction: Items on the IUQ were developed from a review of literature pertaining to imagery in sport and from consulting experts in the fields of motor learning, sports psychology, and questionnaire development techniques (Hall & Barr, 1989).

Reliability: The authors reported that the average test-retest reliability coefficient across all items on a rowing version of the IUQ was .71.

Validity: The IUQ successfully discriminated between novice and elite rowers. Novices indicated seeing themselves rowing incorrectly more often. Elite rowers reported more frequently using kinesthetic imagery. They also had more structure and regularity to their imagery sessions (Hall & Barr, 1989).

Norms: Not cited. Psychometric data were based on the responses to the IUQ of 348 rowers at high school, college, and national team levels (Hall & Barr, 1989).

Availability: Contact Craig Hall, Faculty of Kinesiology, University of Western Ontario, London, Ontario, Canada N6A 3K7. (Phone # 519-679-2111, ext. 8388; FAX # 519-661-2008; E-mail:chall@uwovax. uwo.ca)

References

*Barr, K., & Hall, C. (1992). The use of imagery by rowers. *International Journal of Sport Psychology, 23,* 243-261.

*Erskine, J. W., Maddox, K., & Ashford, B. (1994). The use of imagery by British track and field athletes [Abstract]. *Journal of Sports Sciences, 12,* 191.

Hall, C., & Barr, K. (1989). Imagery use among rowers [Abstract]. *Proceedings of the 20th annual conference of the Canadian Society for Psychomotor Learning and Sport Psychology* (p. 45). Victoria, British Columbia, Canada.

Overby, L. Y. (1993). Imagery use by dancers [Abstract]. *Proceedings of the Association for the Advancement of Applied Sport Psychology annual convention* (p. 13a). Montreal, Canada.

*Rogers, W., Hall, C., & Buckolz, E. (1991). The effects of an imagery training program on imagery ability, imagery use, and figure skating performance. *Journal of Applied Sport Psychology, 3,* 109-125.

 # *Imagery Use Questionnaire for Soccer Players (IUQ-SP)

Jill Salmon, Craig Hall, and Ian Haslam

Source: Salmon, J., Hall, C., & Haslam, I (1994). The use of imagery by soccer players. *Journal of Applied Sport Psychology, 6,* 116-133.

Purpose: To examine the cognitive and motivational use of imagery by soccer players of various skill levels.

Description: The IUQ-SP contains several sections. In addition to assessing demographic information, one section contains questions pertaining to the general use of imagery by soccer players during practice and competition. Another section examines the motivational and cognitive use of imagery by soccer players, based on the theoretical framework proposed by Paivio (1985). A final section contains items concerning soccer players' use of auditory imagery (i.e., talking during a game). Participants respond to each item on a 7-point Likert scale with the anchorings 1 (*never*) to 7 (*always*).

Construction: Items regarding the general use of imagery were extracted from the original Imagery Use Questionnaire (Hall, Rodgers, & Barr, 1990). To develop the remaining sections, an initial draft of the IUQ-SP was reviewed by experts in sport psychology, psychology, coaching, and imagery use. Items were modified or deleted based on the input of these experts.

Reliability: Test-retest reliability coefficients (n=20) across a 2- to 3-week interval ranged from .55 to .92. Internal consistency coefficients pertaining to the cognitive and motivational use of imagery by soccer players ranged from .75 (Cognitive General) to .85 (Cognitive Specific).

Validity: A principal components factor analysis (varimax rotation) supported the 4-cell theoretical framework proposed by Paivio (i.e., Cognitive General, Cognitive Specific, Motivation Specific, and Motivation General) regarding the use of imagery, although the distinction between Cognitive General and Cognitive Specific domains was less well-defined.

It was also found that national and provincial players had significantly higher scores than did local players on the Cognitive Specific and Motivational General domains of imagery use. Further, provincial soccer players scored higher than local soccer players on the auditory use of imagery. National and provincial soccer players were then combined as a group (and labeled elite soccer players) and compared to local soccer players on the IUQ-SP via stepwise discriminant function analysis. It was found that elite soccer players reported using both internal and external imagery more frequently than did local (nonelite) soccer players.

Norms: Not cited. Psychometric data were based on the responses of 90 national, 112 provincial, and 161 local soccer players in Canada. The players (n=126 males; n=74 females) in the first two groups ranged in age from 15 to 30 years. There were 75 males and 86 females representing the local soccer group.

Availability: Contact Craig R. Hall, Faculty of Kinesiology, University of Western Ontario, London, Ontario, Canada N6A 3K7. (Phone 519-679-2111; ext. 8388; FAX # 519-661-2008; E-mail: chall@uwovax. uwo.ca)

References

Hall, C., Rodgers, W., & Barr, K. (1990). The use of imagery by athletes in selected sports. *The Sport Psychologist, 4,* 1-10.

Paivio, A. (1985). Cognitive and motivational functions of imagery use in human performance. *Canadian Journal of Applied Sport Sciences, 10,* 228-285.

 [Mental Imagery Tests] [MIT]
Dorothy L. Moody

Source: Moody, D. L. (1967). Imagery differences among women of varying levels of experience, interests, and abilities in motor skills. *Research Quarterly, 38*, 441-448.

Purpose: To examine individual differences in motor-skill imagery.

Description: Individuals are presented three filmed subtests, involving observations of objects and/or persons in movement. Imagery subtest I involves recognition of four geometric forms in which participants respond to 10 test items. Imagery subtest II requires requires participants to watch a brief movie of a motor act (such as a golf swing) and then identify that act when it is presented as one of four similar motor acts a few seconds later. Imagery subtest III requires participants to watch a brief movie of a motor act and then read and answer a series of five questions on that act. There are 10 test films.

Construction: Not indicated.

Reliability: A corrected split-half odd-even internal consistency coefficient of .87 was obtained (composite score) among 77 college women.

Validity: The three subtests were *not* successful in discriminating between college physical education majors and nonmajors.

Norms: Not reported.

Availability: Unknown.

194 Movement Imagery Questionnaire (MIQ)
Craig Hall and John Pongrac

Source: Hall, C., Pongrac, J., & Buckholz, E. (1985). The measurement of imagery ability. *Human Movement Science, 4*, 107-118.

Purpose: To assess individual differences in visual and kinesthetic imagery of movements.

Description: The MIQ contains 18 items, 9 for the Visual subscale and 9 for the Kinesthetic subscale. Participants are asked to use visual or kinesthetic imagery while performing a variety of arm movements, leg movements, and movements involving the entire body. They are asked to rate how difficult it is to use visual or kinesthetic imagery while performing each movement task. Participants respond to each subscale using a 7-point rating scale. Total scores range from 9 (high score on imagery) to 63.

Construction: An initial pool of 28 items was administered to 74 physical education students. Item analyses led to the retention of 18 items.

Reliability: Cronbach alpha internal consistency coefficients of .87 (Visual subscale) and .91 (Kinesthetic subscale) were reported based on the responses of another sample of 80 physical education students. A test-retest reliability coefficient of .83 was reported among 32 of these students (no time interval specified).

Validity: Not discussed.

Norms: Not cited. Psychometric data are based on the responses of independent samples of 74 and 80 physical education students.

Availability: Contact Craig Hall, Faculty of Kinesiology, University of Western Ontario, London, Ontario, Canada N6A 3K7. (Phone # 519-679-2111, ext. 8388; FAX # 519-661-2008; E-mail: chall@uwovax. uwo.ca)

References

*Atienza, F., Balaguer, I., & Garcia-Merita, M. L. (1994). Factor analysis and reliability of the Movement Imagery Questionnaire. *Perceptual and Motor Skills, 78,* 1323-1328.

*Goss, S., Hall, C., Buckholz, E., & Fishburne, G. (1986). Imagery ability and the acquisition and retention of movements. *Memory and Cognition, 14,* 469-477.

Grovios, G. (1992). On the reduction of reaction time with mental practice. *Journal of Sport Behavior, 15,* 141-157.

*Hall, C., Buckolz, E., & Fishburne, G. (1989). Searching for a relationship between imagery ability and memory of movements. *Journal of Human Movement Studies, 17,* 89-100.

Hardy, L., & Parfitt, G. (1994). The development of a model for the provision of psychological support to a national squad. *The Sport Psychologist, 8,* 126-142.

Jowdy, D. P., & Harris, D. V. (1990). Muscular responses during mental imagery as a function of motor skill level. *Journal of Sport & Exercise Psychology, 12,* 191-201.

*Margolies, M. D., Griffey, D. C., & Fahleson, G. A. (1986).Imagery orientation and meta cognitions of athletes during skill acquisition and performance [Abstract]. *Proceedings of the annual conference of the Association for the Advancement for Applied Sport Psychology* (p.47). Jekyll Island, GA.

Martin, K. A., & Hall, C. R. (1995). Using mental imagery to enhance intrinsic motivation. *Journal of Sport & Exercise Psychology, 17,* 54-69.

*Mumford, B., & Hall, C. (1985). The effects of internal and external imagery on performing figures in figure skating. *Canadian Journal of Applied Sport Sciences, 10,* 171-177.

*O'Halloran, A-M, & Gauvin, L. (1994). The role of preferred cognitive style in the effectiveness of imagery training. International *Journal of Sport Psychology, 25,* 19-31.

*Pargman, D., Juaire, S., & Gill, K. (1987). Comparison of imagery induced arousal effects on performance of a visually distorted, novel ball tossing task in female collegiate athletes of high and low imaging abilities [Abstract].*Research Abstracts* (p. 210). Reston, VA: Proceedings of the American Alliance for Health, Physical Education, Recreation, and Dance annual convention, Las Vegas, NV.

*Rodgers, W., Hall, C., & Buckolz, E. (1991). The effects of an imagery training program on imagery ability, imagery use, and figure skating performance. *Journal of Applied Sport Psychology, 3,* 109-125.

Vividness of Movement Imagery Questionnaire (VMIQ)

Anne Isaac and David F. Marks

Source: Issac, A., Marks, D. F., & Russell, D. G. (1986). An instrument for assessing imagery of movement: The Vividness of Movement Imagery Questionnaire (VMIQ). *Journal of Mental Imagery, 10*(4), 23-30.

Purpose: To assess individual differences in the visual imagery of movement and the imagery of kinesthetic sensations.

Description: The VMIQ contains 24 items. Participants are asked to rate the vividness of imagery for an item obtained watching somebody else and doing it themselves. Items cover basic body movements to movements requiring precision and control in upright, unbalanced, aerial situations. Examples of items include "kicking a ball in the air" and "riding a bike." Participants respond to each item using a 5-point ordinal scale with the anchorings *perfectly clear and as vivid as normal vision* to *no image at all.*

Construction: Not indicated.

Reliability*: A test-retest reliability coefficient of .76 was reported over a 3-week interval among 220 high school and college undergraduate students.

Validity*: Convergent validity was supported in that participants' (*n*=220) responses to the VMIQ and Marks' Vividness of Visual Imagery Questionnaire were correlated. Furthermore, correlation coefficients ranging from .45 to .75 were reported when comparing the responses of independent samples (*n*=25; *n*=25; *n*=16) of trampolinists on the VMIQ with Marks' imagery questionnaire.

Norms*: Not cited. Psychometric data are presented for 170 undergraduate physical education students, 50 high school students, and 56 trampolinists residing in New Zealand.

**Availability: Contact Anne Isaac, School of Aviation, Massey University, Private Bag 11-222, Palmerston North, New Zealand. (Phone # 64 6 3503227; FAX # 64 6 3503200; E-mail: a.isaac@massey.ac.nz)

References

*Campos, A., & Perez, M. J. (1988). Vividness of Movement Imagery Questionnaire: Relations with other measures of mental imagery. *Perceptual and Motor Skills, 67,* 607-610.

*Campos, A. C., & Perez, M. J. (1990). A factor analytic study of two measures of mental imagery. *Perceptual and Motor Skills, 71,* 995-1001.

Eves, F., Barber, A., Hall, L., & Davies, N. (1994). Ability with visual images in swimmers, canoeists, and trampolinists [Abstract]. *Journal of Sports Sciences, 12,* 190.

*Gordon, S., Weinberg, R., & Jackson, A. (1994). Effect of internal and external imagery on cricket performance. *Journal of Sport Behavior, 17,* 60-75.

Hardy, L., & Parfitt, G. (1994). The development of a model for the provision of psychological support to a national squad. *The Sport Psychologist, 8,* 126-142.

Isaac, A. R. (1992). Mental practice. Does it work in the field? *The Sport Psychologist, 6,* 192-198.

*Isaac, A. R., & Marks, D. F. (1994). Individual differences in imagery experience: Developmental changes and specialization. *British Journal of Psychology, 85,* 479-500.

*Tham, E. K., & Richardson, P. A. (1995). Effects of music on vividness of movement imagery [Abstract]. *Journal of Applied Sport Psychology, 7* (Suppl.), S115.

---

*Additional data on reliability and validity, and normative data for 1,202 individuals are presented in the unpublished doctoral dissertation of the first author (A. Isaac, personal communication, March 13, 1990).

White, A., & Hardy, L. (1994). The effects of using different imagery perspectives on the learning and performance of two different motor tasks [Abstract]. *Journal of Sports Sciences, 12,* 214-215.

Williams, L. R. T., & Issac, A. R. (1991). Skill differences associated with movement performance. II. Imagery and kinaesthesis. *Journal of Human Movement Studies, 21,* 129-136

Chapter 14

Leadership

Tests in this chapter assess the perceptions/preferences of athletes for specific leader behaviors from the coach, coach's perceptions of his or her own leader behavior, and satisfaction with various aspects of leadership in sport. Tests also assess the leadership tendencies of soccer players and the leadership qualities of athletic administrators.

196   *Leadership Quality Scale (LQS)
James J. Zhang and Dale G. Pease

Source: Zhang, J. J., & Pease, D. G. (1995). Leadership qualities of athletic administrators: Development of a scale [Abstract]. *Research Quarterly for Exercise and Sport, 66* (Suppl.), A-50.

Purpose: To assess the leadership qualities of intercollegiate athletic administrators.

Description: The LSQ contains 25 items and two subscales: (a) current leadership perceptions of intercollegiate athletic administrators and (b) future leadership preferences for intercollegiate athletic administrators. Participants respond to each item using a 9-point Likert scale.

Construction: A panel of experts (*N*=20) participated in a modified Delphi study that elicited 45 items pertinent to the leadership qualities of intercollegiate athletic administrators. A total of 28 items were retained and evaluated for content validity by this same panel of experts.

Reliability: Cronbach alpha internal consistency coefficients ranged from .59 to .85.

Validity: Exploratory factor analysis (varimax rotation) among 60 participants resulted in four factors: (a) Management Skills (10 items); (b) Personal Integrity (6 items), (c) Creative Ability (5 items), and (d) Social Skills (4 items).

Norms: Not cited. Psychometric data were reported for 10 intercollegiate athletic directors, 10 college physical education professors, 10 intercollegiate administration staff, 10 intercollegiate athletic coaches, and 20 athletic administration or sport management majors.

**Availability: Contact James J. Zhang, Dept. of Health and Human Performance, University of Houston, Houston, TX 77204-5331. (Phone # 713-743-9869; FAX # 713-743-9860; E-mail: educ1b@jetson.uh.edu)

197 Leadership Scale for Sports (LSS)
Packianathan Chelladurai and S. D. Saleh

Source: Chelladurai, P., & Saleh, S. D. (1980). Dimensions of leader behavior in sports: Development of a leadership scale. *Journal of Sport Psychology, 2,* 34-45.

Purpose: The LSS can be used to examine (a) the preferences of athletes for specific leader behavior from the coach, (b) the perceptions of athletes regarding the actual leader behavior of their coach, and (c) the coach's perceptions of his or her own leader behavior.

Description: The LSS is a 40-item questionnaire containing five factors: Training and Instruction, Democratic Behavior, Autocratic Behavior, Social Support, and Positive Feedback. Athletes respond to each item using a 5-point Likert scale. Versions include athletes' preferred leadership and the athletes' perceived leadership.

Construction: A total of 99 items were chosen and modified from existing leadership scales. Factor analysis of the responses of 80 male and 80 female physical education majors led to the retention of 37 items representing five defined factors. In the second stage of development, seven items were added to tap the instruction behavior of a coach; also, six more social support items were added. The revised questionnaire (containing 50 items) was then administered to 102 physical education students and a male sample of 223 college varsity athletes representing four sports at different Canadian universities. Factor analyses of participants' responses led to the retention of five factors as previously noted.

Reliability: Alpha reliability coefficients ranged from .66 (Autocratic Behavior) to .79 (Positive Feedback) among 102 physical education majors. Alpha reliability coefficients were also reported for the 223 athletes who were queried regarding both their preferred and perceived leader behaviors. These coefficients ranged from .45 (Autocratic Behavior) to .83 (Training and Instruction) for the preferred version, and from .79 (Autocratic Behavior) to .93 (Training and Instruction) for the perceived version. Test-retest reliability coefficients among 53 of the physical education majors across a 4-week interval ranged from .71 (Social Support) to .82 (Democratic Behavior).

Validity: Construct validity was supported by demonstrating through factor analyses the emergence of five identical factors (noted above) across both the physical education majors ($n=102$) and the varsity athletes ($n=223$). On the average, these five factors accounted for 45.43% of the variance in participants' responses to the items of the questionnaire.

Norms: Not cited. Descriptive data were reported for 45 male and 57 female physical education majors and 223 varsity athletes representing basketball, track and field, rowing, and wrestling from different Canadian universities. [Also, see Chelladurai, P. (1989), *Manual for the Leadership Scale for Sports,* which is available from the author.]

**Availability: Contact Packianathan Chelladurai, School of HPER, The Ohio State University, 453 Larkins Hall, 337 West 17th Avenue, Columbus, OH 43210-1284. (Phone # 614-292-0816; FAX # 614-688-3432; E-mail: chelladurai.1@osu.edu)

References

*Chelladurai, P. (1990). Leadership in sports: A review. *International Journal of Sport Psychology, 21,* 328-354

*Chelladurai, P., Imamura, H., Yamaguchi, Y., Oinuma, Y., & Miyauchi, T. (1988). Sport leadership in a cross-national setting: The case of Japanese and Canadian university athletes. *Journal of Sport & Exercise Psychology, 10,* 374-389.

*Crespo, M., Balaguer, I., & Atienza, F. (1993). Variables influencing leadership styles in tennis coaches. *Proceedings of the Eighth World Congress of Sport Psychology* (pp. 205-208). Lisbon, Portugal.

*Dwyer, J. J. M., & Fischer, D. G. (1988). Psychometric properties of the coach's version of Leadership Scale for Sports. *Perceptual and Motor Skills, 67,* 795-798.

Dwyer, J. J. M., & Fischer, D. G. (1990). Wrestlers' perceptions of coaches' leadership as predictors of satisfaction with leadership. *Perceptual and Motor Skills, 71,* 511-517.

*Eichas, T. M., & Krane, V. (1993). Relationships among perceived leadership styles, member satisfaction, and team cohesion in high school basketball players [Abstract]. *Research Quarterly for Exercise and Sport, 64* (Suppl.), A-101-102.

*Garland, D. J., & Barry, J. R. (1990). Personality and leader behaviors in collegiate football: A multidimensional approach to performance. *Journal of Research in Personality, 24,* 355-370.

*Hastie, P. A. (1993). Coaching preferences of high school girl volleyball players. *Perceptual and Motor Skills, 77,* 1309-1310.

Isberg, L. (1993). What does it mean to be an elite coach in team sport? *Proceedings of the Eighth World Congress of Sport Psychology* (pp. 233-239). Lisbon, Portugal.

*Kozub, S. A. (1994). The relationship between coaching behavior and player leadership [Abstract]. *Research Quarterly for Exercise and Sport, 65* (Suppl.), A-88.

*Kozub, S. A. (1995). Investigating the determinants of team cohesion [Abstract]. *Journal of Applied Sport Psychology, 7* (Suppl.), S82.

*Laughlin, N., & Laughlin, S. (1994). The relationship between similarity in perceptions and teacher/coach leader behavior and evaluations of their effectiveness. *International Journal of Sport Psychology, 25*, 396-410.

*Pease, D. G., & Kozub, S. A. (1994). Perceived coaching behaviors and team cohesion in high school girls basketball teams [Abstract]. *Journal of Sport & Exercise Psychology, 16* (Suppl.), S93.

*Pease, D. G., & Kozub, S. A. (1994). Role of goal orientations in athlete leadership behavior [Abstract]. *Research Quarterly for Exercise and Sport, 65* (Suppl.), A-90.

*Riemer, H. A., & Chelladurai, P. (1995). Leadership and satisfaction in athletics. *Journal of Sport & Exercise Psychology, 17*, 276-293.

*Salminen, S., & Liukkonen, J. (1993). Coach-athlete relationship and coach's behavior in training sessions. *Proceedings of the Eighth World Congress of Sport Psychology* (pp. 886-889). Lisbon, Portugal.

*Salminen, S., & Liukkonen, J. (1994). The convergent and discriminant validity of the coach's version of the Leadership Scale for Sports. *International Journal of Sport Psychology, 25*, 119-127.

*Serpa, S., Pataco, V., & Santos, F. (1991). Leadership patterns in handball international competition. *International Journal of Sport Psychology, 22*, 78-89.

*Shields, D. L. L., Bredemeier, B. J. L., Gardner, D. E., & Bostrom, A. (1995). Leadership, cohesion, and team norms regarding cheating and aggression. *Sociology of Sport Journal, 12*, 324-336.

*Spink, K. S. (1995). Cohesion and leadership behaviors as predictors of athlete satisfaction [Abstract]. *Journal of Applied Sport Psychology, 7* (Suppl.), S111.

*Spink, K. S. (1995). Examining the effects of cohesion and leadership on the intention to participate of female sport team athletes [Abstract]. *Journal of Sport & Exercise Psychology, 17* (Suppl.), S98.

Summers, R. J. (1983). A study of leadership in a sport setting [Abstract]. *In Psychology of motor behavior and sport-1983* (p.130). Proceedings of the North American Society for the Psychology of Sport and Physical Activity annual convention, East Lansing, MI.

Terry, P. (1984). The coaching preference of elite athletes [Abstract]. *In Proceedings of the 1984 Olympic Scientific Congress* (p. 87). Eugene, OR: College of Human Development and Performance Microform Publications.

*Twardochleb, T., & Spink, K. S (1995). Actual and perceived leadership behaviors as predictors of cohesion in exercise classes [Abstract]. *Journal of Applied Sport Psychology, 7* (Suppl.), S118.

*van Rossum, J. H. A. (1995). Talent in sport: Significant others in the career of top-level Dutch athletes. In M. W. Katzko & F. J. Monks (Eds.), *Nurturing talent: Individual needs and social ability* (pp. 43-57). The Netherlands: Van Forcum. Assen.

*Vealey, R. S., Chabot, H. F., Walter, S. M., & Strait. L. (1993). Personal investment in coaching: Antecedents of coaching ideology behavior, and satisfaction [Abstract]. *Proceedings of the Association for the Advancement of Applied Sport Psychology annual convention* (p. 152). Montreal, Canada.

*Westre, K. R., & Weiss, M. R. (1991). The relationship between perceived coaching behaviors and group cohesion in high school football teams. *The Sport Psychologist, 5*, 41-54.

*Zhang, J., Jensen, B. E., & Mann, B. L. (1994). Modification and revision of the Leadership Scale for Sport [Abstract]. *Research Quarterly for Exercise and Sport, 65* (Suppl.), A-59-60.

198 [Scale of Athlete Satisfaction] [SAS]
Packianathan Chelladurai, Hiroaki Imamura,
Yasuo Yamaguchi, Yoshihiro Oinuma, and
Takatomo Miyauchi

Source: Chelladurai, P., Imamura, H., Yamaguchi, Y., Oinuma, Y., & Miyauchi, T. (1988). Sport leadership in a cross-national setting: The case of Japanese and Canadian university athletes. *Journal of Sport & Exercise Psychology, 10,* 374-389.

Purpose: To assess satisfaction with various aspects of leadership in athletics and the outcomes of athletic participation that can be associated with leadership.

Description: The Scale of Athlete Satisfaction contains 10 items related to leadership in athletics. The respondent is asked to indicate his or her satisfaction with the content of each item using a 7-point Likert scale.

Construction: Items were selected to represent various elements of leadership in athletics. Translations of scale items were made into the Japanese language. Factor analyses of the responses of Canadian (n=100) and Japanese (n=115) male university athletes to the scale revealed two common factors labeled Leadership (64.9% accountable variance) and Personal Outcome (14.1% accountable variance).

Reliability: Alpha reliability coefficients of the Leadership and Personal Outcome factors were .95 and .86, respectively.

Validity: Not discussed.

Norms: Not cited. Descriptive data were reported for 115 Japanese and 100 Canadian male university athletes.

**Availability: Contact Packianathan Chelladurai, School of HPER, The Ohio State University, 453 Larkins Hall, 337 West 17th Ave., Columbus, OH 43210-1284. (Phone # 614-292-0816; FAX # 614-688-3432; E-mail: chelladurai.1@osu.edu)

199 | *Sport Leadership Behavior Inventory (SLBI)
Susan D. Glenn and Thelma S. Horn

Source: Glenn, S. D., & Horn, T. S. (1993). Psychological and personal predictors of leadership behavior in female soccer athletes. *Journal of Applied Sport Psychology, 5,* 17-34.

Purpose: To measure leadership tendencies in soccer athletes.

Description: The SLBI contains 25 items, of which 19 items describe psychological characteristics or behaviors deemed desirable for team leaders in soccer, whereas 6 items are filler items. Participants respond to each item on a 7-point Likert scale in terms of how descriptive the item is of the individual being evaluated. A single measure is derived based on the total score of the 19 items.

Construction: The development of the SLBI began with the selection of a set of 104 words derived from the literature on leadership behavior. These words depicted personal characteristics of leadership. Three sport studies experts were asked to rate each word for appropriateness, comprehension, and descriptiveness. Forty-six words were retained.

Two samples of high school female athletes (*N*=86) and one sample of interscholastic coaches (*N*=30) were asked to evaluate each word in terms of how desirable it would be for a team leader to possess that characteristic. A total of 19 words were included as part of the final version of the SLBI.

Reliability: A Cronbach alpha internal consistency coefficient of .85 and a test-retest reliability coefficient of .74 (across a 14-day interval) were reported. Also, a Cronbach alpha coefficient of .91 was reported when 106 female soccer players self-rated their leadership characteristics using the SLBI.

Validity: Concurrent validity was supported by the low but statistically significant relationships of athletes' (*N*=106) self-ratings on the SLBI and (a) coaches' ratings of their leadership behavior (*r*=.27) and (b) peer ratings of their leadership behavior (*r*=.36).

Norms: Not cited. Psychometric data were reported for 106 female soccer athletes representing seven midwestern interscholastic varsity teams.

Availability: Contact Susan D. Glenn, Department of Exercise and Movement Science, University of Oregon, Eugene, OR 97403-1240. (E-mail: sdglenn@oregon.uoregon.edu)

Chapter 15

Life Adjustment

Tests in this chapter assess life events and stressors, such as injury, that are experienced by athletes and that necessitate adjustment.

Chapter 15. Life Adjustment 325

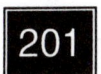
200 [Athletic Adjustment Prediction Scale] [AAPS]
Donald I. Templer and Arthur T. Daus

Source: Templer, D. I., & Daus, A. T. (1979). An athlete adjustment prediction scale. *The Journal of Sports Medicine and Physical Fitness, 19*, 413-416.

Purpose: To evaluate the degree of adjustment/maladjustment among college athletes.

Description: The AAPS contains 43 items including nine items of the MMPI Lie scale. Participants respond using a 7-point Likert scale.

Construction: The items were developed based on the authors' clinical experiences in working with college athletes.

Reliability: Not reported.

Validity: The majority of items on the AAPS failed to discriminate among 18 "lesser" college football players versus 11 "better" players. Twelve of the lesser players were viewed as problem athletes.

Norms: Not cited. Descriptive statistics and psychometric data were cited for 29 college football players.

**Availability: Contact Donald I. Templer, California School of Professional Psychology, 1350 M Street, Fresno, CA 93721. (Phone # 209-486-8420; FAX # 209-486-0734)

201 Athletic Life Experiences Survey (ALES)
Michael W. Passer and Marla D. Seese

Source: Passer, M. W., & Seese, M. D. (1983). Life stress and athletic injury: Examination of positive versus negative events and three moderator variables. *Journal of Human Stress, 9*(4), 11-16.

Purpose: To examine positive and negative life changes among male college athletes.

Description: The ALES contains 70 items (e.g., "conflict with teammates," "troubles with head coach"). Players are asked to report each event they experienced during the last 12 months, whether the event was "good" or "bad" at the time of occurrence, and the impact that the event had on their lives at the time of the occurrence. Scores on the ALES range from +3 (good, great effect) to -3 (bad, great effect).

Construction: The Life Experiences Survey (1977) was modified to be appropriate to assess the events experienced by males participating in college athletics.

Reliability: Not cited.

Validity: NCAA Division II male football players who incurred significant time-loss injuries ($n=9$) had experienced more negative life changes during the previous 12 months than had uninjured players ($n=40$). However, these findings did not hold up when injured ($n=6$) versus noninjured ($n=49$) NCAA Division I football players were compared on the ALES.

Norms: Psychometric data were based on the responses of 104 male collegiate varsity football players representing Division I and Division II teams.

Availability: Contact Michael W. Passer, Department of Psychology, 238 Gutherie, University of Washington, Box 351525, Seattle, WA 98195-1525. (Phone # 206-685-1814; 206-543-2640; FAX # 206-685-3157; E-mail: mpasser@u.washington.edu)

References

*Hanson, S. J., McCullagh, P., & Tonymon, P. (1992). The relationship of personality characteristics, life stress, and coping resources to athletic injury. *Journal of Sport & Exercise Psychology, 14,* 262-272.

*Hardy, C. J., Richman, J. M., & Rosenfeld, L. B. (1991). The role of social support in the life stress/injury relationship. *The Sport Psychologist, 5,* 128-139.

Mueller, D. P., Edwards, D. W., & Yarvis, R. M. (1977). Stressful life events and psychiatric symptomology: Change as undesirability. *Journal of Health and Social Behavior, 18,* 307-317.

Summers, J. & Stewart, E. (1993). The arousal-performance relationship: Examining differing conceptions. *Proceedings of the Eighth World Congress of Sport Psychology,* (pp. 306-309). Lisbon, Portugal.

 ## Life Events Questionnaire (LEQ)
Roeland Lysens, Yves Vanden Auweele, and M. Ostyn

Source: Lysens, R., Vanden Auweele, Y., & Ostyn, M. (1986). The relationship between psychosocial factors and athletic injuries. *Journal of Sports Medicine and Physical Fitness, 26,* 77-89.

Purpose: To assess unique life events germane to physical education students that necessitate major life adjustments.

Description: College students are asked to respond to 74 life events, indicating on a 10-point scale the average degree of social readjustment necessary for each event experienced during their first year at the university. Students can include events not listed.

Construction: Second-year college students were administered questionnaires seeking information on life events experienced during their first year at the university that influenced their personal, athletic, and study life and that resulted in changes in their accustomed living patterns. The LEQ was developed from an evaluation of these responses. The LEQ represents a modification of the Social and Athletic Readjustment Rating Scale (SARRS).

Reliability: Not discussed.

Validity: Concurrent validity was reported by demonstrating positive correlation coefficients ($n=99$) with personality scales measuring neuroticism, hypochondria, state and trait anxiety, and lack of social desirability. However, the LEQ failed to differentiate between students who did or did not experience acute or overuse injuries.

Norms: Not cited. Psychometric data were reported for 66 male and 33 female university freshman physical education students.

Availability: Contact Roeland Lysens, Institute of Physical Education, Katholieke Universiteit Leuven, Tervuursevest, 101, Leuven, B-3001 Heverlee, Belgium. (Phone # +32 16 329 114)

 ***Life Events Survey for Collegiate Athletes (LESCA)**
Trent A. Petrie

Source: Petrie, T. A. (1992). Psychosocial antecedents of athletic injury: The effects of life stress and social support on female collegiate gymnasts. *Behavioral Medicine, 18*, 127-138.

Purpose: To assess life stress among college athletes.

Description: The LESCA is a 69-item life events survey. Athletes are asked to determine which events have occurred in the last year, and then for each occurring event, to indicate the life event's impact at the time of occurrence on an 8-point Likert scale with the anchorings -4 (*extremely negative*) to +4 (*extremely positive*). An example of an item is "major change in playing status on team." Negative, positive, and total life stress scores can be derived.

Construction: Intercollegiate athletes ($N=166$) were administered a two part questionnaire containing (a) life events items from existing instrumentation and (b) instructions to list additional life events that also influenced in a positive or negative manner these individuals' athletic performance/behavior or personal, social, or academic life. Five male and five female doctoral students then evaluated this preliminary list of 109 life events in terms of their relevance to collegiate athletics. A total of 69 life events items were retained. These items were then reviewed by eight collegiate athletes to ensure item clarity and lack of ambiguity.

Reliability: Test-retest reliability coefficients across a one-week interval ($N=65$) were .84 (negative), .76 (positive), and .83 (total). Across an 8-week interval ($N=72$) reported reliability coefficients were .62 (negative), .48 (positive), and .72 (total score).

Validity: Injured ($n=76$) collegiate gymnasts differed from uninjured (*n*=26) gymnasts on the negative score (but not the positive or total derived scores). Further, LESCA negative scores were related to total injuries and days missed among the injured gymnasts. Convergent validity was supported in that these individuals' scores on LESCA were related to their scores on the Social and Athletic Readjustment Rating Scale.

In addition, it was found that social support moderated the life stress-injury relationship. The negative LESCA scores of gymnasts categorized as low in social support were related to experienced minor injuries, total injuries, and number of days missed. Conversely, the positive LESCA scores of the high social support group of gymnasts were also correlated to moderate injuries experienced and number of meets missed. Further support for the discriminant validity of the LESCA was found in that participants' scores were unrelated to their scores on short form of the Marlowe-Crowne Social Desirability scale. Additional validity information can be found in Petrie (1993a, 1993b).

Norms: Not cited. Psychometric data were reported for (a) 75 male and 91 female athletes from 22 sports at a Division 1-A university and (b) 103 female collegiate gymnasts from 8 Division 1-A teams representing four separate regional athletic conferences.

**Availability: Contact Trent A. Petrie, Department of Psychology, University of North Texas, P. O. Box 13587, Denton, TX 76203-6587. (Phone # 817-565-2671; FAX # 817-565-4682; E-mail: petriet@terrill.unt.edu)

References

*Perna, F. M. (1995). Competitive anxiety and sleep quality: An investigation of performance anxiety models in a health domain [Abstract]. *Journal of Applied Sport Psychology, 7* (Suppl.), S98.

*Petrie, T. A. (1993a). Coping skills, competitive trait anxiety, and playing status: Moderating effects on the life stress-injury relationship. *Journal of Sport & Exercise Psychology, 15,* 261-274.

Petrie, T. A. (1993b). The moderating effects of social support and playing status on the life stress-injury relationship. *Journal of Applied Sport Psychology, 5,* 1-16

204 | Social and Athletic Readjustment Rating Scale (SARRS)

Steven T. Bramwell, Minoru Masuda, Nathaniel N. Wagner and Thomas H. Holmes

Source: Bramwell, S. T., Masuda, M., Wagner, N. N., & Holmes, T. (1975).Psychosocial factors in athletic injuries: Development and application of the Social and Athletic Readjustment Rating Scale (SARRS). *Journal of Human Stress, 1*(2), 6-20.

Purpose: To assess life events that influence sport performance in terms of degree of adjustment made.

Description: The SARRS contains 57 life events likely to be experienced by an athlete that may necessitate major life adjustments. Participants are instructed to indicate the magnitude of change for each life event item to be scaled.

Construction: A modification of the Social Readjustment Rating Scale was made to include the addition of 20 new life events unique to athletics. These modifications were made based on preliminary questionnaire responses of collegiate and professional athletes. These athletes were asked to identify life events that impacted their career and sport performance. Modifications were also based on the athletic experience of one of the authors.

Reliability: Not cited.

Validity: Comparison of football players' ($n=66$) responses to the SARRS with an earlier American (nonathlete) sample's responses to the SRRS indicated that the ordering of life events across samples was correlated ($r=.84$) for both instruments. Furthermore, the SARRS successfully discriminated between injured ($n=36$) and noninjured ($n=46$) college football players in terms of stressful life events experienced.

Norms: Not cited. Psychometric data are reported for 66 University of Washington football players.

Availability: Unknown. Test items are available in the source, but require permission to employ.

References

Cryan, P. D., & Alles, W. F. (1983). The relationship between stress and college football injuries. *Journal of Sports Medicine and Physical Fitness, 23,* 52-58.

May, J. R., Veach, T. L., Reed, M. W., & Griffey, M. S.(1984). A psychological study of health, injury, and performance in athletes on the U.S. Alpine Ski Team. *The Physician and Sportsmedicine, 13*(10), 111-115.

Chapter 16

Locus of Control

Tests in this chapter assess individuals' perceptions of internal and/or external factors that control their reinforcements in relation to exercise behavior, sport performance, injury rehabilitation, and career choice.

205 Exercise Objectives Locus of Control Scale (EOLOC)

Marina L. McCready and Bonita C. Long

Source: McCready, M. L., & Long, B. C. (1985). Locus of control, attitudes toward physical activity, and exercise adherence. *Journal of Sport Psychology, 7,* 346-359.

Purpose: To assess individuals' perceptions of what controls their reinforcements in relation to exercise behavior.

Description: The EOLOC consists of three 6-item subscales: Internality, Powerful Others, and Chance. For example, participants respond to the item "I am directly responsible for whether or not I reach my exercise goals" (Internal scale). Participants respond to each item using a 5-point Likert scale with the anchorings *strongly agree* to *strongly disagree.*

Construction: An initial 24-item test pool was developed reflective of the three subdomains (above). Ten graduate students evaluated each item for clarity and content validity. The same 24 items were evaluated through item analysis and internal consistency checks among 60 aerobic fitness class participants (*M* age=30 years; *n*=50 females, *n*=10 males). Six items were eliminated, and two new Chance subscale items were added. The revised 20-item EOLOC was administered to 87 females (*M* age= 30 years) involved in fitness programs. Item analysis led to the elimination of two Chance subscale items resulting in the 18-item EOLOC. Intercorrelation coefficients among subscales were low, although the Internal and Powerful Others subscales were not correlated.

Reliability: Alpha reliability coefficients (*n*=87 females) were .79, .69, and .75 for the Internal, Powerful Others, and Chance subscales, respectively. Test-retest reliability coefficients for this sample (who were participating in the exercise programs) were .32 (Internal), .72 (Powerful Others), and .60 (Chance) across a 3- to 4-month interval.

Validity: The construct validity of the EOLOC was examined through principal component factor analysis (*n*=172 females) in which five factors emerged accounting for 51% of the variance. Factor 5 was not evaluated because it only accounted for 4% of the total variance. Factors 1 and 2 were defined by the all the Internal and Chance items, whereas the Powerful Others items were split between Factors 3 and 4.

Discriminant validity was supported in that participants' responses to the EOLOC were not related to a measure of social desirability.

Norms: Not reported. Psychometric data were cited for 172 female subjects.

**Availability: Contact Bonita C. Long, Department of Counseling Psychology, 2125 Main Mall, University of British Columbia, Vancouver, B. C., Canada V6T 1Z4. (Phone #604-822-4756; FAX # 604-822-2328; E-mail: blong@unixg.ubc.ca)

References
*Dishman, R. K., & Steinhardt, M. (1990). Health locus of control predicts free-living, but not supervised, physical activity: A test of exercise-specific control and outcome-expectancy hypotheses. *Research Quarterly for Exercise & Sport, 61,* 383-394.

*Doganis, G., Theodorakis, Y., & Bagiatis, K. (1991). Self-esteem and locus of control in adult female fitness program participants. *International Journal of Sport Psychology, 22,* 154-164.

Ekkekakis, P., & Zervas, Y. (1993). The effect of a single bout of aerobic exercise on mood: Co-examination of biological and psychological parameters in a controlled field study. *Proceedings of the Eight World Congress of Sport Psychology* (pp. 543-547). Lisbon, Portugal.

Long, B. C., & Haney, C. J. (1986). Enhancing physical activity in sedentary women. Information, locus of control, and attitudes. *Journal of Sport Psychology, 8,* 8-24.

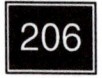 ## [Fitness Locus of Control Scale] (FITLOC)
James R. Whitehead and Charles B. Corbin

Source: Whitehead, J. R., & Corbin, C. B. (1988). Multidimensional scales for the measurement of locus of control reinforcements for physical fitness behaviors. (1988). *Research Quarterly for Exercise and Sport, 59,* 108-117.

Purpose: To assess among individuals locus of control of reinforcement beliefs specific to physical fitness behaviors.

Description: The FITLOC is an 11-item test containing three subscales: Internality (IFit), Powerful Others (PFit), and Chance (CFit). Participants respond to each item using a 6-point Likert format.

Construction: After reviewing the literature on social learning and locus of control theory, items were developed reflecting the three dimensions (internality, powerful others, and chance) of physical fitness behavior reinforcement locus of control beliefs. Four exercise psychology experts reduced the battery of items to 18 items. The 18 trial items were evaluated among 119 freshman students who were also administered concurrently a shortened version of the Marlowe-Crowne Social Desirability scale, 9 ambiguous filler items, Levenson's IPC scales, and the Weight Locus of Control scale. Principal components factor analysis led to the retention of 11 items with moderate alpha reliability. The three subscales correlated positively with the theoretically corresponding IPC and WLOC scales. Correlation coefficients for the IFit, CFit, and PFit subscales with the social desirability scale were statistically significant. An additional sample of 125 freshman undergraduate students was administered either the 11-item FITLOC or the 11-item FITLOC combined with 6 ambiguous filler items. The addition of these six camouflaging items had minimal effect on the psychometric properties of the FITLOC.

Reliability: Alpha reliability coefficients ($n=62$ undergraduate students in freshman composition classes) were .62 (IFit), .74 (PFit), and .84 (CFit). For 133 undergraduate students enrolled in physical education, alpha reliability coefficients were .78 (IFit), .74 (PFit). and .82 (CFit). Test-retest reliability coefficients ($n=60$ freshman composition students) across a 2-week interval were .69 (Ifit), .59 (PFit), and .67 (Cfit).

Validity: Concurrent validity was evident by the correlation of individuals' ($n=115$) scores on the FITLOC subscales with the IPC subscales. Weak support for concurrent validity was evident when participants' ($n=133$) scores on the FITLOC subscales were correlated with self-report estimates of physical activity participation. Construct validity was supported through a series of factor analytic studies that led to the retention of the three subscale factors noted above.

Norms: Not reported. Psychometric data are cited for independent samples ($n=115$; $n=125$; $n=133$) of undergraduate male and female students.

**Availability: Contact James Whitehead, Department of HPER, University of North Dakota, Box 8235. Grand Forks, ND 58202. (Phone # 701-777-4347; FAX # 701-777-3650; E-mail: jwhitehe@plains.nodak.edu)

340

References

*Kimiecik, J., & Burk, C. (1992). Examining the relationship among health and exercise locus of control, health and exercise value, and self-reported exercise behavior [Abstract]. *Proceedings of the North American Society for the Psychology of Sport and Physical Activity annual convention* (p. 156). Pittsburgh, PA.

Tappe, M. K., & Duda, J. L. (1988). Personal investment predictors of life satisfaction among physically active middle-aged and older adults. *Journal of Psychology, 122,* 557-566.

[Locus of Control in Rehabilitation Scale] [LCRS]

Joan L. Duda, Alison E. Smart, and Marlene K. Tappe

Source: Duda, J. L., Smart, A. E., & Tappe, M. K. (1989). Predictors of adherence in the rehabilitation of athletic injuries: An application of personal investment theory. *Journal of Sport & Exercise Psychology,11,* 367-381.

Purpose: To examine the degree to which athletes perceive their successful injury rehabilitation to be either under their personal control or the responsibility of the athletic trainer.

Description: The LCRS contains nine items and includes internal and external locus of control subscales. Individuals respond to each item using a 6-point Likert scale.

Construction: Not discussed.

Reliability: Cronbach alpha reliability coefficients ($n=40$) for the Internal and External subscales were .77 and .75, respectively.

Validity: Stepwise multiple regression analysis indicated that internal locus of control was a significant predictor of the mean percentage of completed exercises across scheduled rehabilitation sessions.

Norms: Not reported. Psychometric data were cited for 40 male and female intercollegiate athletes who had sustained a sport-related injury of at least second-degree severity.

Availability: Contact Joan L. Duda, Department of Health, Kinesiology, and Leisure Studies, 113 Lambert Hall, Purdue University, W. Lafayette, IN 47907. (Phone # 317-494-3172; FAX # 317-496-1239; E-mail: lynne@vm.cc.purdue.edu)

 ***[Physical Fitness Locus of Control Scale] [PFLCS]**

John E. Bezjak and Jerry W. Lee

Source: Bezjak, J. E., & Lee, J. W. (1990). Relationship of self-efficacy and locus of control constructs in predicting college students' physical fitness behaviors. *Perceptual and Motor Skills, 71,* 499-508.

Purpose: To assess participants' locus of control specific to physical fitness settings.

Description: The PFLCS contains 27 items and three subscales: (a) Internal Physical Fitness Locus of Control (e.g., "I alone control the personal behaviors that affect my physical fitness status"), (b) Powerful Other Physical Fitness Locus of Control (e.g., "Other people have the power to make certain that I accomplish my physical fitness goals"), and (c) Chance Physical Fitness Locus of Control (e.g., "If it is meant to be, I will reach my physical fitness objectives"). Participants respond to each item on a 6-point Likert scale with the anchorings 1 (*strongly disagree*) to 6 (*strongly agree*).

Construction: Not discussed.

Reliability: Cronbach alpha internal consistency coefficients ($N=300$ approximately) of .82 (Internal scale), .86 (Chance scale), and .83 (Powerful Other Scale) were reported.

Validity: Construct validity was supported by exploratory and confirmatory factor analyses ($N=209$ approximately), in which a three factor model emerged. However, respondents' ($N=211$) scores on these locus of control scales were not related to their reported frequency and duration of participation in health-related physical fitness.

Norms: Not reported. Psychometric data were reported for approximately 300 undergraduate students (n=161 females; n=139 males), and descriptive statistics and psychometric data were also reported for 211 undergraduate students (n=114 females; n=93 males). Subjects were located at colleges and universities in the Riverside, California, area.

Availability: Last known address: John E. Bezjak, Department of Institutional Research, University of Phoenix, 4615 East Elwood Stree, Phoenix, AZ 85040.

Reference
*Bezjak, J. E., & Langga-Sharifi, E. (1991). Validation of the Physical Fitness Opinion Questionnaire against marathon performance. *Perceptual and Motor Skills, 73*, 993-994.

209 [Sport Career Locus of Control Test] [SCLCT]
M. L. Kamlesh and T. R. Sharma

Source: Kamlesh, M. L. (1989). Internal and external factors affecting sports career. *Indian Journal of Sports Science, 1*(1), 59-67.

Purpose: To identify the most significant internal and external factors influencing the career of a sportsman.

Description: The SCLCT contains 20 items. The test is designed to assess internal factors (superiority in game skill, practice, and ability) and external factors (financial backing, equipment and coaching, luck, and influence of high-ups) as they affect the sports career of an athlete. Participants respond to each item (e.g., "To a great extent, my sports career is controlled by accidental happenings"-luck factor) using a 5-point Likert scale.

Construction: Items and factors were identified through an intensive examination of the sociology and psychology of sport literature and on the basis of experience-oriented observations. An initial battery of 35 items was reduced to 20 items based on review by experts and knowledgeable athletes (M. L. Kamlesh, personal communication, April 13, 1996).

Reliability: A test-retest reliability coefficient (*n*=23) of .65 was reported.

Validity: Not reported.

Norms: Not cited. Descriptive data were cited for 122 male and 81 female randomly selected athletes (ages 20-33 years) from the National Institute of Sports, Patiala, the Laxmibai College of Physical Education, Gwalior, and the Punjab Goverment College of Physical Education, Patiala, in India.

**Availability: Contact M. L. Kamlesh, Lakshmibai National College of Physical Education, Kariavattom P. O., Post Box No. 3, Trivandrum (Kerala) 695 581, India. [Phone # (09) 0471-418712, 418722; FAX # (09) 0471 418769], or National Psychological Corporation 4/230, Kacheri Ghat, Agra- 282004, India.

210 Sport Locus of Control Scale [SLCS]
James Domnick DiFebo

Source: DiFebo, J. D. (1975). Modification of general expectancy and sport expectancy within a sport setting. In D. M. Landers (Ed.), *Psychology of sport and motor behavior II* (pp. 247-254). State College, PA: Penn State HPER Series No. 10.

Purpose: To assess internal and external dimensions of locus of control as expressed in a sport setting.

Description: The SLCS consists of 20 items measuring internal or external locus of control. Participants respond to each item using a 4-point Likert scale.

Construction: Not discussed.

Reliability: An alpha reliability coefficient (*n*=112 college students) of .55 was reported. A test-retest reliability coefficient of .70 was reported across a 2-week interval.

Validity: Concurrent validity was supported in that participants'

(n=112) scores on the SLCS were correlated with their responses to the Rotter Internal-External Locus of Control Scale (r=.36). However, construct validity was not supported in that the instrument failed to detect changes in an intervention program designed to modify locus of control in a physical education setting over 16 weeks.

Norms: Not reported. Psychometric data were cited for 112 freshman college students enrolled in a basic instructional physical education program at a midwestern university.

Availability: Contact James D. DiFebo, 419 Salisbury Street, Meyersdale, PA 15552.

Chapter 17

Miscellaneous

Tests in this chapter examine a potpourri of psychological constructs including the affective responses of athletes to experiencing injury, the athletic identity, attitudes toward sport psychological services, psychological factors related to spectator attendance and allegiance to sport teams, sportsmanship attitudes, officials' role satisfaction, and athletes' superstitious beliefs.

211 *Affect Recovery Process Scale [ARPS]
Kanshi Uemukai

Source: Uemukai, K. (1993). Affective responses and the changes in athletes due to injury. *Proceedings of the Eighth World Congress of Sport Psychology* (pp. 500-503). Lisbon, Portugal.

Purpose: To evaluate the affective responses of athletes to injury.

Description: The ARPS contains 31 items reflecting the categories of Denial, Anger, Bargaining, Depression, Acceptance, and Impatience. Participants respond on a 5-point scale with the anchorings 1 (*not at all true*) to 5 (*extremely true*).

Construction: The ARPS is patterned after the Kübler-Ross (1969) model of death and dying. The subscale of Impatience was added based on interviews with injured athletes. Two injured college athletes evaluated the ARPS for content clarity.

Reliability: Cronbach alpha internal consistency coefficients (*N*=212) ranged from .62 to .87.

Validity: Not discussed.

Norms: Not cited. Psychometric data were reported for 63 female and 149 male injured athletes.

Availability: Last known address: Kanshi Uemukai, Institute of Health and Sport Sciences, University of Tsukuba, Japan.

Reference
Kübler-Ross, E. (1969). *On death and dying*. New York: MacMillan.

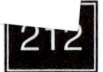

*Athletic Identity Measurement Scale (AIMS)

Britton W. Brewer, Judy. L. Van Raalte, and Darwin E. Linder

Source: Brewer, B. W., Van Raalte, J. L., & Linder, D. E. (1993). Athletic identity: Hercules' Muscles or Achilles' Heel? *International Journal of Sport Psychology, 24,* 237-254.

Purpose: To assess "...the degree to which an individual identifies with the athlete role" (p. 237).

Description: The AIMS contains 10 items (e.g., "I consider myself an athlete" and "Sport is the most important part of my life"). Participants respond to each item using a 7-point Likert-type scale with the anchorings 1 (*strongly disagree*) and 7 (*strongly agree*).

Construction: Initially, 11 items were developed based on input from undergraduate research assistants and former athletes. The items were designed to reflect the social, cognitive, and affective dimensions of athletic identity. Preliminary analyses led to the elimination of one item.

Reliability: Cronbach alpha coefficients ($N=243$; $N=449$; $N=90$) of .93, .87, and .81 were reported, and a test-retest reliability coefficient of .89 was reported across a 14-day period.

Validity: Exploratory principal components factor analysis ($N=243$) supported the unidimensionality of the AIMS. Convergent validity was supported in that participants' scores on the AIMS were highly positively correlated with their scores on the Perceived Importance Profile importance of sports competence scale ($r=.83$), as well as other subscales of this instrument. Furthermore, AIMS scores were higher for participants reporting high levels of athletic involvement.

In a second study, it was found that participants' ($N=449$) AIMS scores were related to their scores on the Self-Role Scale ($r=.61$) and to the subscales of the Sport Orientation Questionnaire. These participants' AIMS scores were not related to their scores on a measure of self-esteem.

In Study 3, it was found that intercollegiate football players' scores on the AIMS were correlated with the Perceived Importance Profile importance of sports competence scale ($r=.42$), but not with various subscales of the Physical Self-Perception Profile.

Norms: Not cited. Psychometric data were reported for two samples of 243 and 449 college students enrolled in introductory psychology classes and 90 male intercollegiate football players.

**Availability: Contact Britton L. Brewer, Center for Performance Enhancement and Applied Research, Department of Psychology, Springfield College, 263 Alden Street, Springfield, MA 01109-3797. (Phone # 413-748-3696; FAX # 413-748-3854; E-mail: britton_brewer@scns.spfldcol.edu). Items are also listed in the *Source*.

References

*Brewer, B. W., Boin, P. D., & Petitpas. A. J. (1993, August). *Dimensions of athletic identity.* Paper presented at the annual meeting of the American Psychological Association, Toronto, Ontario, Canada.

*Brewer, B. W., Denson, E. L., & Jordon, J. M. (1992, May). *Temporal stability of major planning, career planning, and athletic identity in freshman student-athletes.* Paper presented at the Ninth Annual Conference on Counseling Athletes, Springfield, MA.

*Brewer, B. W., & Linder, D. E. (1992). Distancing oneself from a poor season: Divestment of athletic identity [Abstract]. *Proceedings of the Association for the Advancement of Applied Sport Psychology annual convention* (p. 5). Colorado Springs, CO.

*Brewer, B. W., Van Raalte, J. L., & Linder, D. E. (1990, May). *Development and preliminary validation of the Athletic Identity Measurement Scale.* Paper presented at the annual meeting of the North American Society for the Psychology of Sport and Physical Activity, Houston, TX.

*Brewer, B. W., Van Raalte, J. L. , & Linder, D. E. (1991, June). *Construct validity of the Athletic Identity Measurement Scale.* Paper presented at the annual meeting of the North American Society for the Psychology of Sport and Physical Activity, Pacific Grove, CA.

*Buntrock, C. L., & Brewer, B. W. (1994, August). *Social and personal aspects of athletic identity.* Paper presented at the annual meeting of the American Psychological Association, Los Angeles, CA.

*Buntrock, C. L., Brewer, B. W., & Petitpas, A. J. (1994, October). *Distancing oneself from a poor season: A replication and extension.* Paper presented at the annual meeting of the Association for the Advancement of Applied Sport Psychology, Incline Village, NV.

*Cornelius, A. (1995). The relationship between athletic identity, peer and faculty socialization, and college student development. *Journal of College Student Development, 36,* 560-573.

*Good, A. J., Brewer, B. W., Petitpas, A. J., Van Raalte, J. L., & Mahar, M. T. (1993, Spring). Identity foreclosure, athletic identity, and college sport participation. *The Academic Athletic Journal,* pp. 1-12.

352

*Hale, B. D. (1993, June). *A three year evaluation of a life skills developmental drug education program for college athletes.* Paper presented at the 8th World Congress of Sport Psychology, Lisbon, Portugal.

*Hale, B. D. (1995, July). *Exclusive athletic identity: A predictor of positive or negative psychological characteristics?* Paper presented at the IXth European Congress on Sport Psychology, Brussels, Belgium.

*Hale, B. D., & Waalkes, D. (1994). Athletic identity, gender, self esteem, academic importance, and drug use: A further validation of the AIMS [Abstract]. *Journal of Sport & Exercise Psychology, 16* (Suppl.), S62.

*Kendzierski, D., & Furr, R. M. (1995, August). *Correlates of physical activity identities.* Paper presented at the annual meeting of the American Psychological Association, New York, NY.

*Lavallee, D., Gordon, S., & Grove, J. R. (1995, June). *Athletic identity as a predictor of zeteophobia among retired athletes.* Paper presented at the 12th Annual Conference on Counseling Athletes, Springfield, MA.

*Martin, J. J., Adams Mushett, C., & Eklund, R. (1995). Factor structure of the Athletic Identity Measurement Scale with adolescent swimmers with disabilities. *Brazilian Journal of Adapted Physical Education Research, 1,* 87-100.

*Martin, J. J., Adams Mushett, C., & Lynch, K. (1994, October). *Social psychological characteristics of international elite youth swimmers with disabilities.* Paper presented at the annual meeting of the Association for the Advancement of Applied Sport Psychology, Incline Village, NV.

*Martin, J. J., Adams Mushett, C., & Smith, K. L. (1995). Athletic identity and sport orientation of adolescent swimmers with disabilities. *Adapted Physical Activity Quarterly, 12,* 113-123.

*Matheson, H., Brewer, B. W., Van Raalte, J. L., & Andersen, B. (1995). Athletic identity of national level badminton players: A cross-cultural analysis. In R. Reilly, M. Hughes, & A. Lees (Eds.), *Science and racquet sports* (pp. 228-231). London: E & FN Spon.

*Owens, S. S. (1994, October). *The relationship between student athlete identity and career exploration.* Paper presented at the annual conference of the Association for the Advancement of Applied Sport Psychology, Lake Tahoe, NV.

*Petrie, T., & Stoever, S. (1995). Psychosocial antecedents of athletic injury: A temporal analysis [Abstract]. *Journal of Applied Sport Psychology, 7,* S99.

*Van Raalte, N. S., & Cook. R. G. (1991). Gender specific situational influences on athletic identity [Abstract]. *Proceedings of the North American Society for the Psychology of Sport and Physical Activity annual convention* (p. 200). Pacific Grove: CA.

*Wiechman, S. A., & Williams, J. M. (1995). Relationship of ethnicity and other factors to athletic identity in high school athletes [Abstract]. *Journal of Applied Sport Psychology, 7,* S125.

213 *Attitudes Toward Seeking Sport Psychology Consultation Questionnaire (ATSSPCQ)

Scott B. Martin, Craig A. Wrisberg, Patricia A. Beitel, and John Lounsbury

Source: Martin, S. B., Wrisberg, C. A., Beitel, P. A., and Lounsbury, J. (1995, October). *African-American and Caucasian NCAA Division I athletes' attitudes toward seeking sport psychology consultation.* Paper presented at the annual convention of the Association for the Advancement of Applied Sport Psychology, New Orleans, LA.

Purpose: To assess the attitudes and perceptions of college athletes' toward sport psychological skills training and toward seeking sport psychology consultation services.

Description: The ATSSPCQ contains 50 items (e.g., "I do not have much respect for sport psychology consultants," and "Athletes need to develop a mental plan for competition prior to actually competing"). Participants respond to each item employing a 7-point Likert scale.

Construction: Items on the ATSSPCQ were initially evaluated for content validity by five professionals (three psychology or sport psychology professors and two sport psychology doctoral students). A second draft of the ATSSPCQ was then pilot tested with five collegiate basketball players. The ATSSPCQ was then administered to 225 NCAA Division I athletes.

Exploratory principal components factor analysis ($N=225$) with varimax rotation resulted in a three-factor solution accounting for 35 percent of the variance in participants' responses to the ATSSPCQ. All items loaded 0.23 or greater on these three factors and were retained. The three factors described athletes' negative consequences of seeking sport psychology consultation, athletes' confidence in sport psychology consultation, or athletes' interpersonal openness and willingness to try sport psychology consultation.

Reliability: A Cronbach alpha internal consistency coefficient ($N=225$) of .71 was reported for the entire ATSSPCQ. Test-retest reliability coefficients ($N=16$) over an 8-week period, computed for each item separately, ranged from .69 to .98.

Validity: None of the comparisons between the participants' (N=225) responses to the ATSSPCQ and their responses to the Attitude Toward Seeking Professional Psychological Help questionnaire (Fischer & Turner, 1970) produced statistically significant differences.

Norms: Not cited. Descriptive statistics and psychometric data were reported for 48 African-American scholarship athletes (n=14 females; n=34 males) and 177 Caucasian scholarship athletes (n=79 females; n=98 males) attending an NCAA Division I university.

**Availability: Contact Scott B. Martin, Department of Kinesiology, University of North Texas, P. O. Box 13857, Denton, TX 76203-6857. (Phone # 817-565-2651; FAX # 817-565-4904; E-mail: smartin@coefs.coe.unt.edu)

Reference

Fischer, E. H., & Turner, J. L. (1970). Orientations to seeking professional help: Development and research utility of an attitude scale. *Journal of Consulting and Clinical Psychology, 35,* 79-90.

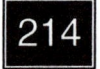 ## *Fan Psychology Scale (FPS)
Dale G. Pease and James J. Zhang

Source: Pease, D. G., & Zhang, J. J. (1995, September). *Dimensions of fan psychology: Development of the Fan Psychology Scale (FPS)*. Paper presented at the annual conference of the Association for the Advancement of Applied Sport Psychology, New Orleans, LA.

Purpose: To assess "... psychological factors that are related to spectator attendance of professional basketball games" (p. 5).

Description: The FPS contains 35 items and four subscales: Fan Identification (e.g., "I feel proud that the team belongs to this city"); Team Image (e.g., "I consider that the players on the team are role models of the community"); Salubrious Attraction (e.g., "I come to the game just for getting away from tension in my life"); and Entertainment Value (e.g., "I take pleasure from the excitement of the audience"). Participants respond to each item using a 5-point Likert scale with the anchorings 1 (*strongly disagree*) to 5 (*strongly agree*).

Construction: Initially, 75 items representing psychological
vant to fan attendance were derived from a review of tł
Based on a review of these items by three university professors in sport
psychology and/or sport management, and two senior NBA team
administrators, a total of 50 items were retained.

Exploratory principal components factor analysis ($N=1,012$) with
varimax rotation led to the retention of four factors accounting for
52.10% of the variance explained.

Reliability: Cronbach alpha coefficients ($N=1012$) were .92 (Fan
Identification), .88 (Team Image), .69 (Salubrious Attraction) and .69
(Entertainment Value).

Validity: Concurrent validity was supported in that attendance frequency was positively related to these fan's ($N=1,012$) scores on the FPS. The
correlation coefficients for the four subscales ranged from .56 to .83.

Norms: Not cited. Psychometric data were reported for 716 male and
296 female spectators ranging in age from 10 to 74 years (M age=33.86
years, $SD=12.57$) who attended six second-half 1993-1994 season home
games of a major NBA Western Conference team. The majority
(75.60%) of these fans were Caucasian.

Availability: Contact Dale G. Pease, Department of Health and Human
Performance, 123 Melcher Gym, University of Houston, Houston, TX
77204-5331. Phone # 713-743-9838; FAX # 713-743-9860; E-mail:
dpease@uh.edu)

215 [Friendship Expectations Questionnaire] [FEQ]

Brian J. Bigelow, John H. Lewko, and Linda Salhani

Source: Bigelow, B. J., Lewko, J. H., & Salhani, L. (1989). Sport-involved
children's friendship expectations. *Journal of Sport & Exercise
Psychology, 11*, 152-160.

Purpose: To assess the characteristics children conceptualize as important to have in a friendship relationship when involved in sport.

Description: The questionnaire assesses eight friendship expectations (FEs)) across five discrete friendship-sport contexts. These FEs include stimulation value, helping, sharing, loyalty and commitment, acceptance, intimacy potential, ego reinforcement, and source of humor. The questionnaire contains a total of 40 items. Children respond to each item using a 7-point Likert scale.

Construction: Not discussed.

Reliability: Corrected internal consistency coefficients (n=40 boys & 40 girls, ages 9-12 years) ranged from .86 to .95 across each of the five sport contexts.

Validity: Not discussed.

Norms: Not presented. Psychometric data were based on the responses of 80 children.

Availability: Contact John H. Lewko, Child and Development Studies, Laurentian University, Sudbury, Ontario, Canada P3E 2C6.

216 *Interventions Perceptions Questionnaire (IPQ)
Britton W. Brewer, Karin E. Jeffers, Albert J. Petitpas, and Judy L. Van Raalte

Source: Brewer, B. W., Jeffers, K. E., Petitpas, A. J., & Van Raalte, J. L. (1994). Perceptions of psychological interventions in the context of sport injury rehabilitation. *The Sport Psychologist, 8,* 176-188.

Purpose: To assess perceptions of psychological interventions used within the context of sport injury rehabilitation.

Description: The IPQ contains seven items that examine perceptions of satisfaction, motivational effects, treatment adherence effects, beliefs/attitudes, and general effectiveness of various psychological interventions. Items are scored using a 7-point Likert-type scale.

Construction: Not discussed.

Reliability: A Cronbach alpha internal consistency coefficient (*N*=161) of .82 was reported.

Validity: Convergent validity was supported in that participants' responses to the IPQ were correlated (*r*=.69) with their scores on the Treatment Acceptability Questionnaire.

Norms: Not cited. Psychometric data were obtained from 161 under-graduate students (*n*=86 females; *n*=75 males) attending a small north-eastern college. Approximately 45% of these students reported having had an athletic injury requiring physical therapy.

**Availability: Contact Britton W. Brewer, Center for Performance Enhancement and Applied Research, Department of Psychology, Springfield College, 263 Alden Street, Springfield, MA 01109-3797. (Phone # 413-748-3696; FAX # 413-748-3854; E-mail: britton_brewer@scns.spfldcol.edu)

217 Job Satisfaction Scale [JSS]
Joe P. Ramsey

Source: Evans, E., Ramsey, J. P., Johnson, D., Renwick, D., & Vienneau, J-G (1986). A comparison of job satisfaction, leadership behavior and job perception between male and female athletic directors. *The Physical Educator, 43*, 39-43.

Purpose: To evaluate the job satisfaction of college athletic directors.

Description: The scale contains 20 items to assess athletic directors' satisfaction with the general work situation. Athletic directors respond to each item using a 5-point ordinal scale.

Construction: Not discussed.

Reliability: An internal consistency coefficient of .81 was reported among 204 college athletic directors.

358

Validity: Not discussed.

Norms: Psychometric data were cited for 171 male and 33 female college athletic directors representing both Divisions IA (*n*=79), II (*n*=28), III (*n*=31) and 31 Canadian colleges and universities.

Availability: Last known address: Joe P. Ramsey, Department of Physical Education, Florida Atlantic University, Boca Raton, FL 33431. (Phone # 305-393-3792)

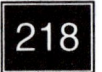 # *Multidimensional Sportsmanship Orientations Scale (MSOS)
Robert J. Vallerand, N. M. Briere, C. Blanchard, and Pierre J. Provencher

Source: Vallerand, R. J., & Losier, G. F. (1995). Self-determined motivation and sportsmanship orientations: An assessment of their temporal relationship. *Journal of Sport & Exercise Psychology, 16*, 229-245.*

Purpose: To assess athletes' orientations toward the sportsmanship dimensions as outlined by Vallerand, Briere, Blanchard, and Provencher (1996).

Description: The MSOS contains five sportsmanship orientation subscales with five items each: (a) one's full commitment toward sport participation, (b) social conventions in sport, (c) rules and officials, (d) the opponent, and (e) negative approach toward one's participation in sport. Participants respond using a 5-ordinal scale with the anchorings 1 (*does not correspond at all to me*) to 5 (*corresponds exactly to me*).

Construction: Initially, 20 items per subscale were developed and then evaluated by two sport psychologists for content validity. Then the 12 best items per subscale were administered to 15 athletes to assess item clarity and ecological relevance. The revised version was then administered to 150 athletes. A factor analysis of these athletes' scores led to the retention of five items per subscale.

*Note: The first author indicated (R. Vallerand, personal communication, April 16, 1996) that the reader should refer to Vallerand, Briere, Blanchard, and Provencher (1996) for an update on the development and validation procedures of the MSOS.

Reliability: An overall mean Cronbach alpha coefficient of .73 (*N*>600) was reported. An average test-retest reliability coefficient of .67 across 5 weeks was also cited.

Validity: Confirmatory factor analysis (*N*>600) supported the five-factor structure of the MSOS. Also, correlation coefficients ranging from .20 to .44 were reported between behavioral intentions and participants' responses to each subscale of the MSOS.

Norms: Not provided. Psychometric data were cited for over 750 athletes.

**Availability: Contact Robert J. Vallerand, Department of Psychology, University of Quebec at Montreal, P. O. Box 8888, Station "Centreville," Montreal, Quebec, Canada H3C 3P8 (Phone # 514-987-4836; FAX # 514-987-7953; E-mail: vallerand.robert_j@uqam.ca)

Reference

*Vallerand, R. J., Briere, N. M., Blanchard, C., & Provencher, P. J. (1996). *The development and validation of the Multidimensional Sportsmanship Orientations Scale.* Paper submitted for publication.

219   Power Value Orientation Test (PVO)
Brenda J. Bredemeier

Source: Bredemeier, B. J. (1980). An instrument to assess the expressive and instrumental power valued in sport and in everyday life. *Research abstracts--American Alliance for Health, Physical Education, Recreation and Dance* (p. 66). Annual convention, Detroit, MI.

Purpose: To assess expressive and instrumental power value orientations in sport and in everyday life.

Description: Not provided.

Construction: Not indicated.

Reliability: Alpha internal consistency coefficients from .86 to .92 were reported among 230 athletes.

Validity: Content validity was established via the use of expert opinion.

Norms: Not cited. Psychometric data were based on 230 male and female athletes representing professional, college varsity, and noncollege varsity levels.

Availability: Contact Brenda J. Bredemeier, Department of Human Biodynamics, 206 Hearst Gymnasium, University of California, Berkeley, CA 94720-4482. (Phone # 510-642-1704; FAX # 510-642-7241; E-mail: brenda@uclink2.berkeley.edu)

---

 *Soccer Officials' Satisfaction Scale [SOS]
Adrian H. Taylor

Source: Taylor, A. H. (1993). Satisfaction among soccer officials: Some antecedents and consequences. In J. R. Nitsch & R. Seiler (Eds.), *Motivation, emotion and stress* (Vol. 1). Sankt Augustin, Germany: Academia Verlag.

Purpose: To assess role satisfaction among soccer officials.

Description: The SOS measures how often a soccer official has felt satisfied with various facets of the role including personal fitness, performance, achievements, support received, pay, social contacts, and the role of officiating in general. A 4-point ordinal scale, with the anchorings 0 (*never*) to 3 (*often*), is used to assess frequency of feelings of satisfaction.

Construction: A review of surveys of occupational satisfaction, extensive interviews with officials in Ontario, Canada, and reviews by a 12-member panel with experience in psychometric construction produced a nine-item measure of satisfaction among officials. All 1,269 registered soccer officials in Ontario were mailed the Ontario Soccer Officials' Survey 3 months into the soccer season and 4 months later at the end of the season. The survey included sections on sources of stress, burnout, satisfaction, intentions to quit, and background variables. Exploratory principal components factor analysis, conducted on the data collected at each time period, produced a unidimensional nine-item scale.

Reliability: Cronbach alpha reliability coefficients were .71 (N=733) and .75 (N=529) for the data collected at each time period, respectively.

Validity: Construct validity was supported in that officials' SOS scores were negatively correlated with intent to quit (r= -.42), actual dropout, and their scores on six of the seven sources of stress identified in the survey. However, the correlation coefficients representing the relationships between their SOS scores and their scores on the sources of stress ranged from -.09 to -.16.

Norms: Not cited. Psychometric data were reported for 529 male soccer officials (M age=38.7 years; SD=11.0) from Ontario, Canada, who had served as officials, on average, for 7.27 years.

**Availability: Contact Adrian H. Taylor, Chelsea School Research Centre, University of Brighton, Gaudick Road, Eastbourne, East Sussex, England BN20 7SP. (Phone # 01273-643743; FAX # 01273-643704; E-mail: aht@bton.ac.uk)

221 Social Comparison Jealousy Scale (SCJ)
Dale G. Pease

Source: Pease, D. G. (1988). Social comparison jealousy and its relationship to group cohesion [Abstract]. *In Psychology of motor behavior and sport* (p. 161). Proceedings of the North American Society for the Psychology of Sport and Physical Activity annual convention. Knoxville, TN.

Purpose: To assess the emotions of jealousy and envy in a sport context.

Description: Not indicated.

Construction: The original scale designed to measure jealousy and envy was reduced from 20 to 12 items. This was based on the conceptual framework that jealousy is a triadic relationship, whereas envy is viewed as a dyadic relationship.

Reliability: An alpha reliability coefficient of .83 was reported for the SCJ among 71 sport participants.

Validity: The hypothesized inverse relationship between respondents' scores on the SCJ and the social subscales of the Group Environment Questionnaire failed to materialize ($N=71$).

Norms: Not reported. Psychometric data were cited for 71 team sport participants.

Availability: Contact Dale G. Pease, Department of Health and Human Performance, 123 Melcher Gym, University of Houston, Houston, TX 77204-5331. (Phone # 713-743-9838; FAX # 713-743-9860; E-mail: dpease@uh.edu)

222 Sport Psychology Consultant Evaluation Form (CEF)
John Partington and Terry Orlick

Source: Partington, J., & Orlick, T. (1987). The Sport Psychology Consultant Evaluation Form. *The Sport Psychologist, 1,* 309-317.

Purpose: To assess the perceptions athletes have of sport psychology consultants, and the amount and type of athlete-consultant contact.

Description: The CEF contains 10 consultant characteristic items that athletes rate on a 11-point ordinal scale. Six additional items relate to the duration of several types of contact between athlete and sport psychology consultant. Perceived consultant effectiveness is also assessed by two rating criteria using an 11-point ordinal scale.

Construction: Item selection was based on interview data on consultant effectiveness gathered from 75 Olympic athletes and 17 national team coaches.

Reliability: An alpha internal consistency coefficient of .68 was reported for 104 Canadian Olympic athletes. The test-retest reliability coefficient for the consultant characteristics total scale score ($n=15$ national team athletes) was .81 across a 2-day interval.

Validity: Concurrent validity of the consultant characteristics scale was evidenced by demonstrating positive correlation coefficients with perceived consultant effectiveness ($r=.68$, effect on you; $r=.57$, effect on team). Stepwise multiple regression analysis indicated that the scale of consultant characteristics accounted for three times more variance in predicting effectiveness than was possible from knowledge of the amounts and types of consultant contacts.

Norms: Not reported. Psychometric data were cited for 104 Canadian Olympic athletes who evaluated 26 sport psychology consultants.

Availability: Contact John Partington, Department of Psychology, Carleton University, Ottawa, Canada, K1S 5B6. (Phone 613-520-2600, ext. 2695)

References

*Gould, D., Murphy, S., Tammen, V., & May, J. (1991). An evaluation of U.S. Olympic sport psychology consultant effectiveness. *The Sport Psychologist, 5*, 111-127.

Hardy, L., & Parfitt, G. (1994). The development of a model for the provision of psychological support to a national squad. *The Sport Psychologist, 8*, 126-142.

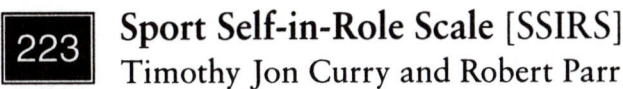

223 Sport Self-in-Role Scale [SSIRS]
Timothy Jon Curry and Robert Parr

Source: Curry, T. J., & Parr, R. (1988). Comparing commitment to sport and religion at a Christian college. *Sociology of Sport Journal, 5*, 369-377.

Purpose: To assess a college student's involvement in the sport role, particularly regarding agenda setting, decision making, and emotional involvement.

Description: The SSIRS contains 13 items. Participants are asked to respond on a 5-point Likert scale to items such as "During the week, I have made several decisions in which my sport involvement has influenced my decision," and "I often dream or daydream about sports."

Construction: Items were selected initially from Jackson's (1981) Social Identity Questionnaire. Five items were eliminated due to extreme response skewness. Three additional items were added that linked thought and identity to the sport role such as "Being an athlete is an important part of who I am."

Reliability: A Cronbach alpha internal consistency coefficient (n=348 male college students) of .92 was reported.

Validity: Concurrent validity was examined in which participants' (n=220) responses to the SSIRS correlated positively with their commitment to sport (r=.64), their enjoyment of sport role (r=.33), and their time spent in sport role (r=.55) (Curry & Weaner, 1987).

Norms: Not cited. Psychometric data were based on the responses of 348 students attending a small, private, church-affiliated institution close to Springfield, Ohio, as well as 220 male college students attending Ohio State University.

Availability: Contact Timothy Jon Curry, Department of Sociology, The Ohio State University, 375D Bricker Hall, 190 North Oval Mall, Columbus, OH 43210. (Phone # 614-292-7560; E-mail: tcurry@magnus.acs.ohio state.edu)

References
*Curry, T. J. (1993). The effects of receiving a college letter on the sport identity. *Sociology of Sport Journal, 10,* 73-87

*Curry, T. J., & Weaner, J. S. (1987). Sport identity salience, commitment, and the involvement of self in role: Measurement issues. *Sociology of Sport Journal, 4,* 280-288.

Curry, T. J., & Weiss, D. (1989). Sport identity and motivation for sport participation: A comparison between American college athletes and Austrian student sport club members. *Sociology of Sport Journal, 6,* 257-268.

Jackson, S. E. (1981). Measurement of commitment to role identities. *Journal of Personality and Social Psychology, 40,* 138-146.

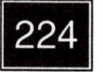 **224** ## Sport Situation Rigidity Test (SSRT)
A. Craig Fisher and Susan K. Borowicz

Source: Fisher, A. C., Borowicz, S. K., & Morris, H. H. (1978). Behavioral rigidity across sport situations. In D. M. Landers & R. W. Christina (Eds.), *Psychology of motor behavior and sport-1977* (pp.359-368). Champaign, IL: Human Kinetics Publishers.

Purpose: To assess an individual's resistance to change across a variety of athletic situations.

Description: The SSRT contains 16 sport situations varying in degree of difficulty of response. Respondents are directed to react to the decision of the coach in the situation (based on their personal coaching philosophy) using a 5-point Likert scale.

Construction: The SSRT was developed with the assistance of several male college coaches and a graduate sport psychology class to ensure that the situations were representative of real-life coaching experiences.

Reliability: Test-retest reliability coefficients ($n=56$ male undergraduate physical education majors) for the 16 sport situations ranged from .08 to .75.

Validity: Principal component factor analysis resulted in the retention of seven factors. (The reliability of situations loading on these factors ranged from .49 to .75.) There was no relationship between participants' ($n=56$) scores on the Test of Behavioral Rigidity and the SSRT, thus failing to support the concurrent validity of the SSRT.

Norms: Not cited. Psychometric data were reported for 56 undergraduate students noted above.

**Availability: Contact A. Craig Fisher, Department of Exercise and Sport Sciences, Ithaca College, Ithaca, NY 14850. (Phone # 607-274-3112; FAX # 607-274-1943; E-mail: cfisher@ithaca.edu)

 **225** ## *Sport Spectator Identification Scale [SSIS]
Daniel L. Wann and Nyla R. Branscombe

Source: Wann, D. L., & Branscombe, N. R. (1993). Sport fans: Measuring degree of identification with their team. *International Journal of Sport Psychology, 24,* 1-17.

Purpose: To assess "individual allegiance or identification with a sports team" (p. 3).

Description: The SSIS contains seven items. The items focus on the level of identification with the University of Kansas men's varsity basketball team (e.g., "How strongly do you see yourself as a fan of the Kansas University basketball team?"). Participants respond to each item using an 8-point ordinal scale.

Construction: Not discussed.

Reliability: Cronbach alpha internal consistency coefficients ($N=188$; $N=358$) of .91 and .93 were reported. A test-retest reliability coefficient ($n=49$) of .60 was reported across a one-year period.

Validity: Exploratory principal components factor analysis ($N=188$) yielded one factor accounting for 66.3% of the variance, thereby supporting the unidimensionality of the SSIS. In addition, individuals who most strongly identified with this basketball team reported more involvement with the team, displayed "a more ego-enhancing pattern of attributions for the team's success," had higher and more positive expectations for the teams' future performances, and were more committed to investing time and resources to watching the team perform.

Norms: Not cited. Psychometric data were reported for independent samples of undergraduate students (Sample 1= 75 males, 113 females; Sample 2= 175 males, 183 females) attending the University of Kansas.

**Availability: Contact Daniel L. Wann, Department of Psychology, Murray State University, 1 Murray Street, Murray, KY 42071-3311 (Phone # 502-762-2860; FAX # 502-762-3424; E-mail: danwann@msumusik. mursuky.edu). Items are also displayed in the *Source*.

References

*Wann, D. L. (1994). The "noble" sports fan: The relationship between team identification, self-esteem, and aggression. *Perceptual and Motor Skills, 78*, 864-866.

*Wann, D. L., & Dolan, T. J. (1994). Influence of spectators' identification on evaluation of the past, present, and future performance of a sports team. *Perceptual and Motor Skills, 78*, 547-552.

*Wann, D. L., Dolan, T. J., McGeorge, K. K., & Allison, J. A. (1994). Relationships between spectator identification and spectators' perceptions of influence, spectators' emotions, and competition outcome. *Journal of Sport & Exercise Psychology, 16*, 347-364.

226 *Sports Injury Clinic Athlete Satisfaction Scale (SICASS)

Sally May and Adrian Taylor

Source*: Taylor, A. H., & May, S. (1995). Development of a sports injury clinic athlete satisfaction scale for auditing patient perceptions. *Physiotherapy Theory and Practice, 11*, 231-238.

Purpose: To assess athletes' satisfaction with the care provided in a sports injury clinic.

Description: The SICASS contains 13 items reflecting satisfaction with three aspects of a consultation with a sports physiotherapist: (a) empathy (EMP), (b) information given (INFO), and (c) competence (COMP). Participants respond to each item using a 5-point Likert scale with the anchorings *strongly agree* to *strongly disagree*.

Construction: Following an extensive review of literature concerned with the evaluation of patient satisfaction, and also open-ended interviews with patients who had attended a sports injury clinic, a pool of 26 items was reworded from the Medical Interview Satisfaction Scale (Wolf, Putnam, James, & Stiles, 1978). Eight individuals with psychometric or sports physiotherapy expertise were then asked to check each item for clarity and place the items under the defined headings of cognitive, affective, and behavioral satisfaction. Sixteen items were retained. Exploratory factor analysis (see validity section) led to the retention of 13 items.

Reliability: Cronbach alpha reliability coefficients of .87 (EMP), .73 (INFO), and .73 (COMP) were reported.

Validity: The SICASS was given to 262 new patients attending one of five sports injury clinics in England; 160 completed responses were received. These participants' scores on the SIRCASS were subjected to exploratory factor analysis with varimax rotation resulting in the retention of a three-factor structure. Three items did not load on any single factor and were removed.

*Note: The first author listed in the *Source* prepared this test summary (A. Taylor, personal communication, April 12, 1996).

Norms: Not cited. Psychometric data were reported for 160 injured athletes (*M* age =32.9 years; *SD*= 11.6).

**Availability: Contact Adrian Taylor, Chelsea School Research Centre, University of Brighton, Gaudick Road, Eastbourne, East Sussex, England BN20 7SP. (Phone 01273-643743; FAX 01273-643704; E-mail: aht@bton.ac.uk)

Reference

Wolf, H. M., Putnam, S. M., James, S. A., & Stiles, W. B. (1978). The Medical Interview Satisfaction Scale (MISS): Development of a scale to measure patient perceptions of physician behavior. *Journal of Behavioral Medicine, 1,* 391-401.

227 [Sportsmanship Questionnaire] [SQ]
W. Wright and S. Rubin

Source: Wright, W., & Rubin, S. (1989). The development of sportsmanship [Abstract]. *Proceedings of the 7th World Congress in Sport Psychology* (p. 155). Singapore.

Purpose: To examine sportsmanship attitudes among athletes.

Description: The SQ contains 12 sport situations, each with a moral dilemma. Participants respond to each situation using a Likert scale.

Construction: Not discussed.

Reliability: Not presented.

Validity: Discriminant validity was supported in that females' sportsmanship was higher than that of males. Also, sportsmanship was higher among older individuals (21-22 years) than younger individuals (14-15 years old).

Norms: Not cited. Psychometric data were based on the responses of 54 athletes and 56 nonathletes ranging in age from 14 to 22 years.

Availability: Last known address: W. Wright, Department of Psychology, Whitman College, Walla Walla, WA.

228 State of Consciousness During Movement Activity Inventory (SCMAI)
Jane Adair

Source: Adair, J. (1987). Development of the State of Consciousness During Movement Activity (SCMAI) and its implications [Abstract]. *Proceedings of of the Association for the Advancement of Applied Sport Psychology annual conference* (p. 22). Newport Beach: CA.

Purpose: To describe the characteristics of states of consciousness that movement performers may experience during participation.

Description: The SCMAI contains two subscales: The Greatest Moment Scale (GMS) describing a Greatest Moment State of Consciousness, and the Worst Moment Scale (WMS) describing a Worst Moment State of Consciousness. Participants are asked to recall a greatest and worst moment from the same movement activity, and respond "to descriptions of phenomena available to consciousness." Participants respond using a 5-point Likert scale in which they are asked to rate the intensity of the experience.

Construction: Items were developed from a review of psychological and sport consciousness theory, practice, and current method of inquiry. In addition, four pilot studies were completed.

Reliability: Cronbach alpha reliability coefficients of .89 (GMS) and .88 (WMS) were reported; an alpha reliability coefficient of .92 was reported for the SCMAI. A test-retest reliability coefficient of .73 was reported ($n=60$).

Validity: The SCMAI was successful in discriminating between groups varying in skill level and intrinsic motivation and between worst and greatest moment states.

Norms: Not cited. The author noted (J. Adair, personal communication, June 8, 1996) that psychometric data were reported for 267 female and 153 male sport and dance participants enrolled in physical education, dance, and psychology classes.

Availability: Contact Jane Adair, Department of Physical Education & Kinesiology, California State University, 1250 Bellflower Boulevard Long Beach, CA 90815. (Phone 310-985-4086; FAX 310-985-8066).

229 *Success Orientation Questionnaire [SOQ]
P. C. Terry

Source: Terry, P. C. (1995). Development of an instrument for assessing the success criteria of tennis coaches [Abstract]. *Journal of Sports Sciences, 13, 77.*

Purpose: "...to assess how coaches judge their own success in tennis" (p. 77).

Description: The SOQ contains 40 items and 10 subscales: Systematic Organization; Competitive Success; Workrate and Discipline, Coaching Reputation, Player Fulfillment, Interpersonal Relationships, External Perceptions, Symbols of Success, Intrinsic Rewards, and Fun for Players.

Construction: The SOQ was developed based on input from the Lawn Tennis Association's Director of Coaching, and 12 Lawn Tennis Association registered professional coaches.

Reliability: Not indicated.

Validity: Exploratory principal components factor analysis ($N=169$) with varimax rotation led to a 10-factor solution accounting for 60.5% of the variance.

Norms: Not cited. Psychometric data were cited for 169 (109 males, 60 females) registered tennis coaches (M age= 37.6 years; SD= 12.8).

Availability: Contact P. C. Terry, Brunel University, Borough Road, Isleworth, Middlesex TW7 5DU, United Kingdom. (Phone # 0181 568 8741, ext. 2892; FAX # 0181 569 9198; E-mail: terry@wlihe.ac.uk)

230 [Superstitious Beliefs and Behavior Scale] [SBBS]
Hans G. Buhrmann, B. Brown, and Maxwell K. Zaugg

Source: Buhrmann, H., Brown, B., & Zaugg, M. (1982), Superstitious beliefs and behavior: A comparison of male and female basketball players. *Journal of Sport Behavior*, 5, 175-185.

Purpose: To examine superstitious beliefs and practices among athletes.

Description: The scale contains 40 items categorized into seven areas: clothing and appearance, fetish, pre-game, game, team ritual, prayer, and coach. Athletes respond to each item using a 5-point Likert scale.

Construction: Not discussed.

Reliability: A test-retest reliability coefficient of .95 was reported among 24 high school basketball players.

Validity: Not discussed.

Norms: Descriptive data were presented for 272 male and 257 female basketball players, ages 12-22.

Availability: Last known address: Hans G. Buhrmann, Department of Physical Education, University of Lethbridge, 4401 University Drive, Lethbridge, Alberta, Canada T1K 3M4.

Reference
*Buhrmann, H. G., & Zaugg, M. K. (1983). Religion and superstitions in the sport of basketball. *Journal of Sport Behavior*, 6, 146-157.

231 *Verrone Athletic Needs Survey (VANS)
Tracy Verrone

Source: Verrone, T. (1990). Sport psychology needs of college athletes [Abstract]. *Proceedings of the Third Southeast Sport and Exercise Psychology Symposium.* Greensboro, NC.

Purpose: To assess areas in which athletes express an interest in psychological assistance.

Description: The VANS contains 54 items and nine subscales: Injury, Aggression, Anxiety/Arousal, Goal Setting, Mental Preparation, Academic/Career, Self-Concept, Relationships, and Time Management.

Construction: A panel of experts ($N=17$) was used to establish content validity.

Reliability: The author reported moderate internal consistency coefficients ($N=129$) for each subscale.

Validity: Exploratory principal component factor analysis with varimax rotation failed to support the hypothesized nine subscales of the VANS ($N=129$).

Norms: Not available. Psychometric data were reported for 129 Division IA male or female college athletes.

Availability: Contact Tracy Verrone, 407 Diamond Avenue, Johnstown, PA 15905.

Chapter 18

Motivation (Exercise)

Tests in this chapter assess reasons for adherence to exercise and injury rehabilitation programs, commitment to exercise and running, perceived benefits/barriers to exercise participation, and the motives/incentives individuals express for participating in running and other forms of exercise. Tests also assess perceived exertion, feeling states that stem from exercising, negative addiction to exercise/running, and stages of exercise behavior change.

232 [Adherence to Exercise Questionnaire] [AEQ]
Donald Siegel, James Johnson, and Caryl Newhof

Source: Siegel, D., Johnson, J., & Newhof, C. (1987). Adherence to exercise and sport classes by college women. *Research Abstracts of the American Alliance for Health, Physical Education, Recreation, and Dance annual convention,* Las Vegas, NV.

Purpose: To assess reasons for adhering to exercise classes by women.

Description: A 20-item questionnaire.

Construction: Not indicated.

Reliability: A test-retest reliability coefficient of .75 was reported over a one-week period.

Validity: Discriminant validity was supported in that college women ($n=135$) who completed exercise classes differed on the questionnaire from those ($n=51$) who dropped out in terms of being more positive about developing and utilizing personal skills, using their minds in physical activity, and being involved in social interactions.

Norms: Not cited. Psychometric data were reported for 186 college women.

Availability: Contact Donald S. Siegel, Exercise and Sport Studies Department, Scott Gymnasium, Smith College, Northampton, MA 01063. (Phone 413-585-3977; E-mail: dsiegel@smith.edu)

233 Barriers to Exercise and Sport Questionnaire (BESQ)
Damon Burton, Tom Raedeke, and Earle Carroll

Source: Burton, D., Raedeke, T., & Carroll, E. (1989). Exercise goals, perceived barriers, and activity patterns of adult exercisers with differential athletic participation backgrounds [Abstract]. In *Psychology of motor behavior and sport* (p. 110). Kent, OH: Proceedings of the North American Society for the Psychology of Sport and Physical Activity annual convention.

Purpose: To assess the barriers individuals perceive regarding participating in exercise and sport.

Description: The BESQ (Form D) assesses nine barriers to exercise/sport participation including Program, Social Support, Resource, Club, Health, Other Commitments, Lethargy, Other Interests, and Program Satisfaction. Individuals respond to 32 items using a 4-point Likert scale.

Construction*: An initial pool of 51 items was developed by identifying barriers commonly reported in the exercise adherence literature. Three judges evaluated the items for syntax, clarity, and face validity resulting in the retention of 39 items (Form A). This form was administered to 112 former college athletes and college nonathletes. Item and factor analyses led to the retention of 21 items (Form B) representing five subscales. Then 18 new or reworded items were added to Form B to develop social support, resource, and other commitments barriers subscales as well as improve health/fitness and program satisfaction subscale items. This new 39-item version (Form C) was administered to 292 current and former adult members of faculty/staff wellness programs from three universities and a community college in the Northwest. Item analyses and factor analyses (exploratory and confirmatory) led to the retention of 32 items representing nine subscales, and this version was labeled Form D.

Reliability: Not indicated.

Validity: Confirmatory factor analysis ($n=292$) supported the construct validity of the BESQ. Also, former male collegiate athletes ($n=58$) differed from former high school athletes/nonathletes ($n=54$) in that the former group perceived health and fitness and motivation to be less of a barrier to participating in exercise than did the latter group. A median split of both groups based on current levels of physical activity participation revealed that the more active group perceived fewer programming, motivation, and ego barriers than did the less physically active group.

---

*Note: From Burton, Raedeke, and Carroll (1990)

Norms: Not indicated. Psychometric data were presented for 58 male former collegiate athletes and 54 high school athletes/ nonathletes, as well as 292 former adult members of faculty/staff wellness programs.

Availability: Contact Damon Burton, Department of Physical Education, 107 PEB, University of Idaho, Moscow, ID 83843 (Phone # 208-885-2186; FAX # 208-885-5929; E-mail: dburton@raven.csrv.uidaho.edu)

References

*Burton, D. (1992). Toward a personal investment model of exercise adherence: A replication and extension employing updated instrumentation [Abstract]. *Proceedings of the North American Society for the Psychology of Sport and Physical Activity annual convention* (p. 139). Pittsburgh, PA.

*Burton, D., Raedeke, T., & Carroll, E.(1990). *Predicting physical activity patterns of adult males with differential sport participation backgrounds.* Manuscript submitted for publication.

Raedeke, T., Burton, D., & Pierce, B. (1991). Examining ageand gender differences in adult exercise behavior: A personal investment perspective [Abstract]. *Proceedings of the North American Society for the Psychology of Sport and Physical Activity annual convention* (p. 189). Pacific Grove, CA.

*Children's Effort Rating Table (CERT)
John G. Williams and Roger G. Eston

Source: Williams, J. G., Eston, R. G., & Furlong, B. (1994). CERT: A perceived exertion scale for young children. *Perceptual and Motor Skills, 79,* 1451-1458.

Purpose: To assess perceptions of exercise effort among children.

Description: Children are asked to rate perceptions of exercise effort on an ordinal scale ranging from 1 (*Very, Very Easy*) to 10 (*So Hard I'm Going to Stop*).

Construction: The scale was developed so as to contain more developmentally appropriate verbal language for children and to better reflect the types of heart rates commonly found among children.

Reliability: An intraclass coefficient of 0.91 was reported (Lamb, 1996) among 9- and 10-year-old children.

Validity: Children's scores on CERT correlated positively with actual heart rate ($r=.76$) and work output ($r=.75$) (Eston, Lamb, Bain, Williams, & Williams, 1994).

Norms: Not cited. Psychometric data were reported for 16 preadolescent children ($n=8$ boys; $n=8$ girls; M age=10.0 years; SD=1.1), recruited from a primary school in Liverpool, England.

**Availability: Contact John G. Williams, Department of Kinesiology, West Chester University, West Chester, PA 19382. (Phone # 610-436-6119; E-mail: jwilliams@wcupa.edu)

References

*Eston, R. G., Lamb, K. L., Bain, A., Williams, A. M., & Williams, J. G. (1994). Validity of a perceived exertion scale for children. *Perceptual and Motor Skills, 78*, 691-97.

*Lamb, K. L. (1996). Children's ratings of effort during cycle ergometry: An examination of the validity of two effort rating scales: *Pediatric Exercise Science, 7*, 407-421.

*Williams, J. G., Furlong, B., Hockley, T. J., & MacKintosh,C. (1993). Rating and regulation of exercise intensity in young children [Abstract]. *Medicine and Science in Sports and Exercise, 25* (Suppl.), S8.

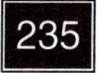

235 Commitment to Physical Activity Scale (CPA)

Charles B. Corbin, A. Brian Nielsen, Laura L. Bordsdorf and David R. Laurie

Source: Corbin, C. B., Nielsen, A. B., Bordsdorf, L. L., & Laurie, D. R.(1987). Commitment to physical activity. *International Journal of Sport Psychology, 18*, 215-222.

Purpose: To assess an individual's commitment to participating in physical activity.

Description: The CPA is a 12-item questionnaire designed to assess commitment to the broad domain of physical activity.

Construction: The CPA was modified from the Commitment to Running scale by substituting the term *physical activity* for the term *running*. Also, slight modifications were made in the wording of some items to make them more readable.

Reliability: Split-half reliabilities were .88 (n=238 males) and .91 (n=212 females). Test-retest reliability coefficients of .76 and .85 were reported for these male and female participants, respectively, across a one-week interval.

Validity: The CPA was successful in discriminating between individuals (n=450) who differed in self-report levels of involvement in physical activity.

Norms: Not cited. Psychometric data were reported for 450 undergraduate students.

Availability: Contact Charles B. Corbin, Department of Exercise Science and Physical Education, Arizona State University, Tempe, AZ 85287-0404. (Phone # 602-965-7652; FAX # 602-965-4716 or 602-965-8108; E-mail: c.b.corbin@asu.edu)

References

*Deeter, T. E. (1988). Does attitudinal commitment predict physical activity participation? *Journal of Sport Behavior, 11,* 177-192.

Deeter, T. E. (1990). Re-modeling expectancy and value in physical activity. *Journal of Sport & Exercise Psychology, 12,* 86-91.

Fung, L. (1992). Commitment to training among wheelchair marathon athletes. *International Journal of Sport Psychology, 23,* 138-139.

*Nielsen, A. B., Borsdorf, L. L., & Corbin, C. B. (1984). Commitment to general and specific physical activity. *Proceedings of the 1984 Olympic Scientific Congress* (p. 85). Eugene, OR: College of Human Development and Performance Microform Publications.

*Nielsen, A. B., Borsdorf, L. L., & Corbin, C. B. (1987). Attitude assessment and term variation in physical education [Abstract]. *Proceedings of the American Alliance for Health, Physical Education, Recreation, and Dance annual convention* (p. 86). Las Vegas, NV.

*Schuster, C. M., McCullagh, P., & Caird, J. K. (1990). Physical activity commitment in college students [Abstract]. *Proceedings of the Association for the Advancement of Applied Sport Psychology annual convention* (p. 107). San Antonio, TX

236 Commitment to Running Scale (CR)
Mary Ann Carmack and Rainer Martens

Source: Carmack, M. A., & Martens, R. (1979). Measuring commitment to running: A survey of runners' attitudes and mental states. *Journal of Sport Psychology, 1,* 25-42.

Purpose: To assess the feelings individuals have about running.

Description: The Commitment to Running (CR) Scale contains 12 items. Participants are asked to respond to each item using a 5-point Likert scale indicating the degree to which the item describes their feelings about running.

Construction: An initial pool of 30 items was developed by scanning the popular literature on running and interviewing local runners. Ten runners and five runner-research colleagues evaluated the content validity of each item. Item discrimination coefficients (n=180) were computed to evaluate the extent to which each item was sensitive to measuring both extremes of the disposition. The resulting analysis led to the retention of 12 items.

Reliability: A reliability coefficient of .93 was computed using analysis of variance. An internal consistency coefficient of .97 was derived using Kuder-Richardson formula 20. These coefficients were based on the responses of 315 runners. Secondary data are cited indicating a test-retest reliability coefficient (n=100 adult males) of .84 across a 2- to 3-month time interval.

Validity: Concurrent validity was supported by showing an association of participants' (n=315) CR scores to length of run, discomfort experienced when a run is missed, and perceived addiction to running. Also, high CR runners were differentiated from low CR runners in terms of the perceived benefits derived from running.

Norms: Descriptive and psychometric data are provided for 315 runners (250 males and 65 females) between the ages of 13 and 60 (M=28.8 years). The sample included runners from competitive road races, regular midday university runners, prospective 1980 Olympic distance and middle-distance runners, runners from a high school track camp, and those participating in community fun runs.

Availability: Contact Rainer Martens, Human Kinetics Publishers, P. O. Box 5076, 1607 North Market Street, Champaign, IL 61825-5076. (Phone # 217-351-5076; FAX # 217-351-2674; E-mail: rainer@hkusa.com)

383

References

Acevedo, E. O., Dzewaltowski, D. A., Gill, D. L., & Noble, J. M. (1992). Cognitive orientations of ultramarathoners. *The Sport Psychologist, 6,* 242-252.

*Chapman, C. L., & De Castro, J. M. (1990). Running addiction: measurement and associated psychological characteristics. *The Journal of Sports Medicine and Physical Fitness, 30,* 283-290.

*Conboy, J. K. (1994). The effects of exercise withdrawal on mood states in runners. *Journal of Sport Behavior, 17,* 188-203.

Dyer, J. B., & Crouch, J. G. (1987). Effects of running on moods: A time series study. *Perceptual and Motor Skills, 64,* 783-789

Feltz, D. L., Lirgg, C. D., & Albrecht, R. R. (1992). Psychological implications of competitive running in elite young distance runners: A longitudinal analysis. *The Sport Psychologist, 6,* 128-138.

Jibaja-Rusth, M. L., Pease, D., & Rudisill, M. (1989). The relationship of goal orientations to running motivation: Commitment and addiction [Abstract]. *Psychology of motor behavior and sport* (p. 140). Proceedings of the North American Society for the Psychology of Sport and Physical Activity annual convention. Kent, OH.

*Labbe, E. E., Welsh, M. C., Coldsmith, B., & Hickman, H. (1991). High school cross country runners: Running commitment, health locus of control and performance. *Journal of Sport Behavior, 14,* 85-91.

*Masters, K. S., & Lambert, M. J. (1989). On gender comparison and construct Validity: An examination of the Commitment to Running Scale in a sample of marathon runners. *Journal of Sport Behavior, 12,* 196-202.

Noble, J. M., Dzewaltowski, D. A., Acevado, E. D., & Gill, D. L. (1989). Sport-specific psychological characteristics and attributions of Leadville Trail 100 ultramarathoners [Abstract]. *Psychology of motor behavior and sport* (p. 147). Proceedings of the North American Society for the Psychology of Sport and Physical Activity annual convention. Kent, OH.

Summers, J. J., Machin, V. J., & Sargent, G. I. (1983). Psychosocial factors related to marathon running. *Journal of Sport Psychology, 5,* 314-331.

237 Exercise and Sport Goal Inventory (ESGI)
Damon Burton, Tom Raedeke, and Earle Carroll

Source: Burton, D., Raedeke, T., & Carroll, E. (1989). Exercise goals, perceived barriers, and activity patterns of adult exercisers with differential athletic participation backgrounds [Abstract]. In *Psychology of motor behavior and sport* (p. 110). Kent, OH: Proceedings of the North American Society for the Psychology of Sport and Physical Activity annual convention.

Purpose: To assess the goals individuals express toward the values of exercise and sport.

Description*: The ESGI (Form D) contains 66 items and assesses 10 exercise/sport goals including Health/Fitness, Performance, Involvement, Outcome, Recognition, Solitude, Social, Mental Health, Muscular Fitness, and "Feel Good." Individuals respond to each item using a 4-point Likert scale.

Construction*: A battery of 208 items was generated to assess eight exercise and sport incentives. This pool of items was derived by (a) using selected items from Duda and Tappe's (1989) Personal Incentives for Exercise Questionnaire, (b) modifying items from several goal inventories, and (c) composing items based on current exercise motivation research. Three judges rated the items for syntax, clarity, and face validity, leading to the retention of 156 items (Form A). Form A was administered to 112 former college athletes and 106 university wellness group members and community aerobic dance participants. Item analyses and factor analyses led to the retention of 72 items (Form B) containing six 12-item subscales. A total of 27 new items were added (Form C) to develop further solitude and involvement subscales and strengthen health/fitness and mental health subscales. This 99-item form was administered to 292 current and former adult members of faculty/staff wellness programs from three universities and a community college in the Northwest. Item analyses and factor analyses (exploratory and confirmatory) of these individuals' responses led to the retention of the current 66-item Form D.

Reliability: Not reported.

Validity: Confirmatory factor analysis ($n=292$) supported the construct validity of the ESGI. In addition, former collegiate male athletes ($n=58$) expressed significantly higher outcome, recognition, and social exercise goals than did former high school athletes/nonathletes ($n=54$). A median split, based on current physical activity participation, revealed that those individuals still highly active had higher performance and social goals and lower outcome goals than did those individuals categorized as less physically active.

Norms: Not presented. Psychometric data provided were based on the responses of 58 former male collegiate athletes and 54 former high school athletes/nonathletes, as well as 292 current and former adult members of faculty/staff wellness programs.

*From Burton, Raedeke, and Carroll (1990).

Availability: Contact Damon Burton, Department of Physical Education, 107 PEB, University of Idaho, Moscow, ID 83843. (Phone # 208-885-2186; FAX # 208-885-5929; E-mail: dburton@raven.csrv.uidaho.edu)

References

*Burton, D. (1992). Toward a personal investment model of exercise adherence: A replication and extension employing updated instrumentation [Abstract]. *Proceedings of the North American Society for the Psychology of Sport and Physical Activity annual convention* (p. 139). Pittsburgh, PA.

Burton, D., Raedeke, T., & Carroll, E. (1990). *Predicting physical activity patterns of adult males with differential sport participation backgrounds.* Manuscript submitted for publication.

Raedeke, T., Burton, D., & Pierce, B. (1991). Examining age and gender differences in adult exercise behavior: A personal investment perspective [Abstract]. *Proceedings of the North American Society for the Psychology of Sport and Physical Activity annual convention* (p. 189). Pacific Grove, CA.

*Exercise Benefits/Barriers Scale (EBBS)
Karen R. Sechrist, Susan Noble Walker, and Nola J. Pender

Source: Sechrist, K. R., Walker, S. N., & Pender, N. J. (1987). Development and psychometric evaluation of the Exercise Benefits/Barriers Scale. *Research in Nursing & Health, 10,* 357-365.

Purpose: "...to measure perceived benefits of and perceived barriers to exercise" (p. 358).

Description: The EBBS contains 43 items and two scales: a 29-item Benefits scale (e.g., "feel relaxed" and "self-concept improved") and a 14 item Barriers scale (e.g., "exercise is hard work" and "family not encouraging"). Individuals respond to each item on the benefits scale using a 4-point Likert scale with the anchorings 1 (*strongly disagree*) to 4 (*strongly agree*). Items on the barriers scale are reverse scored.

Construction: Items were developed primarily from an interview study. One adult in each of 100 randomly selected households in a midwestern community was interviewed to determine his or her beliefs concerning the positive and negative outcomes of controlling weight, managing stress, and exercising regularly. Responses by these individuals to the exercise domain were evaluated for appropriateness as items for inclusion in the initial EBBS. In addition, items were derived from a review of the literature on perceived benefits/barriers to exercise.

A total of 65 items (45 perceived benefits; 20 perceived barriers) were administered to 664 adults, of which the responses of 650 adults to the instrument were used. Item analysis and exploratory factor analysis led to the retention of the 43-item EBBS.

Reliability: Cronbach alpha internal consistency coefficients (N=650) were .96, .87, and .95 for the Benefits scale, Barriers scale, and the entire instrument, respectively. Test-retest reliability coefficients across a 2-week interval computed on an independent sample of 63 adults recruited from the community were .89, .77, and .89 for the Benefits scale, Barriers scale, and the entire instrument, respectively.

Validity: An exploratory principal components factor analysis (varimax rotation) yielded a nine-factor solution accounting for 64.9% of the variance. Five of the factors were identified as benefits factors (e.g., Life Enhancement), and the remaining factors were barrier factors (e.g., Time Expenditure).

Norms: Not cited. Psychometric and descriptive statistics were presented for 650 adults (M age= 38.7 years) of which females composed 60% of the sample.

Availability: Last known address: Karen R. Sechrist, School of Nursing, Northern Illinois University, DeKalb, IL 60115.

Reference

DeVoe, D., Kennedy, C., Harman-Anderson, J. K., & Zimmerman, T. (1995). Home schooling: An assessment of parental attitudes toward exercise and child activity levels. *Physical Educator, 52,* 134-139.

239 [Exercise Motivation Questionnaire] [EMQ]
David A. Dzewaltowski

Source: Dzewaltowski, D. A. (1989). Toward a model of exercise motivation. *Journal of Sport & Exercise Psychology, 11,* 251-269.

Purpose: To assess exercise motivation, based on the theory of reasoned action and social cognitive theory.

Description: The questionnaire assesses self-efficacy and outcome expectations in relation to exercise behavior. For example, self-efficacy scores represented an average of participants' confidence (from 0 to 100) in adhering to an exercise program in spite of their work schedule, when fatigued physically, or when exercise is boring. The questionnaire also assesses constructs from the theory of reasoned action, such as behavioral intention and subjective norm.

Construction: Not discussed.

Reliability: Alpha reliability coefficients (n=328 undergraduate students) ranged from .80 to .97 for all constructs.

Validity: Multiple regression analysis indicated that the social cognitive theory constructs accounted for 14% of the variance in predicting exercise behavior. Attitude and subjective norm accounted for 20% of the variance in behavioral intention using path analysis. Commonality analysis indicated that the theory of reasoned action constructs did not accounted for any unique variance in exercise behavior over the constructs from social cognitive theory.

Norms: Not reported. Psychometric data were cited for 328 undergraduate students.

**Availability: Contact David A. Dzewaltowski, Department of Kinesiology, 8 Natatorium, Kansas State University, Manhattan, KS 66506-0302. (Phone # 913-532-0708; FAX # 913-532-6486; E-mail: dadx@ksu.ksu.edu)

References

Ermler, K. L., Kovar, S. K., & Reinders. S. M. (1993). The effect of three different lifetime fitness class structures on various fitness parameters of college students. *The Physical Educator, 50,* 52-56.

Yordy, G. A., & Lent, R. W. (1993). Predicting aerobic exercise participation: Social cognitive, reasoned action, and planned behavioral models. *Journal of Sport & Exercise Psychology, 15,* 363-374.

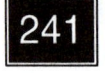

*Exercise Motivation Questionnaire (EMQ)
John M. Silva, Allen Cornelius, and Ellen Carpenter

Source: Silva, J. M., Cornelius, A., & Carpenter, E. (1992). Motive structures for engaging in regular exercise [Abstract]. *Proceedings of the Association for the Advancement of Applied Sport Psychology* (p. 95). Colorado Springs, CO.

Purpose: To examine individuals' motivation structure for participating in regular exercise.

Description: The EMQ contains three subscales: Motivational Orientation (RMSS), Extrinsic Motivation (EMSS), and Intrinsic Motivation (IMSS).

Construction: Not discussed.

Reliability: Cronbach alpha internal consistency coefficients of .77 (RMSS), .66 (IMSS), and .82 (EMSS) were reported for 154 individuals.

Validity: Not discussed.

Norms: Not cited. Psychometric data were reported for 88 males and 66 females who participated in a variety of exercise settings.

Availability: Contact John M. Silva, Department of Physical Education, 203 Fetzer Gymnasium, CB #8700, University of North Carolina, Chapel Hill, NC 27599-8700. (Phone # 919-962-5176; FAX # 919-962-0489; E-mail: usilva@uncmvs.oit.unc.edu)

*Exercise Motivations Inventory (EMI)
David Markland and Lew Hardy

Source: Markland, D., & Hardy, L. (1993). The Exercise Motivations Inventory: Preliminary development and validity of a measure of individual's reasons for participation in regular physical exercise. *Personality & Individual Differences, 15*, 289-296.

Purpose: To assess individuals' participation motives for exercise.

Description: The EMI is a 44-item inventory containing 12 subscales: Stress Management, Weight Management, Re-creation, Social Recognition, Enjoyment, Appearance, Personal Development, Affiliation, Ill-Health Avoidance, Competition, Fitness, and Health Pressures. For each item, participants respond to the stem "Personally, I exercise..." using a 6-point ordinal scale with the anchorings 0 (*not at all true for me*) to 5 (*very true for me*).

Construction: Items were generated from an examination of the literature on exercise adherence and from participants' (*N*=76) responses to an open ended questionnaire in which they were asked to state the three main reasons why they exercised. Items were also borrowed from the Personal Incentives for Exercise Questionnaire (Duda & Tappe, 1989). A total of 76 items were then evaluated by 5 individuals with expertise in exercise psychology, motivational psychology, and test construction; the items were evaluated for clarity, lack of ambiguity, content validity,and ease of understanding. Participants' (*N*=249) responses to the 71 items retained were subjected to exploratory principal components factor analysis with varimax rotation. Following elimination of low-loading and ambiguously loading items, a second principal components factor analysis (equamax rotation) yielded 12 factors accounting for 69.40% of the variance. Following an examination of internal consistency, the EMI was reduced to 44 items with 12 subscales comprising 2-6 items each.

Reliability: Cronbach alpha reliability coefficients (*N*=249) ranged from .63 to .92 for the 12 subscales. Test-retest reliability coefficients (*n*=57) ranged from .59 to .88 across a 4- to 5-week interval.

Validity: The authors reported previously (Markland & Hardy, 1991) that the discriminant validity of the EMI was supported; gender, age, and type of exercise involvement (i.e., competitive versus noncompetitive activities) mediated participants' responses to the EMI. Furthermore, the authors reported that participants' scores on the Enjoyment and Re-creation subscales of the EMI were significantly related to a measure of intrinsic motivation for exercise.

The first author (D. Markland, personal communication, March 27, 1996) provided additional information as follows about the validity of

390

the EMI. Markland, Ingledew, Hardy, and Grant (1992) found that the Re-creation, Enjoyment, Fitness, Personal Development, Affiliation, and Stress Management subscales successfully discriminated between female members of community-based aerobics classes and members of a Weight Watchers group taking part in aerobics as part of the weight reduction programme. In an interesting study by Ingledew, Hardy and de Sousa (1995), Weight Management subscale scores were differentially predicted amongst males and females by body mass index and body shape dissatisfaction.

Norms: Not cited. Psychometric data were reported for 249 individuals including 115 female participants in aerobics classes (*M* age=35.60 years, *SD*=14.84); 91 undergraduate students (*M* age=21.21 years, *SD*=3.65; 35%=female, 65%=male); and 43 members of local sport clubs (*M* age=25.39 years, *SD*=11.38; 81%=male, 19%=female).

**Availability: Contact David Markland, Division of Health and Human Performance, University of Wales, Bangor Gwynedd, United Kingdom LL57 2EN. (Phone # 01248-382756; FAX # 01248-371053; E-mail: pes004@bangor.ac.uk)

References
*Ersen, E., & Fazey, J. A. (1992). Motivation for exercise participation in Turkey: Using English-derived factors [Abstract]. *Journal of Sports Sciences, 10,* 603.

*Ingledew, D. K., Hardy, L., & de Sousa, K. (1995). Body shape dissatisfaction and exercise motivations [Abstract]. *Journal of Sports Sciences, 13,* 60.

*Markland, D., & Hardy, L. (1991). The development of the Exercise Motivations Inventory: A measure of individuals' reasons for participating in physical activity [Abstract]. *Journal of Sports Sciences, 9,* 445.

*Markland, D., Ingledew, D. K., Hardy, L., & Grant, L.(1992). A comparison of exercise motivations of participants in aerobics and Weight Watcher exercisers [Abstract]. *Journal of Sports Sciences, 10,* 609-610.

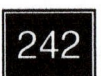 # *Exercise-Induced Feeling Inventory (EFI)
Lise Gauvin and W. Jack Rejeski

Source: Gauvin, L., & Rejeski, W. J. (1993). The Exercise-induced Feeling Inventory: Development and initial validation. *Journal of Sport & Exercise Psychology, 15,* 403-423.

Purpose: "...to assess feeling states that occur in conjunction with acute bouts of physical activity" (p. 403).

Description: The EFI uses 12 adjectives (3 adjectives/state) to assess four distinct feeling states: Revitalization, Tranquility, Positive Engagement, and Physical Exhaustion. Participants respond to each adjective (e.g., calm, worn-out, upbeat) using a 5-point ordinal scale with the anchorings 0 (*do not feel*) to 4 (*feel very strongly*).

Construction: The authors felt that responses to one-word adjectives rather than to sentences or lengthy statements was more appropriate in order to assess participants' self-ratings of the intensity of feeling states during acute exercise. Thus, an initial item pool of over 500 adjectives was derived from an affective lexicon and from previous self report instruments. Three experts in exercise psychology then evaluated the items in terms of relevance to participation in acute exercise. A total of 133 items were retained, and 12 additional items were added based on the recommendations of these experts.

In addition, 77 college students who exercised regularly evaluated each adjective to determine the extent to which these words captured their feelings during acute exercise. All 145 adjectives were retained based on the responses of these subjects.

Items were then grouped by the authors into 15 conceptually homogeneous categories, of which the first 8 clusters were retained for further analyses. These clusters were seen as "... directly related to the stimulus properties of exercise" (p. 407). A total of 24 adjectives were identified as most relevant to these clusters. Preliminary factor analysis, an analysis of linguistic redundancy, and comments from participants led the authors to conclude that these eight clusters could be adequately represented by four clusters (Revitalization, Tranquility, Positive Engagement, and Physical Exhaustion), each containing three adjectives.

Of the 12 items, 6 have appeared in previous self-report questionnaires. However, none of the subscales of the EFI duplicate the subscales of these previous questionnaires.

A principal components factor analysis (varimax rotation) evaluated the factor structure of the EFI based on the responses of 256 university students. These participants were asked to rate their feelings to acute exercise while seated in a classroom prior to exercise. The resulting analyses (in which two solutions were examined) indicated support for

Physical Exhaustion and Tranquility factors, but distinct overlap for the Revitalization and Positive Engagement factors.

However, confirmatory factor analysis using structural equation modeling of participants' ($N=154$) responses to the EFI following an acute bout of exercise lent support to the four-factor a priori model. Intercorrelation coefficients were computed across participants' responses to the four subscales, and, although statistically significant, were low.

Reliability: Cronbach alpha internal consistency coefficients ($N=256$; $N=154$) were .87 and .78 (Revitalizaiton); .91 and .80 (Physical Exhaustion); .82 and .72 (Tranquility); and .82 and .74 (Positive Engagement).

Validity: The convergent validity of the EFI was supported in that individuals' ($n=115$) responses to the Revitalization and Positive Engagement subscales were correlated positively with their scores on the Positive Affect subscale of the Positive Affect Negative Affect Schedule (PANAS); also, their responses to the Revitalization subscale correlated positively with the Energy subscale of the Activation Deactivation Adjective Check List (AD-ACL). In addition, their responses to the Revitalization and Physical Exhaustion subscales correlated with the Tiredness subscale of the AD-ACL.

The construct validity of the EFI was further supported in that participants' responses were influenced by the social context of different exercise interventions. Scores on Positive Engagement and Revitalization were higher following exercise in a real-world group setting than in an isolated, laboratory setting. Also, participants' scores on Tranquility were higher in the laboratory exercise setting than were evident in a classroom prior to exercise.

Norms: Not cited. Psychometric data were reported for samples of 256 students (50% female; M age=19.07 years, $SD=1.74$) attending a large university located in the southeastern United States, 154 students (88% female; M age= 28.03 years, $SD=7.61$) attending a large university in eastern Canada who participated in different exercise classes, and 40 female students (M age=18.31 years, $SD=0.86$) attending a university in the southeastern portion of the United States.

Availability: Contact Lise Gauvin, Department of Exercise Science,

Concordia University, 7141 Sherbrooke Street West, DA 208, Montreal, Quebec, Canada H4B 1R6. (Phone # 514-848-3321; E-mail: gauvinl@vax2.concordia.ca)

References

*Bozoian, S., Rejeski, W. J., & McAuley, E. (1994). Self-efficacy influences feeling states associated with acute exercise. *Journal of Sport & Exercise Psychology, 16*, 326-333.

*Gauvin, L., & Rejeski, W. J. (1994). Exploring fluctuations in exercise-induced feeling states in a community sample of women [Abstract]. *Journal of Sport & Exercise Psychology, 16* (Suppl.), S13.

*Rejeski, W. J., Gauvin, L., & Brawley, L. R. (1994). Symposium: The study of exercise-induced feeling states [Abstract]. *Journal of Sport & Exercise Psychology, 16* (Suppl.), S12-S14.

*Rejeski, W. J., & Gauvin, L. (1994). Dose of exercise and in-task feeling states mediate pre- to post changes in exercise-induced feeling states [Abstract]. *Journal of Sport & Exercise Psychology, 16* (Suppl.), S14.

*Vlachopoulos, S., & Biddle, S. (1995). Attributions and goal orientations as predictors of feelings, expectancy and intrinsic motivation after fitness testing with children [Abstract]. *Journal of Sports Science, 13,* 79.

*[Expected Outcomes and Barriers for Habitual Physical Activity Scales] [EOBHPAS]

Mary A. Steinhardt and Rod K. Dishman

Source: Steinhardt, M. A., & Dishman, R. K. (1989). Reliability and validity of expected outcomes and barriers for habitual physical activity. *Journal of Occupational Medicine, 31,* 536-546.

Purpose: To measure outcome-expectancy values and perceived barriers for physical activity.

Description: A total of 12 items address expected outcomes for participating in physical activity (e.g, "A major benefit of physical activity for me is good health"). Fourteen items address barriers to engaging in physical activity (e.g., "The major reason when I do not exercise is that it is too inconvenient"). Participants respond to each item using a 5-point Likert scale with the anchorings 1 (*strongly disagree*) to 5 (*strongly agree*).

A slightly longer version of this instrument was developed for research with employees of CONOCO World Headquarters.

Construction: Items were derived from epidemiology studies of physical activity patterns in North America and from the literature on supervised exercise programs.

Reliability: Cronbach alpha internal consistency coefficients ($N=243$) for derived (via factor analysis) Psychologic, Body Image, and Health benefits factors were .70, .72, and .78. Test-retest reliability coefficients ($N=75$), computed across a 2-month interval, were .81, .89, and .66 for these factors, respectively. Similarly, for the derived barriers factors of Time, Effort, and Obstacles, the reported alpha coefficients were .78, .73, and .47, respectively. Test-retest reliability coefficients were .74, .73, and .70, respectively.

Validity: Exploratory principal components factor analysis (with orthogonal rotation) produced three benefits factors (Psychologic, Body Image, and Health) accounting for 60.7% of the variance and three barriers factors (Time, Effort, and Obstacles) accounting for 48% of the variance. Using multiple regression analysis, these subscales significantly predicted supervised running and free-living physical activity (estimated by 7-day recall at 2-, 5-, and 9-week intervals).

The slightly longer version of this instrument, administered to employees at CONOCO World Headquarters, led to the findings that participants' responses were related to membership and participation in on-site health and fitness programs.

Norms: Not cited. Psychometric and descriptive statistics were reported for two independent samples ($n=80$; $n=163$) of college students enrolled in two sections of a jogging course and a health-related concepts and physical activity course at the University of Georgia. In addition, 968 employees (M age=38.54, SD=11.32) of CONOCO World Headquarters in Houston, Texas, were evaluated on the longer version of the instrument. A total of 606 of these individuals participated in the on site health and fitness program, and 362 were nonparticipants.

**Availability: Contact Mary A. Steinhardt, Department of Kinesiology and Health Education, University of Texas, Austin, TX 78712. (Phone # 512-471-4405; FAX # 512-471-8914; E-mail: marysteinhardt @mail.utexas.edu)

244 Feeling Scale (FS)
W. Jack Rejeski

Source: Hardy, C. J., & Rejeski, W. J. (1989). Not what, but how one feels: The measurement of affect during exercise. *Journal of Sport & Exercise Psychology, 11,* 304-317.

Purpose: To measure affective feelings of pleasure/displeasure toward a given exercise workload.

Description: The scale is represented by a 11-point bipolar good-bad format. Scores ranged from +5 to -5, with verbal anchors provided at the 0 point and at all odd integers. Respondents are asked to indicate how good or bad they feel during various phases of an exercise bout.

Construction: Not discussed.

Reliability: Internal consistency coefficients for this state measure were not reported.

Validity: Concurrent validity was supported in that participants' (n=68 undergraduate students) FS scores were inversely related (-.56) to their scores on Borg's Ratings of Perceived Exertion Scale, although the authors concluded that that the scores were not isomorphic constructs, particularly at high-intensity work. Furthermore, the authors reported that "... FS ratings were directly related to past and present level of involvement in physical exercise/activity, the number of miles spent in aerobic activity, and the belief that exercise is an important component of one's lifestyle" (p. 310).

Norms: Not cited. Psychometric data were reported for 33 females and 35 males enrolled in health and fitness courses at a southeastern university.

Availability: Contact W. Jack Rejeski, Department of Health and Sport Science, Wake Forest University, Campus Box 7234, 309 Gymnasium, Winston-Salem, NC 27109. (Phone # 919-759-5837; E-mail: rejeski@wfu.edu)

References

*Acevedo, E. O. (1992). Concurrent validity of the Feeling Scale [Abstract]. *Proceedings of the Association for the Advancement of Applied Sport Psychology annual convention* (p. 1). Colorado Springs, CO.

*Acevedo, E. O. (1994). Perceived exertion and affect at varying intensities of running. *Research Quarterly for Exercise and Sport, 65*, 372-376.

*Boutcher, S. H., McAuley, E., & Courneya, K. S. (1992). Positive and negative affective response of trained and untrained subjects during and after exercise [Abstract]. *Proceedings of the North American Society for the Psychology of Sport and Physical Activity annual convention* (p. 135). Pittsburgh, PA.

Boutcher, S. H., & Trenske, M. (1990). The effects of sensory deprivation and music on perceived exertion and affect during exercise. *Journal of Sport & Exercise Psychology, 12*, 167-176.

*Caruso, C. M., Morgan, D. W., & Crews, D. J. (1991). Thoughts, feelings, and RPEs during a prolonged maximal run [Abstract]. *Proceedings of the North American Society for the Psychology of Sport and Physical Activity annual convention* (p. 146). Pacific Grove, CA.

Hardy, C. J., Kirschenbaum, D. S., Heaney, T., & Imhoff, L.R. (1989). Affect as an antecedent variable in exercise behavior: The consequences of pre-exercise affective states [Abstract]. In *Psychology of motor behavior and sport* (p. 87). Kent, OH: Proceedings of the North American Society for the Psychology of Sport and Physical Activity annual convention.

*Kenney, E. A., Rejeski, W. J., & Messier, S. P. (1987). Managing exercise distress: The effect of broad spectrum intervention on affect, RPE, and running efficiency. *Canadian Journal of Sport Sciences, 12*, 97-105.

*McAuley, E., & Courneya, K. (1990). Efficacy, metabolic, and affective perceptions during exercise [Abstract]. *Proceedings of the Association for the Advancement of Applied Sport Psychology annual convention* (p. 75). San Antonio, TX.

*Noble, J. M., McCullagh, P., & Byrnes, W. C. (1993). Perceived exertion and Feeling Scale ratings before and after six months of aerobic exercise training [Abstract]. *Journal of Sport & Exercise Psychology, 15* (Suppl.).

*Parfitt, G., & Bowey, J. (1995). The effect of training on the rating of perceived exertion and psychological affect [Abstract]. *Journal of Sports Science, 13*, 70-71.

*Parfitt, G., & Eston, R. (1995). Changes in ratings of perceived exertion and psychological affect in the early stages of exercise. *Perceptual and Motor Skills, 80*, 259-266.

Parfitt, G., Holmes, C., & Markland, D. (1992). The interpretation of physical exertion in exercisers and non-exercisers [Abstract]. *Journal of Sports Sciences, 10*, 619-620.

*Parfitt, G., Markland, D., & Holmes, C. (1994). Responses to physical exertion in active and inactive males and females. *Journal of Sport & Exercise Psychology, 16*, 178-186.

Rejeski, W. J. (1989). The measurement of in-task affect during exercise related tasks [Abstract]. In *Psychology of motor behavior and sport* (p. 86). Kent, OH: Proceedings of the North American Society for the Psychology of Sport and Physical Activity annual convention.

*Rejeski, W. J., Best, D., Griffith, P., & Kenney, E. (1987). Sex-role orientation and the responses of men to exercise stress. *Research Quarterly, 58*, 260-264.

Rejeski, W. J., Hardy, C. J., & Shaw, J. (1991). Psychometric confounds of assessing state anxiety in conjunction with acute bouts of exercise. *Journal of Sport & Exercise Psychology, 13*, 65-74.

 General Affect Scale [GAS]
Shirley A. Hochstetler, W. Jack Rejeski, and
Deborah L. Best

Source: Hochstetler, S. A., Rejeski, W. J., & Best, D. L. (1985). The influence of sex-role orientation on ratings of perceived exertion. *Sex Roles,* *12,* 825-835.

Purpose: To assess feelings of comfort and confidence prior to treadmill exercise.

Description: The GAS consists of 13 bipolar adjectives arranged on a 7-point Likert scale (e.g., tense-relaxed, positive-negative, good-bad).

Construction: Not discussed.

Reliability: A Cronbach alpha internal consistency coefficient of .96 was reported among 33 females.

Validity: Not discussed.

Norms: Not cited. Psychometric data were based on the responses of 33 female undergraduate students from Wake Forest University, Winston-Salem, North Carolina.

Availability: Contact W. Jack Rejeski, Department of Health and Sport Science, Campus Box 7234, 309 Gymnasium, Wake Forest University, Winston-Salem, NC 27109. (Phone # 919-759-5837; E-mail: rejeski@wfu.edu)

246 *[Health Belief Model Questionnaire] [HBMQ]
Bert Hayslip, Daniel Weigand, Robert Weinberg,
Peggy Richardson, and Allen Jackson

Source: Hayslip, B., Weigand, D., Weinberg, R., Richardson, P., & Jackson, A. (in press). The development of new scales for the assess-

398

ment of Health Belief Model constructs in adulthood. *Journal of Aging and Physical Activity.*

Purpose: To assess among younger and older adults various constructs of the Health Belief Model related to exercise participation and adherence.

Description: The HBMQ contains five scales: (a) perceived susceptibility to serious health problems (16 items); (b) expected benefits of exercise (13 items); (c) barriers to exercise (17 items); (d) significant others in support of exercise (11 items); and (e) cues to action (12 items). Participants' responses to all items are assessed using 5-point Likert type scales.

Construction: Items were developed based on a review of the literature on aging and physical activity.

Reliability: Cronbach alpha reliability coefficients, with two exceptions, were above .80 for both a sample of 86 younger adults and a sample of 58 older adults. Alpha coefficients for the five HBM scales, for the younger and older samples, respectively, were (a) Susceptibility to Health Problems (.88, .92); Benefits of Exercise (.90, .87); Barriers to Exercise (.81, .79); Social Support From Others (.77, .85); Cues to Action (.87, .88). For both samples combined, alpha reliabilities were .90 (Susceptibility to Health Problems); .89 (Benefits of Exercise); .80 (Barriers to Exercise); .80 (Social Support From Others); and .87 (Cues to Action).

Validity: Discriminant validity was supported in that the older adult sample, when compared to the younger adult sample, reported fewer cues to exercise, less social support for exercise, but perceived fewer barriers to exercise. Further, individuals who reported having participated in more diverse fitness-related activities in the past perceived greater benefits of such activities, reported more cues to action, and greater support from others to engage in exercise. Persons who reported having participated in either more diverse sport-related or pleasure-related activities perceived more barriers to exercise and more support from others for exercise

Norms: Not cited. Psychometric data were reported for 86 younger adults (*M* age= 21.5 years; *SD*= 2.4), of which 56 were female participants, and 58 community-residing older adults (*M* age=71.8 years; *SD*=6.4 years), of which 38 were female participants.

**Availability: Contact Bert Hayslip, Jr., Department of Psychology, University North Texas, P. O. Box 13587 Unt Station, Denton, TX 76203. (Phone # 817-565-2675; FAX # 817-565-4682; E-mail: fc13@vm.acs.unt.edu)

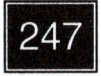 **[Motivation for Participation in Physical Activity Questionnaire] [MPPAQ]**
B. C. Watkin

Source: Watkin, B. C. (1978). Measurement of motivation for participation in physical activity. In U. Simri (Ed.), *Proceedings of the International Symposium on Psychological Assessment in Sport* (pp.188-194). Netanya, Israel: Wingate Institute for Physical Education and Sport.

Purpose: To assess the motives individuals express for participating in physical activity.

Description: The questionnaire contains 19 motivators for participation in physical activity. Individuals respond to each motivator using a 4-point Likert scale.

Construction: Previous attitudinal inventories (such as the Attitudes Toward Physical Activity Inventory), together with discussion with students and colleagues, led to the selection of 14 motivator items. Based on the responses of 181 male and female Grade 10 students in Brisbane, Australia, 7 motivator items were retained. Consequently, a revised questionnaire containing a more extensive list of 19 motivators was developed and tested.

Reliability: Test-retest reliability coefficients for a derived composite motivation score were .74 (*n*=30 male undergraduate students) and .80 (*n*=30 female undergraduate students) across a 7-week interval.

Validity: The total number of hours spent participating in physical activity the previous week was correlated with the composite motivation score, .50 (n=80 male undergraduate students) and .63 (n=158 female undergraduate students). Furthermore, scores on this questionnaire successfully discriminated between undergraduate students electing or not electing to participate in physical education classes.

Norms: Not cited. Psychometric data were provided for 80 male and 158 female freshman students enrolled at Wollongong Institute of Education in Australia.

Availability: Last known address: B. C. Watkin, Department of Human Movement and Sport Science, Institute of Education, University of Wollongong, Wollongong, NSW, Australia 2500.

 Motivation for Physical Activity Questionnaire [MPAQ]
Risto Telama and Martti Silvennoinen

Source: Telama, R., & Silvennoinen, M. (1979). Structure and development of 11- to 19-year-olds' motivation for physical activity. *Scandinavian Journal of Sports Science, 1,* 23-31.

Purpose: To assess the reasons young adults participate in physical exercise and leisure-time physical activity.

Description: The MPAQ contains 33 items focusing on the conscious reflection of physical activity interests, the advance planning of physical activities, and the influence of weather and friends on one's own physical activities. Individuals respond using a 3-point ordinal scale.

Construction: Previous empirical research on motivation for physical activity was drawn upon in constructing the items and measurement methods.

Reliability: Not discussed.

Validity: Principal component factor analysis (n=3,106) followed by varimax rotation supported an eight-factor solution accounting for

23.0% of the variance. The factors were labeled as Fitness Related to Self-Image, Relaxation, Sociability, Preference For Outdoor Activities, Normative Health, Competition and Achievement, Improving One's Physique, and Functional Health.

Norms: Not cited. Psychometric data were reported for 3,106 students residing in Finland. These students were selected through stratified random cluster sampling and represented grades 2-3, 5-6 and 8-9.

Availability: Contact Risto Telama, Department of Physical Education, University of Jyvaskyla, PL 35, SF-40351, Jyvaskyla 10, Finland. (Phone # +358 4160 2115; FAX # +358 4160 2101; E-mail: telama@pallo.jyu.fi)

Motivations of Marathoners Scales (MOMS)
Kevin S. Masters, Benjamin M. Ogles, and Jeffrey A. Jolton

Source: Masters, K. S., Ogles, B. M., & Jolton, J. A. (1993). The development of an instrument to measure motivation for marathon running: The Motivations of Marathoners Scales (MOMS). *Research Quarterly for Exercise and Sport, 64,* 134-143.

Purpose: To identify " ...and measure the motivations of marathon runners as they pertain to training and running a marathon" (p. 135).

Description: The MOMS contains 56 items. Subscales include Life Meaning, Psychological Coping, Self-esteem, Health Orientation, Weight Concern, Personal Goal Achievement, Competition, Affiliation, and Recognition/Approval. Marathon runners are asked to respond to each item in terms of how important it is as a reason for why they trained for and ran a marathon (e.g., "To improve my self-esteem"). Participants respond to each item on a 7-point ordinal scale with the anchorings 1 (*not a reason*) to 7 (*a most important reason*).

Construction: Four general reasons for running were derived from a review of the literature: psychological, physical, social, and achievement. Nine specific reasons (e.g., "maintaining or enhancing self-esteem") were catalogued under these four categories. A total of 120 reasons for running a marathon were included on the initial 9-scale MOMS. These items were submitted to 12 local marathon runners, some of whom had graduate training in psychometrics and/or sport psychology. They were asked to add reasons that were not included and to otherwise evaluate the instrument. As a result of their comments, the instrument was reduced to 96 questions by deleting items very similar in content and by rewording some items.

The responses to this version among 387 male and 95 female participants at three midwestern marathons were evaluated. Items with corrected item-to-total score correlations above .60 on each scale were selected to constitute the final version of the instrument. A total of 56 items were retained.

Reliability: Coefficient alpha internal consistency coefficients ($N=482$) ranged from .80 to .92. For a second sample ($N=712$) of marathon runners, alpha coefficients ranged from .80 to .93.

A total of 113 participants (drawn from the first sample of marathon runners) were used to establish test-retest reliability across a 3- to 4-month interval. Intraclass correlations reported were Health Orientation (.81); Weight Concern (.87); Psychological Coping (.84); Life Meaning (.86); Self-Esteem (.71); Affiliation (.81); Recognition (.87); Competition (.90); Personal Goal Achievement (.82).

Validity: Confirmatory factor analysis (LISREL 7) ($N=712$) supported the construct validity of the MOMS. Participants' scores on the Competition and Personal Goal scales were negatively correlated with their average and best marathon finish times and positively correlated with training miles per week and their responses to the three scales of the Sport Orientation Questionnaire. (Their responses to the Personal Goal scale, as hypothesized, correlated more highly to the Goal and Competitiveness scales of the Sport Orientation Questionnaire than to the Win scale of this instrument.) Scores on the Personal Goal also correlated positively with responses to the Attentional Focusing Questionnaire.

In addition, individuals' ($N=712$) responses to the Affiliation scale correlated positively with the number of marathon runners each person knew and the number of times per week visits were made with other marathon runners and correlated negatively with the percentage of time spent training alone. Also, their responses to the psychological scales of the MOMS correlated positively with dissociative strategies, and their responses to the Weight Concern scale related positively to their use of running as a means of burning calories and negatively to their scores on body satisfaction.

Thus, there was support overall for the convergent validity of the MOMS. Furthermore, scores on the MOMS were not related to a social desirability measure and to most measures where, theoretically, statistically significant correlation coefficients were not expected, thus supporting the discriminant validity of the MOMS.

Norms: Not presented. Psychometric data were based on the responses of two independent samples of marathon runners. Sample 1 contained 387 male and 97 female marathon runners with a mean age of 37.5 years ($SD=9.21$). Twenty percent of these runners were participating in their first marathon. Sample 2 included 601 male and 111 female marathon runners, 20% of whom were running in their first marathon.

Availability: Contact Kevin S. Masters, Department of Psychology, University of Utah, Salt Lake City, UT 84112. (Phone 801-581-6826; E mail: kevin.masters@m.cc.utah.edu)

References

Masters, K. S., & Lambert, M. J. (1989). The relations between cognitive coping strategies, reasons for running, injury, and performance of marathon runners. *Journal of Sport & Exercise Psychology, 11,* 161-170.

*Masters, K. S., & Ogles, B. M. (1990, August). *Development and validation of the Masters-Ogles Marathon Scale.* Paper presented at the 98th convention of the American Psychological Association, Boston, MA.

*Masters, K. S., & Ogles, B. M. (1995). An investigation of the different motivations of marathon runners with varying degrees of experience. *Journal of Sport Behavior, 18*(1), 69-79.

*Ogles, B. M., Masters, K. S., & Richardson, S. A. (1995). Obligatory running and gender: An analysis of participative motives and training habits. *International Journal of Sport Psychology, 22,* 233-248.

250 ***Negative Addiction Scale** [NAS]
Barbara Jo Hailey and Leisa A. Bailey

Source: Hailey, B. J., & Bailey, L. A. (1982). Negative addiction in running: A quantitative approach. *Journal of Sport Behavior, 5,* 150-154.

Purpose: To assess the psychological aspects of negative addiction to running.

Description: The NAS contains 14 items, and was included as part of a larger questionnaire that "...assessed perceptions about running, cognitive style while running, running strategies, and motivation for running" (p. 151). Participants respond to the majority of items using a 5-point Likert scale with the anchorings 1 (*strongly agree*) to 5 (*strongly disagree*).

Construction: Not discussed.

Reliability: Not presented.

Validity: Runners (*N*=12) who ran less than one year evidenced less negative addiction to running than did runners (*n*=16) with over 4 years' running experience.

Norms: Not cited. Psychometric data were reported for 60 male runners (*M* age=32.8 years) who completed a five-mile race.

Availability: Contact Barbara Jo Hailey, University of Southern Mississippi, Southern Station Box 9371, Hattiesburg, MS 39406-9371. (Phone 601-266-4588; E-mail: jo_hailey@bull.cc.usm.edu) Items are listed in the *Source*.

References

*Furst, D. M., & Germone, K. (1993). Negative addiction in male and female runners and exercisers. *Perceptual and Motor Skills, 77*, 192-194.

Pierce, E. F., Eastman, N. W., Tripathi, H. L., Olson, K. G., & Dewey, W. L. (1993). B-endorphin response to endurance exercise: Relationship to exercise dependence. *Perceptual and Motor Skills, 77*, 767-770.

251   *Obligatory Exercise Questionnaire [OEQ]
Larry Pasman and J. Kevin Thompson

Source: Pasman, L., & Thompson, J. K. (1988). Body image and eating disturbance in obligatory runners, obligatory weightlifters, and sedentary individuals. *International Journal of Eating Disorders, 7*, 759-769.

Purpose: To assess the extent to which individuals can be classified as obligatory exercisers.

Description: The OEQ contains 21 items. Participants respond to each item using a 4-point ordinal scale.

Construction: The OEQ represents a modification of the Obligatory Running Questionnaire.

Reliability: A Cronbach alpha coefficient of .96 was reported.

Validity: Participants' responses to the OEQ were related to their responses to two 5-point Likert scales that measured subjective level of anxiety if unable to exercise ($r=.87$) and probability of exercising despite painful injury ($r=.72$). Also, obligatory runners ($N=30$) and obligatory weightlifters ($N=30$) had greater eating disturbances than did sedentary controls ($N=30$).

Norms: Not cited. Contact the second test author for information on characteristics of the sample used to derive validity and reliability data.

Availability: Last known address: J. Kevin Thompson, Department of Psychology, University of South Florida, Tampa, FL 33620.

References

*Coen, S. P., & Ogles, B. M. (1993). Psychological characteristics of the obligatory runner: A critical examination of the anorexia analogue hypothesis. *Journal of Sport and Exercise Psychology, 15*, 338-354.

Johnson, C., Diehl, N., Petrie, T., & Rogers, R. (1995). Social physique anxiety and eating disorders: What's the connection? [Abstract]. *Journal of Applied Sport Psychology, 7* (Suppl.), S76.

252 *Obligatory Running Questionnaire [ORQ]
James A. Blumenthal, Leslie C. O'Toole, and Jonathan L. Chang

Source: Blumenthal, J. A., O'Toole, L. C., & Chang, J. L. (1984). Is running an analogue of anorexia nervosa? *The Journal of the American Medical Association, 252*, 520-523.

Purpose: To assess the extent to which individuals can be classified as obligatory runners.

Description: The ORQ contains 21 true-false items (e.g., "When I don't exercise I feel guilty" and "When I miss a scheduled exercise session I may feel tense, irritable, or depressed").

Construction: Not discussed.

Reliability: Not reported.

Validity: Participants ($N=67$) were categorized into two groups based on a median split of their scores on the ORQ. The two groups did not differ in their responses to the Minnesota Multiphasic Personality Inventory.

Norms: Not cited. Psychometric data were reported for 24 anorectic patients and 43 obligatory runners (22 males; 21 females; M age=31.65 years).

**Availability: Contact James A. Blumenthal, Behavioral Physiology Laboratory, Box 3119, Duke University Medical Center, Durham, NC 27710 (Phone # 919-684-3828; FAX # 919-684-8629; E-mail: blume003@mc.duke.edu)

Personal Incentives for Exercise Questionnaire (PIEQ)
Joan L. Duda and Marlene K. Tappe

Source: Duda, J. L., & Tappe, M. K. (1989). The Personal Incentives for Exercise Questionnaire: Preliminary development. *Perceptual and Motor Skills, 68,* 1122.

Purpose: To evaluate the personal incentives individuals express for participating in exercise.

Description: The PIEQ (4th version) assesses 10 categories of personal incentives related to the exercise context: flexibility/agility, appearance, competition, weight management, mastery, affiliation, social recognition, health benefits, mental benefits, and fitness (strength/endurance). Individuals respond to 48 items using a 5-point Likert scale.

Construction: Based on the Theory of Personal Investment, the open-ended responses of 165 adult exercise participants, and a review of the exercise psychology literature, 85 items were developed and administered to 212 male and 313 female undergraduates from a large midwestern university. Principal component factor analyses (oblique and orthogonal rotations) led to the retention of nine factors. Based on additional analyses, 48 items were retained and administered to samples of 135 male and 217 female college students. Factor analyses supported a stable factor structure across the two samples.

Reliability: Cronbach alpha reliability coefficients ranged from .74 to .94 (*n*=135 college males) and from .77 to .92 (*n*=217 female college students). Test-retest reliability coefficients ranged from .58 to .86 across a 2-week interval (*n*=106).

Validity: Construct validity was supported through factor analyses as noted above.

Norms: Not presented. Psychometric data were reported for 135 male and 217 college females.

**Availability: Contact Joan L. Duda, Department of Health, Kinesiology, and Leisure Studies, 113 Lambert Hall, Purdue University, West Lafayette, IN 47907. (Phone # 317-494-3172; FAX # 317-496-1239; E-mail: lynne@vm.cc.purdue.edu)

References

Duda, J. L., & Tappe, M. K. (1989). Personal investment in exercise among adults: The examination of age and gender-related differences in motivational orientation. In A. C. Ostrow (Ed.), *Aging and motor behavior* (pp. 239-256), Indianapolis, IN: Benchmark Press.

*Finkenberg, M. E., DiNucci, J. M., & McCune, S. L., & McCune, E. D. (1994). Analysis of course type, gender, and personal incentives to exercise. *Perceptual and Motor Skills, 78,* 155-159.

*McCullagh, P., Matzkanin, K. T., & Figge, Jr. (1990).Personal investment in exercise: An examination of adult swimmers [Abstract]. *Proceedings of the Association for the Advancement of Applied Sport Psychology annual convention* (p. 77). San Antonio, TX.

Stainback, R., Ondrea, P., & Hunter, G. (1989). Development and evaluation of an exercise program for outpatient alcoholics [Abstract]. *Proceedings of the Association for the Advancement for Applied Sport Psychology annual convention* (p. 100). Seattle, WA.

*Tappe, M. K., & Duda, J. L. (1988). Personal investment predictors of life satisfaction among physically active middle-aged and older adults. *Journal of Psychology, 122,* 557-566.

Tappe, M. K., Duda, J. L., & Menges-Ehrnwald, P. (1990). Personal investment predictors of adolescent motivational orientation toward exercise. *Canadian Journal of Sport Sciences, 15,* 185-192.

 254 # *Processes of Change Questionnaire (PCQ)
Bess H. Marcus, Joseph S. Rossi, Vanessa C. Selby, Raymond S. Niaura, and David B. Abrams

Source: Marcus, B. H., Rossi, J. S., Selby, V. C., Niaura, R. S., & Abrams, D. B. (1992). *Health Psychology, 11,* 386-395.

Purpose: To evaluate the cognitive and behavioral processes individuals employ during the acquisition and maintenance of exercise adoption.

Description: The PCQ contains 39 items used to evaluate 10 processes of change: Consciousness Raising, Counterconditioning, Dramatic Relief, Environmental Reevaluation, Helping Relationships, Reinforcement Management, Self-Liberation, Self-Reevaluation, Social Liberation, and Stimulus Control. Participants are asked to think back over the past month and rate the frequency of occurrence of each item using a 5-point Likert-type scale with the anchorings 1 (*never*) to 5 (*repeatedly*). An example of an item is "I react emotionally to warnings about an inactive life style" (Dramatic Relief).

Construction: An initial pool of 110 items was developed based on definitions from the model of stages and processes of change, and was also modified from items used in smoking cessation research. Three doctoral-level judges were used to establish content validity by categorizing the items according to the conceptual definitions of 10 change processes. Sixty-five items were retained. Evaluation of item distributions (*n*= 561) led to the elimination of five items. Measurement analyses of the remaining 60 items using the LISREL VI structural modeling program led to the retention of 39 items.

Reliability: Cronbach alpha internal consistency coefficients ($n=540$; $n=561$)) ranged from .62 (Social Liberation) to .89 (Self-Reevaluation).

Validity: Exploratory and confirmatory factor analysis ($n=561$; $n=540$) supported the construct validity of the PCQ.

Norms: Not cited. Psychometric data were provided for 1,101 male or female employees of two worksites, randomly split in half for initial development and cross-validation analyses of the PCQ. Approximately two-thirds of the participants were female, and the average age of the participants was 37.2 years ($SD= 14.2$ years).

Availability: Contact Bess H. Marcus, Division of Behavioral Medicine, The Miriam Hospital, Brown University School of Medicine, RISE Building, 164 Summit Avenue, Providence, RI 02906. (Phone # 401-331-8500, ext. 3707; FAX # 401-331-2453)

255 Ratings of Perceived Exertion (RPE)
Gunnar A. V. Borg

Source: Borg, G. A. V., & Noble, B. J. (1974). Perceived exertion. In J. H. Wilmore (Ed.), *Exercise and sport sciences reviews* (pp. 131-153). New York: Academic Press.

Purpose: To evaluate individual perceptions of effort and exertion during exercise.

Description: The RPE scale consists of 15 grades from 6 (very, very light) to 20 (very, very hard). These gradations correspond roughly to 1/10 the heart variation from 60 to 200 in healthy, middle-aged individuals. The participant is asked to estimate the degree of exertion he or she feels and select the appropriate number on the scale corresponding to this perception of exertion.

Construction: The RPE scale was constructed to follow heart rate for work on the bicycle ergometer among healthy, middle-aged men performing moderate-to-hard exercise. Thus, heart rate should be about 10 times the RPE value.

410

Reliability: Test-retest reliability coefficients of .80 to .98 were reported over a 2- to 4-week period among 21 male and 15 female participants.

Validity: Correlation coefficients of .65 and .68 were reported with heart rate.

Norms: Not cited.

Availability: A copy of the scale appears in the *Source* identified above.

References

*Acevedo, E. O. (1994). Perceived exertion and affect at varying intensities of running. *Research Quarterly for Exercise and Sport, 65,* 372-376.

*Arnold, R., Ng., N., & Pechar, G. (1992). Relationship of related perceived exertion to heart rate and workload in mentally retarded young adults. *Adapted Physical Activity Quarterly, 9,* 47-53.

*Borg, G. A. V. (1982). Psychophysical bases of perceived exertion. *Medicine and Science in Sports and Exercise, 14,* 377-381.

*Borg, G. (1985). *An introduction to Borg's RPE scale.* Ithaca, NY: Mouvement Publications.

Bozoian, S., Rejeski, W. J., & McAuley, E. (1994). Self-efficacy influences feeling states associated with acute exercise. *Journal of Sport & Exercise Psychology, 16,* 326-333.

Brewer, B. W., Van Raalte, J. L., & Linder, D. E. (1990). Effects of pain on motor performance. *Journal of Sport & Exercise Psychology, 12,* 353-365.

*Carton, R. L., & Rhodes, E. C. (1985). A critical review of the literature on ratings scales for perceived exertion. *Sports Medicine, 2,* 198-222.

*Caruso, C. M., Morgan, D. W., & Crews, D. J. (1991). Thoughts, feelings, and RPEs during a prolonged maximal run [Abstract]. *Proceedings of the North American Society for the Psychology of Sport and Physical Activity annual convention* (p. 146). Pacific Grove, CA.

*Ceci, R., & Hassmen, P. (1991). Self-monitored exercise at three different RPE intensities in treadmill versus field running. *Medicine and Science in Exercise and Sport, 23,* 732-738.

*Courneya, K. S., & McAuley, E. (1994). Factors affecting the intention-physical activity relationship: Intention versus expectation and scale correspondence. *Research Quarterly for Exercise and Sport, 65,* 280-285.

*Eston, R. G., & Williams, J. G. (1988). Reliability of ratings of perceived effort regulation of exercise intensity. *British Journal of Sports Medicine, 22,* 153-155.

Garcia, A. W., & King, A. C. (1991). Predicting long-term adherence to aerobic exercise: A comparison of two models. *Journal of Sport & Exercise Psychology, 13,* 394-410.

*Hanin Y., & Syrja, P. (1995). Performance affect in junior ice hockey players: An application of the individual zones of optimal functioning model. *The Sport Psychologist, 9,* 169-187.

*See Carton and Rhodes (1985) for a more recent update on the psychometric properties of RPE scales.

Ljunggren, G., & Hassmen, P. (1991). Perceived exertion and physiological economy of competition walking, ordinary walking and running. *Journal of Sports Sciences, 9,* 273-283.

*Marriott, H. E., & K. L. Lamb (1995). The use of ratings of perceived exertion for regulating exercise levels in rowing [Abstract]. *Journal of Sports Sciences, 13,* 38.

*McAuley, E., & Courneya, K. (1990). Efficacy, metabolic, and affective perceptions during exercise [Abstract]. *Proceedings of the Association for the Advancement of Applied Sport Psychology annual convention* (p. 75). San Antonio, TX.

*Morgan, W. P. (1981). Psychophysiology of self-awareness during vigorous physical activity. *Research Quarterly for Exercise and Sport, 52.* 385-427.

*Morgan, W. P., & Borg, G. A. V. (1976). Perception of effort in the prescription of physical activity. In T. T. Craig, (Ed.), *The humanistic and mental health aspects of sports, exercise and recreation* (pp. 126-129). Chicago, IL: American Medical Association.

Murphy, S. M., Fleck, S. J., Dudley, G., & Callister, R. (1990). Psychological and performance concomitants of increased volume training in elite athletes. *Journal of Applied Sport Psychology, 2,* 34-50.

*Parfitt, G., & Bowey, J. (1995). The effect of training on the rating of perceived exertion and psychological affect [Abstract]. *Journal of Sports Science, 13,* 70-71.

*Parfitt, G., & Eston, R. (1995). Changes in ratings of perceived exertion and psychological affect in the early stages of exercise. *Perceptual and Motor Skills, 80,* 259-266.

*Parfitt, G., Markland, D., & Holmes, C. (1994). Responses to physical exertion in active and inactive males and females. *Journal of Sport & Exercise Psychology, 16,* 178-186.

*Russell, W. D., & Weeks, D. L. (1994). Attentional style in ratings of perceived exertion during physical exercise. *Perceptual and Motor Skills, 78,* 779-783.

Siegel, D., & Johnson, J. (1992). A preliminary study of pacing in cycling. *Journal of Sport Behavior, 15,* 75-86.

Smith, L. L., Brunetz, M. H., Chenier, T. C., McCammon, M. R., Houmard, J. A., Franklin, M. E., & Israel, R. G. (1995). The effect of static and ballistic stretching on delayed onset muscle soreness and creatine kinase. *Research Quarterly for Exercise and Sport, 64,* 103-107.

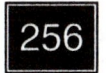 **256** # *Reasons for Exercise Inventory [REI}
Lisa R. Silberstein, Ruth H. Striegel-Moore, Christine Timko, and Judith Rodin

Source: Silberstein, L. R., Streigel-Moore, R. H., Timko, C., & Rodin, J. (1988). Behavioral and psychological implications of body dissatisfaction: Do men and women differ? *Sex Roles, 19,* 219-232.

Purpose: To assess the reasons people identify for exercising.

Description: The REI contains 24 items and includes seven domains:

exercise for weight control, for fitness, for health, for improving body tone, for improving overall physical attractiveness, for improving one's mood, and for enjoyment. Participants respond to each item using a 7-point ordinal scale with the anchorings 1 (*not at all important*) to 7 (*extremely important*).

Construction: Not indicated.

Reliability: Cronbach alpha coefficients ranged from .67 (Enjoyment) to .81 (Weight Control).

Validity: A low, positive relationship ($r=.36$) was found between individuals' ($N=92$) scores on the REI and a scale designed to assess disregulated eating behaviors.

Norms: Not cited. Psychometric data were reported for 45 female and 47 male undergraduate students attending Yale University.

Availability: Last known address: Lisa R. Silberstein, Department of Psychology, Yale University, Box 11A, Yale Station, New Haven, CT 06520. Items are identified in the *Source*.

References

*Cash, T. F., Novy, P. L., & Grant, J. R. (1994). Why do women exercise? Factor analysis and further validation of the Reasons for Exercise Inventory. *Perceptual and Motor Skills, 78*, 539-544.

*Crawford, S., & Eklund, R. C. (1994). Social physique anxiety, reasons for exercise, and attitudes toward exercise settings. *Journal of Sport & Exercise Psychology, 16*, 70-82.

*Eklund, R. C., & Crawford, S. (1994). Active women, social physique anxiety, and exercise. *Journal of Sport & Exercise Psychology, 16*, 431-448.

*Silberstein, L. R., Mishkind, M. E., Striegel-Moore, R. H., Timko, C., & Rodin, J. (1989). Men and their bodies: A comparison of homosexual and heterosexual men. *Psychosomatic Medicine, 51*, 337-346

257 Reasons for Running Scale (RFR)
James M. Robbins and Paul Joseph

Source: Robbins, J. M., & Joseph, P. (1985). Experiencing exercise withdrawal: Possible consequences of therapeutic and mastery running. *Journal of Sport Psychology, 7*, 23-39.

Purpose: A self-report measure of why runners continue to run regularly.

Description: Runners are asked to respond to 21 items using a 7-point ordinal scale with the anchorings *very important* (7 points) to *not at all important* (1 point). Examples of items include "opportunities to relax" and "chance for association and friendship."

Construction: Not discussed.

Reliability: Not cited.

Validity: Construct validity was examined through principal component factor analysis. Five factors emerged accounting for 63.20% of the variance: Mastery, Recognition, Escape, Novelty, and Health.

Norms: Not cited.

Availability: Last known address: James M. Robbins, Department of Psychiatry, Jewish General Hospital, 4333 Chemin de la Cote Ste-Catherine, Montreal, Quebec, Canada H3T 1E4. (Phone # 514-340-8210)

 Rehabilitation Adherence Questionnaire [RAQ]
A. Craig Fisher and Mary A. Domm

Source: Fisher, A. C., Domm, M. A., & Wuest, D. A. (1988). Adherence to sports-injury rehabilitation programs. *The Physician and Sportsmedicine, 16*(6), 47-54.

Purpose: To identify the personal and situational factors related to rehabilitation adherence among athletes.

Description: The RAQ contains six scales: Perceived Exertion, Pain Tolerance, Apathy, Support From Significant Others, Scheduling of Rehabilitation, and Environmental Conditions. For example, participants are asked to respond to the item "I worked out until I felt pain and then stopped" (Pain Tolerance). Participants respond to the 40-item

414

questionnaire using a 4-point Likert scale with the anchors *strongly agree* to *strongly disagree.*

Construction: Items were derived from an analysis of the content of the adherence literature.

Reliability: Not reported.

Validity: Discriminant validity was supported in that the RAQ differentiated between college athlete adherents (*n*=21) and nonadherents (*n*=20), with the adherents perceiving they worked harder at rehabilitation, were more self-motivated, and made a greater effort to fit rehabilitation into their schedules.

Norms: Not reported. Psychometric data were cited for 41 college athletes (*n*=21 males; *n*=20 females) who had been injured in sports.

**Availability: Contact A. Craig Fisher, Department of Exercise and Sport Sciences, Ithaca College, Ithaca, NY 14850. (Phone # 607-274-3112; FAX # 607-274-1943; E-mail: cfisher@ithaca.edu)

References

*Brewer, B. W., Daly, J. M., Van Raalte, J. L., & Petitpas. A. J. (1994). A psychometric evaluation of the Rehabilitation Adherence Questionnaire [Abstract]. *Journal of Sport & Exercise Psychology, 16* (Suppl.), S34.

*Byerly, P. N., Worrell, T., Gahimer, J., & Domholdt, E. (1994). Rehabilitation compliance in an athletic training environment. *Journal of Athletic Training, 29,* 352-355.

*Fields, J., Murphey, M., Horodyski, M., & Stopka, C. (1995). Factors associated with adherence to sport injury rehabilitation in college-age recreational athletes. *Journal of Sport Rehabilitation, 4,* 172-180.

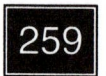 ***Running Addiction Scale (RAS)**
Ellen B. Rudy and Patricia J. Estok

Source: Rudy, E. B., & Estok, P. J. (1989). Measurement and significance of negative addiction in runners. *Western Journal of Nursing Research, 11,* 548-558.

Purpose: To assess aspects of addictive behavior associated with running.

Description: The RAS contains 17 items (e.g., "Do you find that you run even when injured?"). Participants respond using a 3-point ordinal scale ("frequently," "occasionally," "no").

Construction: Form 1 of the RAS contained 14 items and was scored dichotomously with a total score range of 0 to 14. Item analyses and reliability assessment ($N=95$) reduced the RAS to 10 items.

Form 2 evolved from an evaluation of case studies and further analysis of the literature. Fourteen of the original items plus 5 new items were included in this form. However, item analysis led to the elimination of 2 items, resulting in the current 17 item- form.

Reliability: A Cronbach alpha internal consistency coefficient of .66 ($N=220$) was reported. A test-retest reliability coefficient of .71 ($N=15$) was reported across a 2-week interval.

Validity: Convergent validity estimates indicated that, as hypothesized, participants' ($N=186$) responses to the RAS were negatively correlated with self-esteem scores ($r=-23$) and positively correlated with anxiety scores ($r=.48$). Furthermore, participants' level of running addiction was related to the frequency of torn ligament and hematuria injuries.

Norms: Not cited. Psychometric data were reported for 112 men and 108 women, ages 18 to 69 years, participating in a marathon event. Approximately 57% of the men and 46% of the women had been running 5 years or longer.

**Availability: Contact Ellen B. Rudy, School of Nursing, 3500 Victoria Street, University of Pittsburgh, Pittsburgh, PA 15261. (Phone #412-624-2400; FAX # 412-624-2401; E-mail: ebr@med.pitt.edu.).

Reference

*Estok, P., & Rudy, E. (1986). Physical, psychosocial, menstrual changes/risks and addictions in female marathon and nonmarathon runners. *Health Care of Women International, 7*, 187-202.

260 *Running Addiction Scale (RAS)
Carol Lee Chapman and John M. De Castro

Source: Chapman, C. L., & De Castro, J. M. (1990). Running addiction: Measurement and associated psychological characteristics. *Journal of Sports Medicine and Physical Fitness, 30,* 283-290.

Purpose: To evaluate the characteristics associated with running addiction.

Description: The RAS contains 11 items (e.g., "I would run with intense pain"). Participants respond on a Likert scale with the anchorings *strongly agree* to *strongly disagree.*

Construction: Eighteen statements were written regarding the characteristics of running addiction such as withdrawal effects and feelings of a need to run. The statements were pilot tested among five runners and two prominent researchers. In addition, an item analysis was conducted using 49 individuals, leading to the retention of 11 items.

Reliability: A Cronbach alpha internal consistency coefficient (N=49) of .82 was reported.

Validity: Concurrent validity was supported in that participants' scores on the RAS correlated positively with a self-rating measure of running addiction (r=.66 for 32 males; r=.75 for 17 females) and a measure of discomfort (r=.48 for 37 males). Participants' (N=49) scores also correlated positively (r=.80) with their scores on the Commitment to Running Scale and with the number of runs taken per week and the average length of the run (minutes).

Norms: Not cited. Psychometric data were reported for 32 males (ages 24 to 57 years) and 17 females (ages 25 to 29 years).

Availability: Contact John M. De Castro, Department of Psychology, Georgia State University, 200a, Kell Hall, Atlanta, GA 30303. (Phone # 404-651-1623; E-mail: psyjdc@gsusgi2.gsu.edu) Items are also listed in the *Source.*

261 Self-Motivation Inventory (SMo)
Copyright © 1978 by Rod K. Dishman

Source: Dishman, R. K., Ickes, W., & Morgan, W. P. (1980). Self-motivation and adherence to habitual physical activity. *Journal of Applied Social Psychology, 10,* 115-132.

Purpose: To assess the tendency to persist in a vigorous physical activity regardless of extrinsic reinforcement.

Description: The SMo consists of 40 items. Participants are asked to respond to each item using a 5-point Likert format.

Construction: An original pool of 60 items was administered to 399 undergraduate students. Examination of item-total score correlation coefficients led to the retention of 48 items. Factor analysis of participants' responses resulted in the retention of 40 items loading on 11 factors and accounting for 40.5% of the total variance.

Reliability: An alpha reliability coefficient of .91 (standard error=5.84) was reported for the 399 undergraduate students. A second independent sample of undergraduate students produced an alpha coefficient of .86 and a test-retest reliability coefficient of .92 over a one-month interval.

Validity: Concurrent validity was evidenced by the correlation of the SMowith a self-report assessment of exercise frequency ($r=.23$; $n=399$). Also, participants' scores on the SMo correlated ($r=.63$) with their responses to the Thomas-Zander Ego-Strength Scale. However, participants' responses to the SMo also correlated (weakly) with the Marlowe-Crowne Social Desirability Scale.

Support for the construct validity of the scale was demonstrated in two field studies that indicated individuals' responses to the SMo were significantly associated with adherence to programs of physical exercise. Participants were middle-aged adult males involved in a health-oriented exercise program and college females participating in a crew training program.

Norms: Psychometric data were reported for 399 male and female undergraduate students enrolled in introductory psychology classes, 64 female intercollegiate athletes, and 66 middle-aged adult males.

418

Availability: Contact Rod K. Dishman, Department of Exercise Science, University of Georgia, 300 River Road Athens, GA 30602-3654. (Phone # 706-542-9840; FAX # 706-542-3148; E-mail: rdishman@uga.cc.uga.edu)

References

*Biddle, S., & Brooke, R. (1992). The Self-Motivation Inventory modified for children: Psychometric properties and relationships with exercise performance [Abstract]. *Journal of Sports Sciences, 10,* 608.

*Boyce, B. A., & Wayda, V. K. (1994). The effects of assigned and self set goals on task performance. *Journal of Sport & Exercise Psychology, 16,* 258-269.

*Bull, S. J. (1990). Personal and situational influences on adherence to mental skills training. *Journal of Sport & Exercise Psychology, 13,* 121-132.

*Clifford, P. A., Tan, S. Y., & Gorsuch, R. L. (1991). Efficacy of a self-directed behavioral health change program: Weight, body composition, cardiovascular fitness, blood pressure, health risk, and psychosocial mediating variables. *Journal of Behavioral Medicine, 14,* 303-323.

*Dishman, R. K., & Steinhardt, M. A. (1988). Reliablity and concurrent validity for a 7-d re-call of physical activity in college students. *Medicine and Science in Sports and Exercise, 20,* 14-25.

Garcia, A. W., & King, A. C. (1991). Predicting long-term adherence to aerobic exercise: A comparison of two models. *Journal of Sport & Exercise Psychology, 13,* 394-410.

*Gibbs, K., Kennedy, C., DeVoe, D., Linnell, S, & Casey, K. (1995). The effects of self-motivation and financial incentives on participation in a hospital employee wellness program. *Research Quarterly for Exercise and Sport, 66* (Suppl.), A38-39.

*Heiby, E. M., Onorato, V. A., & Sato, R. A. (1987). Cross-validation of the self-motivation inventory. *Journal of Sport Psychology, 9,* 394-399.

*Jackson, C., Kambis, N. K., & Jackson, C. W. (1993). Verification of shorter self-motivation inventories [Abstract]. *Proceedings of the Association for the Advancement of Applied Sport Psychology annual convention* (p. 77). Montreal, Canada.

*Jambor, E. A., & Weekes, E. M. (1994). Self-motivation, expectations, and the influence of education in exercisers and non-exercisers [Abstract]. *Journal of Sport & Exercise Psychology, 16* (Suppl.), S68.

Jambor, E. A., & Weekes, E. M. (1995). Leadership differences between males and females [Abstract]. *Journal of Applied Sport Psychology, 7* (Suppl.), S75.

*Keil Loper, D. A., & Scheer, J. K. (1993). The effects of three counseling methods, locus of control, and self-motivation on exercise adherence of college students [Abstract]. *Research Quarterly for Exercise and Sport , 64* (Suppl.), A-42-43.

*Knapp, D., Gutmann, M., Foster, C., & Pollock, M. (1984). Self-motivation among 1984 Olympic speed skating hopefuls and emotional response and adherence to training [Abstract]. *Proceedings of the 1984 Olympic Scientific Congress.* Eugene, OR: College of Human Development and Performance Microform Publications.

*McCullagh, P., Matzkanin, K. T., & Figge, Jr., J. K. (1990). Personal investment in exercise: An examination of adult swimmers [Abstract]. *Proceedings of the Association for the Advancement of Applied Sport Psychology annual convention* (p. 77). San Antonio, TX.

*Pain, M. D., & Sharpley, C. F. (1986). Some psychometric data on predictive validity of self-motivation inventory. *Perceptual and Motor Skills, 63,* 294.

*Raglin, J. S., Morgan, W. P., & Luchsinger, A. E. (1990). Mood and self-motivation in successful and unsuccessful female rowers. *Medicine and Science in Sports and Exercise 22,* 849-853.

Robertson, J., & Mutrie, N. (1989). Factors to adherence to exercise. *Physical Education Review, 12,* 138-146.

Smith, R. A., & Biddle, S. J. H. (1990). Exercise adherence: An empirical study [Abstract]. *Journal of Sports Sciences, 8,* 283-284.

*Steinhardt, M. A., Young, D. R. (1992). Psychological attributes of participants and non-participants in a worksite health and fitness center. *Behavioral Medicine, 18*(1), 40-46.

Tappe, M. K., & Duda, J. L. (1988). Personal investment predictors of life satisfaction among physically active middle-aged and older adults. *Journal of Psychology, 122,* 557-566.

*Wankel, L. M., Yardley, J. K., & Graham, J. (1985). The effects of motivational interventions upon the exercise adherence of high and low self-motivated adults. *Canadian Journal of Applied Sport Sciences, 10,* 147-156.

*Weber, J., & Wertheim, H. (1989). Relationships of self-monitoring, special attention, body fat percent, and self-motivation to attendance at a community gymnasium. *Journal of Sport & Exercise Psychology, 11,* 105 114.

*Wilder, K. C. (1995). Adherence to a walking program: A comparison of social cognitive theory and trait theory [Abstract]. *Journal of Applied Sport Psychology, 7* (Suppl.), S125.

*Wilson, M. G. (1989). Factors associated with initial participation in workplace behavior change programs. *Wellness Perspectives: Research, Theory and Practice. 6*(2), 32-49.

*Yoo, J. (1993). Analyses of multidimensional factors influencing adherence to exercise. *Proceedings of the Eighth World Congress of Sport Psychology* (pp. 906-910). Lisbon, Portugal.

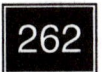 *Self-Motivation Inventory for Children (SMI-C)
Stuart Biddle

Source: Biddle, S., Akande, D., Armstrong, N., Ashcroft, M., Brooke, R., & Goudas, M. (in press). The Self-Motivation Inventory modified for children: Evidence on psychometric properties and its use in physical exercise. *International Journal of Sport Psychology.*

Purpose: To assess the self-motivation of children.

Description: The SMI-C contains 20 items and is a modification of the Self-Motivation Inventory (Dishman, Ickes, & Morgan, 1980) reported previously in this chapter. Children respond to each item using a 5-point Likert scale.

Construction: Items were selected from the SMI randomly; also, items were not considered that were viewed as inappropriate in content or wording for children. The wording of the remaining 20 items was simplified further for use with children 10-16 years old.

Reliability: Cronbach alpha internal consistency coefficients ranged from .70 to .87 for British subjects (N=1019), but the SMI-C failed to demonstrate internal consistency among African children (N=363). A test-retest reliability coefficient of .86 was reported over a 5-week period among 19 children.

Validity: The author (S. Biddle, personal communication, April 8, 1996) summarized evidence for the validity of the SMI-C. Participants' responses to the SMI-C were positively correlated with their shuttle running performance (r=.70, n=24; r=.33, n= 257). In addition, convergent validity was supported in that these children's scores on the SMI-C were positively correlated with their responses to the curiosity, intrinsic mastery motivation, and challenge subscales of the Motivational Orientation in Sport Scale, as well as enjoyment as measured by the Physical Activity Enjoyment Scale. Low, but statistically significant correlation coefficients were found with task and ego goal orientations, as measured by the Task and Ego Orientation in Sport Questionnaire. Factorial validity was demonstrated by a Comparative Fit Index for a one factor model of .969 using confirmatory factor analysis through the EQS program.

Norms: Not cited. Psychometric data were reported for independent samples (Sample 1: N= 434 11- to 15-year-olds; Sample 2 (N= 167 10- to 12-year-olds; Sample 3: N=24 12-year-old boys; Sample 4: N= 257 12- to 14-year-olds; Sample 5: N= 64 12- to 13-year-olds) of children residing in Great Britain.

**Availability: Contact Stuart Biddle, School of Education, University of Exeter, Heavitree Road, Exeter, United Kingdom EX1 2LU. (Phone: +44 01392 264751; FAX +44 01392 264792; E-mail: s.j.h.biddle@exeter.ac.uk)

Reference

*Biddle, S., & Brooke, R. (1992). The Self-Motivation Inventory modified for children: Psychometric properties and relationships with exercise performance [Abstract]. *Journal of Sports Sciences. 10,* 608.

 **263** ***Sport Injury Rehabilitation Adherence Scale (SIRAS)**

Britton W. Brewer, Judy L. Van Raalte, Albert J. Petitpas, Joseph H. Sklar and Terry D. Ditmar

Source: Brewer, B. W., Van Raalte, J. L., Petitpas, A. J., Sklar, J. H., & Ditmar, T. D. (1995, September). *A brief measure of adherence during sport injury rehabilitation sessions.* Paper presented at the annual meeting of the Association for the Advancement of Applied Sport Psychology, New Orleans, LA.

Purpose: "...to assess adherence during clinic-based sport injury rehabilitation sessions" (p. 1).

Description: The SIRAS is a three-item scale. Sport rehabilitation professionals rate the intensity with which a client completes the rehabilitation exercises, the frequency with which the client follows their advice and instructions, and the extent to which a patient is receptive to changes in the rehabilitation program.

Construction: Items for the SIRAS were derived from the adherence literature.

Reliability: The authors reported a Cronbach alpha internal consistency coefficient of .82 (*N*=145).

Validity: Participants' (*N*=145) scores on the SIRAS were significantly correlated (*r*=.21, *p*<.05) with their attendance at rehabilitation sessions. Participants' age, gender, and level of athletic involvement were not related to their SIRAS scores.

Norms: Not indicated. Psychometric data were reported for 145 consecutive patients at an orthopedic physical therapy clinic specializing in sports medicine. These individuals attended at least three rehabilitation sessions.

**Availability: Contact Britton W. Brewer, Center for Performance Enhancement and Applied Research, Department of Psychology, 263 Alden Street, Springfield College, Springfield, MA 01109-3797. (Phone: 413-748-3696; FAX 413-748-3854; E-mail: britton_brewer @scns.spflcol.edu)

References

*Brewer, B. W., Daly, J. M., Van Raalte, J. L., Petitpas, A. J., & Sklar, J. H. (1994). A psychometric evaluation of the Rehabilitation Adherence Questionnaire [Abstract]. *Journal of Sport & Exercise Psychology, 16,* S34.

*Daly, J. M., Brewer, B. W., Van Raalte, J. L., Petitpas, A. J., & Sklar, J. H. (1995). Cognitive appraisal, emotional adjustment, and adherence to rehabilitation following knee surgery. *Journal of Sport Rehabilitation, 4,* 23-30.

*Laubach, W. J., Brewer, B. W., Van Raalte, J. L., & Petitpas. A. J. (1996). Attributions for recovery and adherence to sport injury rehabilitation. *Australian Journal of Science and Medicine in Sport, 28,* 29-33.

264 *Sports Injury Rehabilitation Beliefs Survey (SIRBS)

Sally May and Adrian Taylor

Source: Taylor, A. H., & May, S. (1993). Development of a survey to assess athletes' sports injury rehabilitation beliefs [Abstract]. *Proceedings of the VIIth Conference of the European Health Psychology Society.* Brussels, Belgium.

Purpose: To assess athletes' perceptions of the sports injury rehabilitation process following treatment at a sports injury clinic.

Description: The SIRBS contains 18 items reflecting four subscales: (a) Self-Efficacy (SE), (b) Treatment Efficacy (TE), (c) Susceptibility (SUS), and (d) Severity (SEV). Participants respond to each item using a 5-point Likert scale with the anchorings *strongly agree* to *strongly disagree.*

Construction: Following an extensive review of models to explain health behavior and open-ended interviews with patients attending sports injury clinics, a pool of 46 items was constructed. Eight individuals with psychometric or sports physiotherapy expertise were then asked to check each item for clarity, and place the items under the defined headings of self-efficacy, treatment efficacy, perceived susceptibility, seriousness, and motivation for rehabilitation. These constructs were drawn from the Protection Motivation Theory and the Self-Motivation Theory. Twenty items were retained. Exploratory factor analysis (see validity section) led to the retention of 18 items.

Reliability: Cronbach alpha reliability coefficients of .79 (SE), .83 (TE), .83 (SUS), and .63 (SEV) were reported.

Validity: The SIRBS was given to 446 injured athletes attending one of seven sports injury clinics in southeast England; 264 completed responses were received. These athletes' scores on the SIRBS were subjected to exploratory factor analysis with varimax rotation resulting in the retention of a four-factor structure. Seven items did not load on any single factor, and the apparent conceptual overlap between the self-efficacy and motivation items led to the removal of the latter subscale.

Norms: Not cited. Psychometric data were reported for 264 injured athletes (*M* age=30.6 years, *SD*=11.3), of which 59% of the sample were male athletes.

**Availability: Contact Adrian Taylor, Chelsea School Research Centre, University of Brighton, Gaudick Road, Eastbourne, East Sussex, England BN20 7SP. (Phone # 01273-643743; FAX # 01273-643704; E-mail: aht@bton.ac.uk)

Reference

* Taylor, A. H., & May, S. M. (in press). Threat and coping appraisals as determinants of compliance to sports injury rehabilitation: An application of Protection Motivation Theory. *Journal of Sports Science.*

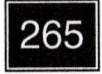

*Stages of Exercise Behaviour Change (SEBC)
Bess H. Marcus, Vanessa C. Selby, Raymond S. Niaura, and Joseph S. Rossi

Source: Marcus, B. H., Selby, V. C., Niaura, R. S., & Rossi, J. S. (1992). Self efficacy and the stages of exercise behavior change. *Research Quarterly for Exercise and Sport, 63,* 60-66.

Purpose: To evaluate the stages that individuals progress through in terms of readiness for exercise participation.

Description: The SEBC contains five items used to evaluate the five stages of change for exercise behavior: Precontemplation,

Contemplation, Preparation, Action, and Maintenance. Participants respond to items such as "I currently do not exercise," or "I intend to exercise in the next 6 months." Participants are assigned to the stage based on evaluating the pattern of items they endorse using a true-false format.

Construction: Items for the SEBC were developed from a similar measure for smoking cessation, but modified to describe exercise behavior. A preparation stage (item) was added after an evaluation of 1,063 participants' responses revealed that many responses clustered in the Action and Maintenance stages.

Reliability: Test-retest reliability ($N=20$) over a 2-week period, using the kappa index of reliability, was computed to be .78.

Validity: Not discussed.

Norms: Descriptive statistics were presented for 1,063 employees at a Rhode Island division of a government agency of which 70% were males (M age=41.1 years; $SD=10.8$), and 420 employees of a Rhode Island medical center, 85% of whom were women (M age=40.5 years; $SD=11.0$). A third sample ($N=20$) of employees of a Rhode Island Medical Center was used to establish reliability estimates.

**Availability: Contact Bess H. Marcus, Division of Behavioral Medicine, the Miriam Hospital/Brown University, School of Medicine, RISE Building, 164 Summit Avenue., Providence, RI 02906 (Phone # 401-331-8500; Ext. 3707; FAX # 401-331-2453)

References

*Buxton, K. E., Mercer, T. H., Hale, B., Wyse, J. P., & Ashford, B. (1994). Evidence for the concurrent validity and measurement reliability of a Stages of Exercise Behaviour Change instrument [Abstract]. *Journal of Sport & Exercise Psychology, 16* (Suppl.), S35.

*Buxton, K. E., Mercer, T. H., Hale, B., Wyse, J. P. & Ashford,B. (1994). Preliminary validation of a Stages of physical activity Behaviour Change Scale (SPABC) [Abstract]. *Journal of Sport & Exercise Psychology, 16* (Supple.), S36.

*Buxton, K. E., Wyse, J. P., Mercer, T. H., & Hale, B. D. (1995). Assessing the stages of exercise behaviour change and the stages of physical activity behaviour change in a British worksite sample [Abstract]. *Journal of Sports Sciences, 13,* 50-51.

*Courneya, K. S., (1995). Perceived severity of the consequences of physical inactivity and stages of change in older adults. *Journal of Sport & Exercise Psychology, 17,* 447-457.

*Gorely, T., & Gordon, S. (1995). An examination of the transtheoretical model and exercise behavior in older adults. *Journal of Sport & Exercise Psychology, 17*, 312-324.

*Loughlan, C., & Mutrie, N. (1995). Recruitment of sedentary NHS staff for a workplace exercise programme using an adapted 'stages-of-change' exercise questionnaire [Abstract]. *Journal of Sports Sciences, 13*, 63-64.

*Marcus, B. H., Eaton, C. A., Rossi, J. S., & Harlow, L. L. (1994). Self-efficacy, decision-making, and stages of change: An integrative model of physical exercise. *Journal of Applied Social Psychology, 24*, 489-508.

*Marcus, B. H., & Owen, N. (1992). Motivational readiness, self-efficacy and decision-making for exercise. *Journal of Applied Social Psychology, 22*, 3-16.

*Marcus, B. H., Pinto, B. M., Simkin, L. R., Audrain, J. E., & Taylor, E. R. (1994). Application of theoretical models to exercise behavior among employed women. *American Journal of Health Promotion, 9*, 49-55.

*Marcus, B. H., Rossi, J. S., Selby, V. C., Niaura, R. S., & Abrams, D. B. (1992). The stages and processes of exercise adoption and maintenance in a worksite sample. *Health Psychology, 11*, 386-395.

*Marcus, B. H., & Simkin, L. R. (1993). The stages of exercise behavior. *The Journal of Sports Medicine and Physical Fitness, 33*, 83-88.

*Naylor, P. J., & McKenna, J. (1995). Stages of change, self-efficacy and behavioural preferences for exercise among British university students [Abstract]. *Journal of Sports Sciences, 13*, 68.

*Naylor, P. J., McKenna, J., Barnes, K., & Christopher, M. (1995). Decision balance and self-reported physical activity levels: Validating the stages of change for exercise in British university students [Abstract]. *Journal of Sports Sciences, 13*, 68-69.

266 | *Subjective Exercise Experience Scale (SEES)
Edward McAuley and Kerry S. Courneya

Source: McAuley, E., & Courneya, K. S. (1994). The Subjective Exercise Experience Scale: Development and preliminary validation. *Journal of Sport & Exercise Psychology, 16*, 163-177.

Purpose: To assess the subjective affective responses to exercise from a multidimensional perspective.

Description: The SEES contains 12 items, with four items per subscale. The subscales include Positive Well-Being, Psychological Distress, and Fatigue. Individuals respond to each item on a 7-point Likert scale with the verbal anchors *not at all* (1) and *very much so* (7).

Construction: An initial pool of 367 items, extracted from a wide variety of affective measures, was evaluated by seven expert researchers in the area of psychosocial responses to exercise. The experts were asked to evaluate the suitability of each item as a subjective experience that could be impacted negatively or positively by exercise participation. A total of 46 items were retained.

These items were then administered to 454 undergraduate students (n=189 males; n=265 females) who were asked to indicate the extent to which exercise participation (i.e., the exercise bout) influenced either positively or negatively these 46 subjective states. A total of 412 usable responses were subjected to a principal axis factor analysis (varimax rotation). A three-factor solution emerged (65.6% accountable variance), with four items retained per factor. The first factor was labeled Positive Well-Being (PWB), the second factor, Psychological Distress (PD), and the third factor was labeled Fatigue (F).

Reliability: Cronbach alpha coefficients were reported as .86 (PWB), .85 (PD, and .88 (F) for the sample of 412 undergraduate students. Among a sample of 51 middle-aged adults participating in an exercise program for previously sedentary individuals, internal consistency coefficients ranged from .84 to .92.

Validity: The construct validity of the SEES was supported through confirmatory factor analysis (n=100). Furthermore, following a graded exercise test, these 100 middle-aged participants reported less Psychological Distress and enhanced Positive Well-Being and increased Fatigue.

Also, among an additional sample of 51 middle-aged individuals enrolled in an exercise program for sedentary individuals, support for the convergent validity of the SEES was found. Participants' responses to the PWB subscale (following an exercise bout) correlated positively, as hypothesized with their responses to the Feeling Scale and the positive affect scale of the Positive and Negative Affect Schedule (PANAS). Similarly, their responses to the PD subscale of the SEES correlated positively with the negative affect scale of the PANAS.

In addition, support for the discriminant validity of the SEES was found. These individuals' (N=51) responses to the Fatigue subscale of the SEES were not correlated, as hypothesized, with their responses to the PANAS and Feeling Scale.

Norms: Not cited. Psychometric data were reported for 454 undergraduate students (n=189 males; n=265 females) enrolled in 13 physical activity classes at a large, comprehensive university; 100 middle-aged adults (*n*=49 males; *n*=51 females; *M* age=54.34 years) participating in a submaximal cycle ergometer graded exercise test; and 51 middle-aged adults (*n*=27 males; *n*=24 females) participating in a structured exercise program for previously sedentary individuals.

Availability: Contact Edward McAuley, Department of Kinesiology, University of Illinois, Freer Hall, 906 South Goodwin Avenue, Urbana, IL 61801. (Phone # 217-333-6487; FAX # 217-244-7322; E-mail: a-mc3@staff.uiuc.edu)

Reference

Hong, S., & McAuley, E. (1995). Subjective responses to acute exercise in college females [Abstract]. *Journal of Sport & Exercise Psychology, 17* (Suppl.), S61.

267 Test of Endurance Athlete Motives (TEAM)
Keith Johnsgard

Source: Johnsgard, K. (1985). The motivation of the long distance runner: II. *The Journal of Sports Medicine and Physical Fitness, 25,* 140-143.

Purpose: To assess the relative strength of 10 motives that appear to encompass the major reasons for endurance training.

Description: The TEAM involves a paired-comparison procedure with individuals required to make 45 forced choices between motives paired randomly. These motives include addictions, afterglow, centering, challenge, compete, feels good, fitness, identity, slim, and social. The test is scored by adding up the number of times each motive is selected. No motive can have a score greater than 9, and the total of the 10 scores must be 45.

Construction: Not discussed.

Reliability: Test-retest reliability coefficients (149 male and 31 female members of the Fifty-Plus Runners' Association) across a one-week interval were .74 (retrospective) and .78 (current). *Retrospective* referred to the initial motives for entering endurance training, whereas *current* referred to the motives for currently being involved in endurance training.

Validity: Not discussed.

Norms: Not cited. Psychometric data were presented for 149 male runners (*M* age= 56.3 years) and 31 female runners (*M* age= 52.5 years).

Availability: Last known address: Keith Johnsgard, Department of Psychology, San Jose State University, One Washington Square, San Jose, CA 95192-0120. (Phone # 408-924-5641)

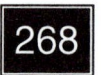 *Time Barriers Towards Exercise Scale (TBTE)
Adrian H. Taylor and Jenny Keith

Source: Taylor, A. H., & Keith, J. (1992). The mediating effect of perceived time barriers in the health locus of control and exercise relationship among corporate executives [Abstract]. *Journal of Sports Sciences, 10,* 625-626.

Purpose: The TBTE assesses perceived time barriers that may restrict involvement in exercise.

Description: The TBTE contains 10 items that reflect perceived time barriers associated with work, facility convenience, and family and social activities that restrict involvement in exercise. The items are prefaced with the statement "I am restricted in the amount of exercise that I can do because...." Participants respond on a 6-point Likert scale with the anchorings 0 (*strongly disagree*) to 5 (*strongly agree*).

Construction: Research literature that has examined barriers towards physical activity participation was initially reviewed. Six items were adopted from the Exercise Benefits/Barrriers Scale (Sechrist, Walker, & Pender, 1987); four additional items were developed. The TBTE, together with measures of health locus of control and physical activity, were administered to six corporate executives to confirm face validity and to check for item ambiguity. All three assessments were then mailed to 100 randomly selected British executives (from an oil industry mailing list). Data from 72 male executives were analyzed.

Reliability: A Cronbach alpha internal consistency coefficient ($N=72$) of .75 was reported.

Validity: Multiple regression analysis revealed that TBTE scores were not related to physical activity levels in the past 7 days. However, a hypothetical question about how an extra hour in the day would be spent was strongly related to TBTE. Those with low TBTE scores (below the median) would choose to spend, on the average, 7.7 minutes ($SD=14.1$) exercising, and those with high TBTE scores would spend, on the average, 20.0 minutes ($SD=21.7$) exercising.

Norms: Not reported. Psychometric data were cited for 72 male executives (M age=43.0 years, $SD=12.9$)

**Availability: Contact Adrian Taylor, Chelsea School Research Centre, University of Brighton, Trevin Towers, Eastbourne, East Sussex, England BN20 7SP. (Phone # 01273-643743; FAX # 01273-643704; E-mail: aht@bton.ac.uk)

Reference

Sechrist, K. R., Walker, S. N., & Pender, N. J. (1987). Development and psychometric evaluation of exercise benefits/barriers scale. *Research in Nursing and Health, 10,* 357-365.

Chapter 19

Motivation (Sport)

Tests in this chapter assess the motives individuals express for participating in sport, the degree of satisfaction derived from sport participation, and the reasons that inhibit people from engaging in sport. Tests also assess spectator motivation, sport commitment, flow states in sport, and perceptions of psychological momentum.

*Background and Sport Enjoyment Questionnaire [BSEQ]

Clay P. Sherman and Dennis Selder

Source: Sherman, C. P., & Selder, D. (1995). A comparison of enjoyment sources between participants of two different sport types [Abstract]. *Journal of Applied Sport Psychology*, 7 (Suppl.), S108.

Purpose: To evaluate the level of enjoyment experienced by sport participants.

Description: Not indicated.

Construction: Not indicated.

Reliability: Not indicated.

Validity: Factor analysis (*N*=140) supported an hypothesized two-dimensional theoretical framework for sport enjoyment

Norms: Not cited. Psychometric data were reported for 105 male and 135 female youth sport participants, ages 10 thru 18 years.

Availability: Contact Dennis Selder, Department of Exercise and Nutritional Sciences, San Diego State University, San Diego, CA 92182. (Phone # 619-594-1920; FAX # 619-594-6553; E-mail: dselder@sciences.sdsu.edu)

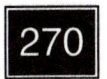

Coaching Orientation Inventory (COI)

Rainer Martens and Daniel Gould

Source: Martens, R., & Gould, D. (1979). Why do adults volunteer to coach children's sports? In G. C. Roberts & K. M. Newell (Eds.), *Psychology of motor behavior and sports-1978* (pp. 79-89). Champaign, IL: Human Kinetics Publishers.

Purpose: To assess the general orientations or motives adults express for coaching youth sport teams.

Description: The COI contains seven items, with each item having three response alternatives (i.e., the three orientations). The respondent is asked to indicate the most and least preferred alternative for each item.

Construction: The COI was modified from the Bass Orientation Inventory. The content validity of the COI was verified by 12 prominent sport psychologists with 98% confirmation that the alternatives for each item correctly assessed the intended orientation.

Reliability: Test-retest reliability coefficients across a one-week interval were .86 (Self Orientation), .77 (Affiliation Orientation), and .84 (Task Orientation).

Validity: Not presented.

Norms: Not cited. Descriptive data were presented for 423 youth sport coaches representing eight sports in communities of three different sizes in Illinois and Missouri.

Availability: Contact Rainer Martens, Human Kinetics Publishers, Box 5076, 1607 North Market Street, Champaign, IL 61825-5076. (Phone # 217-351-5076; FAX # 217-351-2674; E-mail: rainer@hkusa.com)

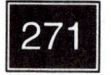 *Flow State Scale (FSS)
Susan A. Jackson and Herbert W. Marsh

Source: Jackson, S. A., & Marsh, H. W. (1995). Development and validation of a scale to measure optimal experience: The Flow State Scale. *Journal of Sport & Exercise Psychology, 18,* 17-35

Purpose: "To assess flow state in sport and physical activity settings" (p. 18).

Description: The FSS contains 36 items and nine subscales: Challenge-Skill Balance, Action-Awareness Merging, Clear Goals, Unambiguous Feedback, Concentration on Task at Hand, Sense of Control, Loss of Self Consciousness, Transformation of Time, Autotelic Experience. Participants respond to each item using a 5-point Likert scale with the anchorings 1 (*strongly disagree*) to 5 (*strongly agree*).

Construction: The FSS is based on Csikszentmihalyi's conceptualization of the dimensions of flow and qualitative research with athletes (Jackson, 1992) that focused on understanding the components of flow from athletes' perspectives. The FSS was reduced from 54 to 36 items based on confirmatory factor analysis of the responses of 394 participants in 41 sports and physical activities.

Reliability: Cronbach alpha coefficients ranged from .80 to .86 across the nine subscales.

Validity: Confirmatory factor analysis indicated that the best solution was a 36-item scale, with 4 items per subscale. Goodness-of-fit indices supported a nine first-order (truly unrelated) factor model, and a model with nine first-order factors and one higher order factor.

Norms: Not cited. Psychometric data were based on the responses of 394 athletes (57% male, 33% female) representing a total of 41 sports and physical activities.

**Availability: Contact Susan A. Jackson, Department of Human Movement Studies, The University of Queensland, Brisbane, Australia 4072 (Phone # 61-7-3365-6845; FAX # 61-7-3365-6877; E-mail: sue-jac@hms01.hms.uq.oz.au)

Reference
*Jackson, S. A. (1992). *Elite athletes in flow: The psychology of optimal sport experience*. Unpublished doctoral dissertation, University of North Carolina, Greensboro, NC.

272 | *Goal Importance Scale (GIS)
Rebecca Lewthwaite

Source: Lewthwaite, R. (1990). Threat perceptions in competitive trait anxiety: The endangerment of importance scales. *Journal of Sport & Exercise Psychology, 12,* 280-300.

Purpose: To assess the perceptions young athletes have about the importance of various goals in the competitive sport context.

Description: The GIS contains 28 items reflecting (a) mastery achievement goals (e.g., "How important is it to you that you learn and improve your skills as an athlete?"); (b) competitive achievement goals (e.g., "How important is it to you that you win your games [don't lose when you play sports]?"); (c) effort goals (e.g., "How important is it to you that you try hard all the time when you play sports?"); (d) affiliation goals (e.g., "How important is it to you that you enjoy being with your friends and teammates when you play sports?"); (e) goals related to the achievement/attainment of others' self-esteem (e.g., "How important is it to you that people who are important to you think you are a good athlete?"); (f) acceptance goals (e.g., "How important is it to you that people who are important to you like you as a person [are not ashamed of you when you play sports]?"; and (g) experiential goals (e.g, "How important is it to you that you feel action and excitement when you play sports?"). Participants respond to each item on a 7-point Likert scale with the anchorings from 1 (*not important at all to me*) to 7 (*very important to me*).

Construction: The GIS was developed by examining previous literature on sport goal orientation and participation motivation.

Reliability: Not discussed.

Validity: An iterated principal axis factor analysis ($N=102$) produced four factors labeled Avoidance of Negative Social Evaluation, Effort and Mastery Achievement, Positive Experiences and Social Evaluation, and Competitive Achievement. These factors accounted for 12.06%, 12.25%, 13.23%, and 11.40% of the variance in the factor analytic model employed.

Norms: Not cited. Psychometric data were reported for 102 male soccer players, ages 9 to 15, representing 11 teams in the Los Angeles area.

Availability: Last known address: Rebecca Lewthwaite, Department of Human Kinetics, University of Wisconsin-Milwaukee, Enderis 411, P. O. Box 413, Milwaukee, WI 53201. (FAX # 414-229-5100)

273	**[Incentive Motivation Inventory] [IMI]**
	Richard B. Alderman and Nancy L. Wood

Source: Alderman, R. B., & Wood, N. L. (1976). An analysis of incentive motivation in young Canadian athletes. *Canadian Journal of Applied Sport Sciences, 1,* 169-176.

Purpose: To evaluate the inventives perceived by young athletes as being available and attractive to them through competitive sport participation.

Description: The inventory contains 70 items and assesses seven major incentive systems including Independence, Power, Affiliation, Arousal, Esteem, Excellence, and Aggression. Participants respond using a 4-point ordinal scale.

Construction: Based on Birch and Veroff's (1966) classification of incentive systems and items from several well-known personality assessment instruments, a pool of 500 items was developed. Face validity was determined by the investigators, several graduate students, and interested coaches. Item analyses led to the retention of 70 items.

Reliability: Kuder-Richardson formula 20 internal consistency coefficients ranged from .27 (Arousal) to .67 (Aggression) when evaluated among 425 youth ice hockey players, ages 11-14 years.

Validity: Not discussed.

Norms: Not available. Psychometric data based on 425 youth ice hockey players, ages 11-14 years.

Availability: Last known address: Richard B. Alderman, Department of Physical Education and Sport Studies, University of Alberta, Edmonton, Alberta, Canada T6G 2H9. (FAX # 403-492-2364)

References

Birch, D., & Veroff, J. (1966). *Motivation--A study of action.* Belmont, CA: Brooks/Cole.

Buxton, K. E., & Ashford, B. (1994). Participation motives and physical self-perceptions in high- and low-frequency aerobic dance participants [Abstract]. *Journal of Sports Sciences, 12,* 184.

Pongrac, J. (1984). Sports participation incentives, locus of control and competitive trait anxiety [Abstract]. *Proceedings of the annual conference of the Canadian Society of Psychomotor Learning and Sport Psychology* (p. 9). Kingston, Ontario, Canada.

274   Minor Sport Enjoyment Inventory (MSEI)
Leonard M. Wankel and Philip S. J. Kreisel

Source: Wankel, L. M., & Kreisel, P. S. J. (1982). Factors underlying enjoyment and lack of enjoyment in minor sport: Sport and age group comparisons. In L. M. Wankel & R. B. Wilberg (Eds.), *Psychology of sport and motor behavior: Research and practice* (pp. 19-43). Edmonton, Alberta: University of Alberta.

Purpose: To assess the reasons underlying sport enjoyment among youth sport participants.

Description: The MSEI contains 10 items such as being with friends or pleasing others. Using a Thurstonian paired comparison approach to scaling, children are asked to select the preferred enjoyment factor from each of the 45 possible pairs of items.

Construction: Items for the inventory were derived from an extensive review of the literature on intrinsic motivation and on youth sport motivation, and from open-ended interviews of 50 youth sport participants. The items generated were reviewed by five experts. Pilot testing (*n*=20) of the 10 retained items was conducted to ensure item clarity and the suitability of the items for the targeted age groups. One item was subsequently discarded, and one item was separated into two items. (Wankel & Kreisel, 1985a)

Reliability: Item-to-item test-retest reliability over a one-week interval was 73% among 7- to 12-year-old boys (*n*=23). Item-to-item test-retest reliability over a 2-day interval was 86% among an older sample (*n*=25; *M* age=16.0 years) (Wankel & Kreisel, 1985a).

Validity: Not discussed.

Norms: Psychometric data were reported for 822 male youth sport participants, ages 7-14 years, representing soccer (*n*=310), hockey (*n*=338), and baseball (n=174). A representative sample was obtained from 20 schools in a large western Canadian city. In addition, Wankel (1983a) provided comparative data for 949 female youth sport participants representing softball (n=260), soccer (n=223), volleyball (n=92), basketball (n=94), gymnastics (n=227), and other activities (e.g., ringette, track and field; n=53).

Availability: Contact Leonard M. Wankel, Department of Physical Education and Sport Studies, University of Alberta, P 320A Van Vliet Center, Edmonton, Alberta, Canada T6G 2H9. (Phone # 403-492-2831; FAX # 403 492-2364; E-mail: lwankel@per.ualberta.ca)

References

*Wankel, L. M. (1983a). Factors influencing girls' enjoyment of sport. Report submitted to Fitness and Amateur Sports Canada (Project No.217, 1982-1983). Ottawa: Fitness and Amateur Sport.

*Wankel, L. M. (1983b). Girls' enjoyment of sport: Age and sport group differences [Abstract]. *In Psychology of motor behavior and sport-1983* (p. 135). Proceedings of the North American Society for the Psychology of Sport and Physical Activity annual convention. Michigan State University, East Lansing.

*Wankel, L. M., & Kreisel, P. S. J. (1985a). Factors underlying enjoyment of youth sports: Sport and age group comparisons. *Journal of Sport Psychology, 7,* 51-64.

Wankel, L. M., & Kreisel, P. S. J. (1985b). Methodological considerations in youth sport motivation research: A comparison of open-ended and paired comparison approaches. *Journal of Sport Psychology, 7,* 65-74.

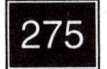

Motivational Orientation in Sport Scale [MOSS]
Maureen R. Weiss, Brenda Jo Bredemeier, and Richard M. Shewchuk

Source: Weiss, M. R., Bredemeier, B. J., & Shewchuk, R. M. (1985). An intrinsic/extrinsic sport motivation scale for the youth sport setting: A confirmatory factor analysis. *Journal of Sport Psychology, 7,* 75-91.

Purpose: To assess the motivational orientations of children within a physical education or sport environment.

Description: Children respond to five motivational orientation subscales containing six items each: (a) Challenge, (b) Curiosity, (c)

Mastery, (d) Judgment, and (e) Criteria. They are first asked to decide for each item whether the statement on the left or the right side was most descriptive and then to indicate whether the statement selected was really true or just sort of true for him or her. Items are scored on a four-point ordinal scale with the anchorings 1 (*extrinsic orientation*) to 4 (*intrinsic orientation*).

Construction: The IESMS represents a modification of Harter's (1981) Motivational Orientation in the Classroom scale in which items were reworded to be compatible with a physical education or sport setting. Exploratory factor analyses (*n*=155) resulted in the retention of six preliminary subscales accounting for 83.3% of the variance.

Reliability: Cronbach alpha internal reliability coefficients for the six subscales (*n*=155) were .81 (Challenge), .61 (Curiosity/Interest), .64 (Mastery), .64 (Judgment), .75 (Criteria), and .65 (Curiosity/Improve skills).

Validity: Not discussed.

Norms: Not cited. Psychometric data were presented for 86 male and 69 female youth sport participants, ranging in age from 8 to 12 years.

Availability: Contact Maureen R. Weiss, Department of Exercise and Movement Science, 1240 Esslinger Hall, University of Oregon, Eugene, OR 97403-1240. (Phone # 541-346-4108; FAX # 541-346-2841; E-mail: mrw@oregon.uoregon.edu)

References
*Black, S. J., & Weiss, M. R. (1992). The relationship among perceived coaching behaviors, perceptions of ability, and motivation in competitive age-group swimmers. *Journal of Sport & Exercise Psychology, 14,* 309-325.

Harter, S. (1981). A new self-report scale of intrinsic versus extrinsic orientation in the classroom: Motivational and informational components. *Developmental Psychology, 17,* 300-312.

*Lawson, R. J., & Fazey, D. (1995). Girls' age, accuracy of perceived swimming competence and motivational orientation [Abstract]. *Journal of Sports Science, 13,* 63.

*Theeboom, M., De Knop, P., & Weiss, M. R. (1995). Motivational climate, psychological responses, and motor skill development in children's sport: A field-based intervention study. *Journal of Sport & Exercise Psychology, 17,* 294-311.

Weiss, M. R., & Horn, T. S. (1990). The relation between children's accuracy estimates of their physical competence and achievement-related characteristics. *Research Quarterly for Exercise and Sport, 61,* 250-258.

276 [Motives for Competition Scale] [MCS]
David Youngblood and Richard M. Suinn

Source: Youngblood, D., & Suinn, R. M. (1980). A behavior assessment of motivation. In R. M. Suinn (Ed.), *Psychology in sports* (pp. 73-77). Minneapolis, MN: Burgess Publishing Company.

Purpose: To identify the motivational characteristics of athletes.

Description: The scale contains 95 items and 19 categories such as social approval, competition, self-mastery, fear of failure, status, heterosexuality, and emotional release. Items within each category can be answered using a yes-no format or a 5-point rating scale format.

Construction: The authors developed a list of needs that might influence the personal choice to be involved in athletics. The list was reviewed by 17 psychology faculty, 22 college-level coaches, and 16 members of the physical education faculty who had prior participation or experience in coaching. A final list of 19 categories resulted.

Reliability: A test-retest reliability coefficient for the total score was .93, with the median test-retest reliability for the subscales of .76, on data from 25 female college swimmers and divers.

Validity: There was a significant correlation coefficient between these (n=25) female athletes' total scores on the scale and their coaches' ratings of their level of motivation at four different times during the season.

Norms: Not cited.

**Availability: Contact Richard M. Suinn, Department of Psychology, Colorado State University, Fort Collins, CO 80523. (Phone # 970-491-1351; FAX # 970-491-1032; E-mail: suinn@lamar.colostate.edu)

References
*Raugh, D., & Wall, R. (1987). Measuring sports participation motivation. *International Journal of Sport Psychology, 18,* 112-119.

*Straub, W. (1984). The motives of athletes [Abstract]. In *Proceedings of the 1984 Olympic Scientific Congress* (p. 106). Eugene, OR: College of Human Development and Performance Microform Publications.

277 [Motives for Participating in Gymnastics] [MPG]

Kimberley A. Klint and Maureen R. Weiss

Source: Klint, K. A. , & Weiss, M. R. (1987). Perceived competence and motives for participating in youth sports: A test of Harter's competence motivation theory. *Journal of Sport Psychology, 9,* 55-65.

Purpose: A self-report questionnaire used to determine motives for participating in gymnastics.

Description: This test contains 32 items; each item is rated on a 5-point Likert scale.

Construction: The test is a modification of instruments developed by Gill, Gross, and Huddleston (1983) and Gould, Feltz, and Weiss (1985). It was adopted specifically to evaluate the reasons children participate in gymnastics.

Reliability: Cronbach alpha reliability coefficients were reported for seven derived subscales. Coefficients ranged from .53 to .86 among a sample of 27 boys and 40 girls (*M* age = 11.4 years, *SD* = 2.3 years).

Validity: Content validity was established by asking seven experts (coaches, teachers, researchers) to evaluate each item based on their understanding of children's experiences and motives in sport.

Norms: Not available. Item descriptive statistics were reported for the 67 children.

Availability: Contact Maureen R. Weiss, Department of Exercise and Movement Science, 1240 Esslinger Hall, University of Oregon, Eugene, OR 97403-1240. (Phone # 541-346-4108; FAX # 541-346-2841; E-mail: mrw@oregon.uoregon.edu)

References

Gill, D. L., Gross, J. B., & Huddleston, S. (1983). Participation motivation in youth sport. *International Journal of Sport Psychology, 14,* 1-14.

Gould, D., Feltz, D., & Weiss, M. (1985). Motives for participating in competitive youth swimming. *International Journal of Sport Psychology, 16,* 126-140.

278 Participation Motivation Questionnaire [PMQ]

Diane L. Gill, John B. Gross, and Sharon Huddleston

Source: Gill, D. L., Gross, J. B., & Huddleston, S. (1983). Participation motivation in youth sports. *International Journal of Sport Psychology, 14,* 1-14.

Purpose: To assess the motives children express for participating in youth sport.

Description: Children are asked to respond to 30 reasons for participating in sports including "I like to win," and "I like to meet new friends." Children respond to each item using a 3-point ordinal scale with the response categories "very important," "somewhat important," and "not at all important."

Construction: The original 37-item questionnaire was developed based on a review of the youth sport literature and from the results of two pilot projects administered to participants at a summer sports school. General categories or dimensions of participation motivation were derived through factor analysis and resulted in the 30-item questionnaire.

Reliability: Cronbach alpha internal consistency coefficients ($n=1,138$) for the eight derived factors (see Validity section) accounting for participation motivation ranged from .30 (Friends) to .78 (Team).

Validity: Factor analyses of the responses of 720 boys and 418 girls to the PMQ suggested that the reasons these children participated in youth sport centered on basic orientations such as achievement, team, friendship, fitness, energy release, skill development, and fun. Success orientation accounted for the largest percent of the variance (19.4%), with all eight factors accounting for 100% of the variance in the factor analytic model utilized. The authors noted, however, that "... considerable psychometric work is needed before the items or factors can be accepted as reliable, valid and comprehensive measures of participation motivation in youth sports" (p. 12).

446

Norms: Not indicated. Psychometric data were cited for 720 boys (ages 9-18 years) and 418 girls (ages 8-18 years) attending the University of Iowa Summer Sports School.

Availability: Contact Diane L. Gill, Exercise and Sport Science Department, University of North Carolina, Greensboro, NC 27412-5001. (Phone # 910-334-5744; FAX # 910-334-3238; E-mail: gilldl@iris.uncg.edu)

References

Ashford, B., & Rickhuss, J. (1992). Life-span differences in participating in community sport and recreation [Abstract]. *Journal of Sports Sciences, 10,* 626.

*Brodkin, P., & Weiss, M. R. (1990). Developmental differences in motivation for participating in competitive swimming. *Journal of Sport & Exercise Psychology, 12,* 248-263.

Buonamano, R., Cei, A., & Mussino, A. (1995). Participant motivation in Italian youth sport. *The Sport Psychologist, 9,* 265-281.

*Chapin, G. K., Ewing, M. E., & Seefeldt, V. D. (1992). A factor analytic study of participants' motives for involvement in youth sport programs [Abstract]. *Proceedings of the North American Society for the Psychology of Sport and Physical Activity annual convention* (p. 142). Pittsburgh, PA.

Flood, S. E., & Hellstedt, J. C. (1991). Gender differences in motivation for intercollegiate athletic participation. *Journal of Sport Behavior, 14,* 159-167.

*Gould, D., Feltz, D., & Weiss, M. (1985). Motives for participating in competitive youth swimming. *International Journal of Sport Psychology, 16,* 126-140.

*Hare, M. (1995). Participation motivation in elite junior tennis players [Abstract]. *Journal of Sports Sciences, 13,* 58.

Mahoney, C. A., Kremer, J., & Scully, D. M. (1994). The evaluation of mental skills training in swimming [Abstract]. *Journal of Sports Sciences, 12,* 200.

*Passer, M. W. (1982). Participation motives of young athletes as a function of competitive trait anxiety, self-esteem, ability, and age [Abstract]. In *Psychology of Motor Behavior and Sport-1982* (p. 103). Proceedings of the annual convention of the North American Society for the Psychology of Sport and Physical Activity, University of Maryland, College Park.

*Ryckman, R. M., & Hamel, J. (1993). Perceived physical ability differences in the sport participation motives of young athletes. *International Journal of Sport Psychology, 24,* 270-283.

*Shi, J., & Ewing, M. E. (1994). A cross-cultural study of participation motivation in table tennis [Abstract]. *Journal of Sport & Exercise Psychology, 16* (Suppl.), S105.

*White, S. A., & Duda, J. L. (1994). The relationship of gender, level of sport involvement, and participation motivation to task and ego orientation. *International Journal of Sport Psychology, 25,* 4-18.

*Wong, E. H., Bridges, L. J., & Talken, T. (1993). Participation motives among youth soccer participants: Similarities and differences across divisions [Abstract]. *Proceedings of the Association for the Advancement of Applied Sport Psychology annual convention* (p. 165). Montreal, Canada.

279 *[Perceptions of Psychological Momentum Questionnaire] [PPMQ]
Steve Miller and Robert Weinberg

Source: Miller, S., & Weinberg, R. (1991). Perceptions of psychological momentum and their relationship to performance. *The Sport Psychologist*, 5, 211-222.

Purpose: To evaluate psychological factors related to perceptions of momentum in volleyball.

Description: The PPMQ contains four scenarios involving two volleyball teams in which psychological momentum and situation criticality are manipulated. Participants are asked to rate on an 11-point Likert scale the degree to which each team would feel momentum, confidence, control, anxiety, and/or discouragement.

Construction: Not discussed.

Reliability: Test-retest reliability coefficients across a 3-week interval (*n*=29 undergraduate students) were .88 (Scenario 1), .93 (Scenario 2), .94 (Scenario 3), and .90 (Scenario 4).

Validity: Respondents (*n*=280) perceived momentum situations as significantly different from nonmomentum situations. Teams coming from behind were viewed as exhibiting "...increased confidence, more momentum, and control of the game while leaving opponents more discouraged and more anxious" (p. 218). Momentum impacted critical game situations more significantly than noncritical game situations.

Norms: Not cited. Psychometric data were based on the responses of 160 Division I volleyball players from 18 teams and 120 students in beginning volleyball classes.

Availability: Contact Robert Weinberg, Department of Physical Education, Health, and Sport Studies, Miami University, Phillips Hall, Oxford, OH 45056. (Phone # 513-529-2700; FAX # 513-529-5006; E-mail: rweinber@miamiu.muohio.edu)

280 *Spectator Decision-Making Inventory (SDMI)

James J. Zhang, Dale G. Pease, Stanley C. Hui, and Thomas J. Michaud

Source: Zhang, J. J., Pease, D. G., Hui, S. C., & Michaud, T. J. (1995). Variables affecting the spectator decision to attend NBA games. *Sport Marketing Quarterly, 4*(4), 29-39.

Purpose: To quantitatively assess variables that affect the decision of spectators to attend professional basketball games.

Description: The SDMI contains 14 items and four variables: Game Promotion, Home Team, Opposing Team, and Schedule Convenience. Participants respond to each item using a 5-point ordinal scale with the anchorings 1 (*none*) to 5 (*very much*).

Construction: Based on a review of the literature and interviews with four administrators of National Basketball Association (NBA) teams, 20 variables were identified that affect the decisions of spectators to attend professional basketball games. Each variable was phrased into a 5-point ordinal scale test item. A panel of five experts (3 university professors in sport management and/or sport psychology and 2 senior NBA team administrators) evaluated the items for content validity. The experts were asked to review "(a) the appropriateness of the format and content, (b) the adequacy and representativeness of test items, and (c) the accuracy of a phrased statement" (p. 31). Based on their analyses, 17 items were retained. Exploratory principal component factor analysis with varimax rotation (N=861) led to the retention of 14 items and four factors (Game Promotion, Home Team, Opposing Team, and Schedule Convenience) accounting for 65.2% of the variance.

Reliability: Cronbach alpha internal consistency coefficients (N=861) were .88, .92., .86, and .63 for Game Promotion, Home Team, Opposing Team, and Schedule Convenience subscales, respectively.

Validity: Stepwise multiple regression analysis indicated that participants' (N=861) responses to the SDMI (except for the Schedule Convenience subscale) were positively related to the number of NBA games attended during the present season. Responses to the Home Team subscale were positively related to the number of seasons in which participants attended NBA games.

Norms: Not indicated. Descriptive and psychometric data are presented for 861 spectators (*M* age= 33.32 years; *SD*= 14.08), selected using random cluster sampling procedures, who were in attendance at six second-half 1993-1994 season home games of a major NBA Western Conference team.

**Availability: Contact James J. Zhang, Department of Health and Human Performance, University of Houston, Houston, TX 77204-5331. (Phone # 713-743-9869; FAX # 713-743-9860; E-mail: educ1b@jetson.uh.edu)

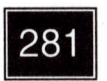 ## *Sport Commitment Model Scales (SCM)
Tara K. Scanlan, Jeffrey P. Simons, Paul J. Carpenter, Greg W. Schmidt, and Bruce Keeler

Source: Scanlan, T. K., Carpenter, P. J., Simons, J. P., Schmidt, G. W., & Keeler, B. (1993). The Sport Commitment Model: Measurement development for the youth-sport domain. *Journal of Sport & Exercise Psychology, 15*, 16-38

Purpose: To assess the determinants of sport commitment, "a psychological construct representing the desire and resolve to continue sport participation" (p. 18). These determinants include an athlete's sport enjoyment, the attractiveness of involvement alternatives, personal investments in participation, social constraints to continue participating in the sport activity, and involvement opportunities afforded by continued participation.

Description: Psychometric evaluation currently supports the appropriateness of items to measure sport commitment (4 items), sport enjoyment (4 items), social constraints (3 items), and involvement opportunities (3 items). Five-point Likert scales are used to assess participants' responses to each item, with the foil for 1 being a form of *not at all/none or nothing* and 5 being a form of *very much or a lot*. For example, participants are asked: "Are you happy playing in (program) this season?" (Sport Enjoyment).

Construction: Survey items were selected so as to be understood by subjects who were representative of diverse sociocultural backgrounds, some of whom were as young as 9-10 years of age. The items also had to be relevant to young athletes participating in a variety of sports and levels of competition. Items were selected, based on reviews of previous literature on commitment and on youth sport, and based on the constitutive definitions established.

Four experts evaluated the content, format, wording, and response foils of each item. Four elementary and two junior high school teachers and several fifth- thru seventh-grade athletes evaluated the items selected by the experts for age-group and ethnic appropriateness. Based on these evaluations, 26 items were retained for the six model constructs proposed (i.e., Sport Commitment, Sport Enjoyment, Involvement Alternatives, Personal Investments, Social Constraints, and Involvement Opportunities).

In Phase 1, the individual-item characteristics, internal consistency of the scales, and discriminant validity were examined among 140 athletes ($n=71$ males; $n=67$ females; $n=2$ not declared) from two youth sport programs. Items for the Sport Commitment Model were part of a larger battery of measures administered to these athletes as part of the Athletes' Opinion Survey. Cronbach alpha internal consistency coefficients of .88 (Sport Commitment), .90 (Sport Enjoyment), .91 (Involvement Alternatives), .87 (Social Constraints), .77 (Personal Investments), and .83 (Involvement Opportunities) were reported. Principal factors extraction with iterations (oblique and orthogonal rotations) led to the verification of the five-factor solution specified. Although some modifications were made to the items of the Involvement Alternatives construct, the majority of items examined in Phase I were retained for further analyses.

Phase 2 attempted to replicate and extend the findings of Phase 1 among 178 athletes ($n=95$ females; $n=83$ males) participating in a suburban Little League program. Individual-item characteristics were judged acceptable, and Cronbach alpha coefficients of .89 (Sport Commitment), .95 (Sport Enjoyment), .88 (Social Constraints), and .80 (Involvement Opportunities) were computed. The Involvement Alternatives and Personal Investments scales evidenced marginal internal consistency. Principal factors extraction with oblique rotation, orthogonal factor analysis, and confirmatory factor analysis again supported the hypothesized five-factor solution. However, the Involvement Alternatives items were viewed as problematic with only one item being retained for further analyses. The investigators also reduced the number of items in the Sport Commitment and Social Constraints scales to facilitate a shorter survey instrument without substantially lowering the internal consistency of these two scales.

Phase 3 examined further the psychometric characteristics of the retained items across several diverse samples (N=1,342) in terms of age, gender, and ethnic background differences. Confirmatory factor analysis via a structural-equation program was used to assess and refine the scales of the Sport Commitment Model. Four runs of the measurement model led to the support of the retained items to measure sport commitment, sport enjoyment, social constraints, and involvement opportunities constructs.

Reliability: Acceptable Cronbach alpha coefficients were reported for the four scales retained (see Construction section).

Validity: Confirmatory factor analyses across diverse samples supported the validity of items to measure the sport commitment, sport enjoyment, social constraints, and involvement opportunities constructs (see Construction section).

Norms: Not presently available. Psychometric properties were evaluated for samples diverse in age, gender, ethnicity, and type of sport participation. These samples included 140 predominantly Caucasian or Asian athletes from two youth-sport programs; 178 predominantly Caucasian athletes participating in a suburban Little League program (M age=12.49 years; SD=1.69); and 1,342 participants of diverse ethnic backgrounds involved in three different youth sport programs (n=553 male football players; M age=12.3 years) (n=322 males and n=294 female youth soccer players; M age=15.7 years) (n=173 female volleyball players; M age=13.0 years).

Availability: Contact Tara K. Scanlan, Department of Psychology, University of California, 1285 Franz Hall, Box 951563, Los Angeles, California 90095-1563. (FAX 310-206-5895; E-mail: scanlan@psych.sscnet.ucla.edu)

References

Scanlan, T. K., & Carpenter, P. J. (1993). Key ingredients to commitment in sport. In J. R. Nitsch & R. Seiler (Eds.), *Motivation, emotion, stress: Proceedings of the VIII European Congress of Sport Psychology* (pp. 21-31, Vol. 1). Sankt Augustin, Germany: Academia Verlag.

Scanlan, T. K., Carpenter, P. J., Schmidt, G. W., Simons, J. P. & Keeler, B. (1993). An introduction to the Sport Commitment Model. *Journal of Sport & Exercise Psychology, 15*, 1-15.

*Scanlan, T. K., Carpenter, P. J., Simons, J. P., & Keeler, B. (1990). Stages of involvement and commitment to a youth sport program [Abstract], *Proceedings of the Association for the Advancement of Applied Sport Psychology annual convention* (p. 106). San Antonio, TX.

*Yin, Z., Boyd, M., & Callaghan, J. (1992). Canonical analysis of goal orientation and its related variables [Abstract]. *Proceedings of the North American Society for the Psychology of Sport and Physical Activity annual convention* (p. 195). Pittsburgh, PA.

*Sport Fan Motivation Scale (SFMS)
Daniel L. Wann

Source: Wann, D. L. (1995). Preliminary validation of the Sport Fan Motivation Scale. *Journal of Sport & Social Issues. 19*, 377-396.

Purpose: To assess motivations for involvement as a sport fan.

Description: The SFMS is a 23-item scale and assesses eight motivations for involvement as a sport fan: eustress, self-esteem, escape, entertainment, economic, aesthetic, group affiliation, and family reasons. Participants respond to each item using an 8-point ordinal scale with the anchorings 1 (*this is not at all descriptive of me*) to 8 (*this is very descriptive of me*). All subscales contain three items except the family reasons subscale, which contains two items.

Construction: Subscales were derived from a review of the literature on the motivations of sport fans. Initially, a 38-item scale was developed. Exploratory principal components factor analysis ($N=272$) led to the retention of seven factors. However, although there were only two items that loaded on the family reasons subscale, this subscale was retained in the final SFMS.

Reliability: Cronbach alpha internal consistency coefficients ($N=272$) ranged from .89 (Eustress) to .63 (Family); an overall alpha coefficient of .90 was reported for the entire scale.

Validity: Confirmatory factor analyses (N=272) supported the hypothesized eight-factor model. Furthermore, the convergent validity of the SFMS was supported in that these participants' responses to the SFMS were positively correlated with their scores on the Sport Spectator Identification Scale. In other words, scores on the SFMS were related to level of identification as a sport fan.

Norms: Not cited. Descriptive statistics and psychometric data were reported for 166 university students and 106 participants in a recreational softball league. There were 100 males and 172 females (M age=22.9 years) who served as participants.

**Availability: Contact Daniel L. Wann, Department of Psychology, Murray State University, 1 Murray Street, Murray, KY 42071-3311. Phone # 502-762-2860; FAX # 502-762-3424; E-mail: danwann@ msumusik.mursuky.edu). Items are also cited in the *Source*.

Reference

*Wann, D. L. (1994). Development of the Sport Spectator Motivation Scale [Abstract]. *Journal of Sport & Exercise Psychology*, 16 (Suppl.), S120.

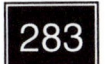 *Sport Motivation Scale (SMS)
Luc G. Pelletier, Michelle S. Fortier, Robert J. Vallerand, Kim M. Tuson, Nathalie M. Briere, and Marc R. Blais

Source: Pelletier, L. G., Fortier, M. S., Vallerand, R. J., Tuson, K. M., Briere, N. M., & Blais, M. R. (1995). Toward a new measure of intrinsic motivation, extrinsic motivation, and amotivation in sports: The Sport Motivation Scale (SMS). *Journal of Sport & Exercise Psychology*, 17, 35-53.

Purpose: To assess various components of intrinsic motivation and extrinsic motivation, and amotivation toward sport.

Description: The SMS contains seven subscales that assess three types of intrinsic motivation (Intrinsic Motivation to Know; Intrinsic Motivation Toward Accomplishments; and Intrinsic Motivation to

Experience Stimulation) and three forms of regulation for extrinsic motivation (Introjection; Identification; and External Regulation). The SMS also contains an Amotivation subscale.

The SMS focuses on the perceived reasons for engaging in sport by asking participants to respond to the question "Why do you practice your sport?" Participants are presented with 28 items (e.g., "For the prestige of being an athlete" and "For the pleasure I feel in living exciting experiences") and are asked to rate each item using a 7-point ordinal scale. There are four items per subscale.

Construction: The SMS was originally constructed in French, and preliminary and validation studies were conducted with approximately 600 athletes (M age= 18.4 years) representing eight different sports. A mean Cronbach alpha internal consistency coefficient of .82 was reported, and a mean test-retest reliability coefficient of .69 was found across a one-month interval. Confirmatory factor analysis (with LISREL) supported the hypothesized seven-factor structure of the instrument. Convergent validity was supported using measures of interest toward sport, sport satisfaction, positive emotions experienced during sport practice. The French version of the SMS was also able to predict sport dropout. The current report (referenced as the *Source* above) details efforts to translate the instrument into English (titled as the Sport Motivation Scale) and to assess its psychometric properties.

Reliability: Cronbach alpha internal consistency coefficients (N=593) ranged from .63 (Identification scale) to .80 (Intrinsic Motivation to Know; Intrinsic Motivation Toward Accomplishments) with a mean alpha coefficient of .75 reported. Internal consistency coefficients ranged from .71 to .85 on a pretest and from .69 to .85 on a posttest of the SMS given to 51 soccer players. Test-retest reliability coefficients ranged from .58 to .84 (M test-retest reliability coefficient of .70) for these same soccer athletes across a 5-week interval.

Validity: Confirmatory factor analysis (LISREL 7) using the scores of 593 university athletes supported the hypothesized seven-factor structure of the SMS. Also, intercorrelation coefficients among the three intrinsic motivation subscales were moderate, and intercorrelations among the seven scales displayed a simplex pattern, thus supporting the construct validity of the SMS.

The convergent validity of the SMS was supported in that participants'

(N=593) responses to the SMS were related to their responses on measures of perceived competence and to four forms of coaches' interpersonal behavior (e.g., caring). Also, these participants' responses to the SMS were related to measures of motivational consequences (i.e., distraction during the activity, effort, and future intentions of practicing the activity).

Norms: Not cited. Psychometric data were reported for 319 male and 274 female university athletes (M age=19.2 years) representing nine sports who resided in Ontario, Canada.

**Availability: Contact Luc G. Pelletier, School of Psychology, University of Ottawa, P. O. Box 450, Station A, Ottawa, Ontario, Canada K1N 6N5. (Phone # 613-562-5800, ext. 4201; FAX # 613-562-5147). Items are also listed in the *Source*.

References

*Fortier, M. S., Vallerand, R. J., Briere, N. M., & Provencher, P. J. (1995). Competitive and recreational sport structures and gender: A test of their relationship with sport motivation. *International Journal of Sport Psychology, 26,* 24-39.

*Li, F., & Harmer, P. (1994). Testing the simplex assumption underlying the Sport Motivation Scale [Abstract]. *Journal of Sport & Exercise Psychology, 16* (Suppl.), S79.

*Li, F., & Harmer, P. (1995). Sport motivation in physical activity: A confirmatory factor analysis [Abstract]. *Research Quarterly for Exercise and Sport, 66* (Suppl.), A-76.

284 Sport Non-Participation Questionnaire (SNQ)
Jane McNally and Terry Orlick

Source: McNally, J., & Orlick, T. (1977). The Sport Non-Participation Questionnaire: An exploratory analysis. In Human performance and behavior (pp. 111-117). *Proceedings of the 9th Canadian Psycho-motor Learning and Sport Psychology Symposium.* Banff, Alberta, Canada.

Purpose: To assess the relative importance of various reasons that inhibit sport participation.

Description: The SNQ contains 55 items. Participants respond to each item using a 10-point ordinal scale.

Construction: A review of the literature, discussions with teachers, coaches, and several sport psychologists, and a pilot study of 144 females who responded to open-ended questions about their perceived reasons for not playing more sports led to the formation of 18 categories depicting reasons that inhibit sport participation. These categories included Significant Others, Ability, Facilities, Health, Sexuality, Self-Concept, Competition, Cosmetic, Physique, Injury, Time, Coaching, Self-Consciousness, Models, Socialization, Organization, Learning, and Aggression. Fifty-five items were developed depicting these 18 areas of concern.

Reliability: Not reported.

Validity: Exploratory factor analysis was conducted among 310 female and 407 male high school students to examine construct validity. Two factors emerged, labeled Self-Esteem/Competitive Threat and Socio-Cosmetic.

Norms: Not cited. Descriptive and psychometric data were presented for 717 high school students.

Availability: Contact Terry Orlick, School of Human Kinetics, University of Ottawa, 125 University, Ottawa, Canada, K1N 6N5. (Phone # 613-562-5800, ext. 4272; FAX # 613-564-7689)

---

285 *[Sport Participation Motivation Questionnaire] [SPMQ]
A. P. McKee, C. A. Mahoney, and J. Kremer

Source: McKee, A. P., Mahoney, C. A., & Kremer, J. (1994). The development of a sport participation motivation questionnaire for use with an adult population in Northern Ireland [Abstract]. *Journal of Sports Sciences, 12,* 201.

Purpose: To assess motives for sport participation among adult populations.

Description: The SPMQ contains 121 items that evaluate four motives for participation in sport among adults: (a) Competition, (b) Psychophysiological health, (c) Affiliation, and (d) Significant Others. Participants respond to each item using a 5-point Likert scale with the anchorings *very untrue* for me to *very true for me.*

Construction: Items for the SPMQ were derived from lengthy face-to-face interviews with individuals (N=22) involved in a variety of sports at various competitive levels; interviews with individuals (N=20) who had chosen not to participate in sport; extensive library research; and item analyses of existing participation motivation questionnaires.

Reliability: Cronbach alpha reliability coefficients for the four factors ranged from .77 to .94 (N=201).

Validity: A principal axis factor analysis supported a four-factor model structure in which 37% of the variance in participants' (N=201) responses to the SPMQ was accounted. (The "competition" factor accounted for 23% of the variance.)

Norms: Not presented. Psychometric data were reported for 201 individuals (n=121 males; n=80 females) actively involved in a wide variety of individual and team sports.

Availability: Last known address: A. P. McKee, Physical Education and Health Unit, The Queen's University of Belfast, Botanic Gardens, Belfast BT7 5EX, Ireland.

286 Sport Satisfaction Inventory (SSI)
N. R. Whittall and Terry D. Orlick

Source: Whittall, N. R., & Orlick, T. D. (1979). The Sport Satisfaction Inventory. In G. C. Roberts & K. M. Newell (Eds.), *Psychology of motor and sport-1978* (pp. 144-155). Champaign, IL: Human Kinetics Publishers.

Purpose: To assess the degree of satisfaction an individual derives from participating in sport.

458

Description: The SSI assesses six dimensions of sport satisfaction: the Sport or game itself, Practice, Coach, Teammates, Opposition, and Personal Ability and Performance. Individuals respond to this 84-item inventory using a 5-point Likert scale.

Construction: Initial categories of sport satisfaction were developed after an extensive review of the sport and industrial psychology literature. An evaluation of the open-ended responses of 44 athletes by four judges led to the creation of seven categories of sport satisfaction. An additional 91 sport participants assisted in the creation of items reflective of each category. Item analyses of the responses of 80 additional athletes representing eight teams led to the retention of 84 items.

Reliability: Internal consistency coefficients (n=120 males and 32 females from 14 teams) ranged from .81 to .93 using the corrected split-half method, and averaged .85 across the six dimensions. Test-retest reliability coefficients (n=23 males and 10 females from 3 teams) ranged from .42 to .91 across a one-week interval; the average test-retest reliability coefficient was .81 when the lowest test-retest reliability coefficient (for the Opposition dimension) was not considered.

Validity: Not discussed.

Norms: Psychometric data were presented for 400 male and female sport participants, ages 10 to 39 years, representing a wide range of athletic abilities (excluding the professional level). These athletes represented 13 different sports.

Availability: Contact Terry D. Orlick, School of Human Kinetics, University of Ottawa, 125 University, Ottawa, Canada, K1N 6N5. (Phone # 613-562-5800, ext. 4272; FAX # 613-564-7689)

 287 *Trampoline Motivation Questionnaire [TMQ]
Jean Whitehead

Source: Whitehead, J. (1976). Trampoline motivation: A short questionnaire. *British Journal of Physical Education, 7*(5), v-vi.

Purpose: To assess one's motivation for trampolining.

Description: The TMQ contains 16 Likert-type items constituting four subscales: Achievement, Fear, Pleasure, and Interest. Participants respond on a 5-point scale to items such as: "Doing this would make me very happy" and "I am not keen to succeed in this."

Construction: A preliminary 50-item questionnaire, appropriate for 11- to 12-year-old beginners and containing 10 subscales, was constructed. Items were developed based on interviews with beginners in trampoline (N=13). Five subscales were derived from Sumner's (1965) conceptual framework for motivation for children's reasons for working hard at school, and five contrasting subscales tapped negative motives. Principal components factor analysis led to the retention of four 10-item sub-scales suitable for responding to by young children. These scales were improved by piloting 40 items for each scale to obtain the 10 items that best discriminated between high and low scorers on the test (J. Whitehead, personal communication, April 10, 1996). The *Source* above describes a shortened version of the TMQ appropriate for college students.

Reliability: Corrected split-half internal consistency coefficients ranged from .96 (N=76 U. S. college students) to .87 (N=126 United Kingdom college students).

Validity: Biserial correlation coefficients of .85 to .88 were obtained between TMQ total scores and students' interest (yes/no) in participating in a trampoline club or class.

Norms: Not cited. Psychometric data were reported for 57 female students attending the University of Oregon trampoline classes and 126 male or female physical education students in their first year at Bedford College of Higher Education in England.

**Availability: Items are listed in the *Source*. For further information, contact Jean Whitehead, Chelsea School Research Centre, University of Brighton, Gaudick Road, Eastbourne, East Susex, BN20 7SP England. (Phone # 01273-600900; FAX # 01273-643704; E-mail: jw73@bton.ac.uk)

460

References

Sumner, R. (1965). *The relationship between school attainment in craft subjects and a test of craft skills.* Unpublished master's thesis, University of Manchester, England.

*Whitehead, J. (1975). Questionnaire on motivation for trampolining. *British Journal of Physical Education, 6*(2), v-vi.

[Women's Sports Orientation Scales] [WSOS]

Donald Siegel and Caryl Newhof

Source: Siegel, D., & Newhof, C. (1984). The sport orientation of female collegiate basketball players participating at different competitive levels. *Perceptual and Motor Skills, 59,* 79-87.

Purpose: To evaluate the reasons given for athletic participation among female athletes.

Description: Sixteen concepts related to the reasons generally given for athletic participation (e.g., self-improvement, excitement) were presented in a semantic differential format using 15 bipolar adjective scales. Scale responses ranged from 1 ("extremely negative feelings") to 4 ("neutral feelings") to 7 ("extremely positive feelings"). The semantic differential factors of evaluation, potency, and activity were represented by five adjective pairs each.

Construction: Concepts related to the reasons generally given for athletic participation were derived from a review of literature. A total of 25 coaches and physical education graduate students eliminated or revised concepts thought to be ambiguous.

Reliability: Alpha internal consistency coefficients (*n*=258 female basketball players) were only acceptable for the evaluative factor (and not for the potency and activity factors). The coefficients ranged from .64 (physical fitness) to .94 (power) with a mean alpha coefficient of .88 reported across the 16 concepts.

Validity: Exploratory factor analysis (*n*=258) of the evaluative component produced three factors accounting for 48.3% of the variance. Factor 1 (27.9% accountable variance) represented the more personal, noncompetitive types of rewards related to sport participation. Factor 2 (10.9% accountable variance) related to competitive achievement, whereas Factor 3 (9.5% accountable variance) appeared to represent pressure from family and friends to participate in athletics.

Norms: Not cited. Psychometric data were reported for female varsity basketball players participating in AIAW programs in Divisions I (n=76), II (n=90), and III (n=92).

Availability: Contact Donald Siegel, Exercise and Sport Studies Department, Scott Gymnasium, Smith College, Northampton, MA 01063. (Phone # 413-585-3977; E-mail: dsiegel@smith.edu)

Chapter 20

Multidimensional

Tests in this chapter assess multiple personality traits, attitudes, motives, beliefs, or psychological skills evident among individuals participating in sport or exercise.

289 | *Athletic Coping Skills Inventory (ACSI-28)
Ronald E. Smith, Robert W. Schutz, Frank L. Smoll, and J. T. Ptacek

Source: Smith, R. E., Schutz, R. W., Smoll, F. L., & Ptacek, J. T. (1995). Development and validation of a multidimensional measure of sport-specific psychological skills: The Athletic Coping Skills Inventory-28. *Journal of Sport & Exercise Psychology, 17,* 379-398.

Purpose: "...to measure individual differences in psychological skills within a sport context" (p. 381).

Description: The ACSI-28 contains 28 items and seven subscales: (a) Coping With Adversity (e.g. "I maintain emotional control no matter how things are going for me"); (b) Peaking Under Pressure (e.g., "The more pressure there is during a game, the more I enjoy it"); (c) Goal Setting/Mental Preparation ("I set my own performance goals for each practice"); (d) Concentration (e.g, "I handle unexpected situations in my sport very well"); (e) Freedom From Worry (e.g, "I put a lot of pressure on myself by worrying how I will perform"); (f) Confidence and Achievement Motivation (e.g., "I feel confident that I will play well"); and (g) Coachability (e.g., "When a coach or manager criticizes me, I become upset rather than helped"). Participants respond to each item using a 4-point ordinal scale with the anchorings 0 (*almost never*) to 3 (*almost always*).

Construction: An earlier version of the ACSI (Smith, Smoll, & Ptacek, 1990) "...was developed in the mid-1980s as part of a research project on psychosocial vulnerability and resiliency factors related to athletic injury" (p. 381). The ACSI was based on a conceptual model that life stress, social support, and psychological coping skills evidenced a causal relationship to sport performance and injury. The ACSI was developed to assess specific psychological coping skills such as concentration and control of worry.

Initially, 87 items were intuitively derived and administered to 637 male or female athletes representing 41 high school teams in three sports and 135 Division I college football players. Exploratory principal components factor analysis with varimax rotation led to the retention of eight factors and 42 items accounting for 49% of the response variance.

Cronbach alpha coefficients for these eight subscales ranged from .64 to .81. Further cross-validation research with 579 male or female high school athletes supported this eight-factor structure. However, confirmatory factor analysis supported a seven-factor model containing 28 items; follow-up principal components analyses indicated that these seven factors accounted for 53% and 58% of the response variance among male and female samples, respectively.

Reliability: Cronbach alpha internal consistency coefficients, computed from the responses of 594 male and 433 female varsity high school athletes to the ACSI-28, ranged from .62 (Concentration) to .78 (Peaking Under Pressure). A total (Personal Coping Resources) score internal consistency coefficient of .86 was reported.

One-week test-retest reliability coefficients ($N=94$) ranged from .47 (Coachability) to .87 (Peaking Under Pressure). The median test-retest reliability coefficient was .82.

Validity: Convergent validity was supported in that participants' ($N=295$ to 771) total scores on the ACSI-28 were positively correlated ($r=.44$) with their scores on the Self-Control Schedule, a measure of cognitive behavioral skills. Participants' responses to the Freedom From Worry subscale correlated negatively ($r=-.59$) with their responses to the worry factor of the Sport Anxiety Scale (SAS), but their scores on the Freedom From Worry subscale did not correlate with their responses to the somatic or concentration disruption factors of the SAS; thus, there is support for both the convergent and discriminant of this subscale. However, participants' responses to the Concentration subscale of the ACSI-28 did not correlate with their responses to the concentration disruption scale of the SAS.

Further support for the convergent validity of the ACSI-28 was reported based on the positive correlation coefficients reported with the Self-Efficacy Scale; the ACSI-28 total score evidenced a correlation coefficient of .58 with the Self-Efficacy scale. Also, participants' responses to several subscales of the ACSI-28 were positively related to their scores on a measure of general self-esteem. However, the authors also reported that there was some evidence of social desirability contamination, in that participants' responses to the ACSI-28 were positively related to their scores on the Crowne-Marlowe Social Desirability Scale.

The authors also reported evidence for the predictive validity of the ASCI-28. Athletes ($N=762$) categorized as overachievers, normal achievers, or underachievers, based on the discrepancy between coaches' ratings of their physical abilities and their subsequent ratings of these athletes' actual performance during the competitive season, were compared on the ACSI-28. Whereas the normal achievers and underachievers did not differ on the ACSI-28, overachievers scored highest on all subscales of the ACSI-28; on several of the subscales they differed significantly ($p<.05$) from at least one of the other two groups.

Further support for the predictive validity of the ACSI-28 was found in relation to performance measures obtained for 104 professional minor league baseball players (Smith & Christensen, 1995). Hierarchical regression analyses revealed that these participants' psychological skills, based on their responses to the ASCI-28 assessed during spring training, were predictive of their batting and pitching skills during the season following spring training; these findings were evident when physical skill differences among these professional athletes were partialed out.

Norms: Descriptive and psychometric statistics were presented for a variety samples including 594 male and 433 female varsity high school athletes (internal consistency data); 94 male or female college participants in intramural and club sport (test stability data); 295 to 771 male or female varsity high school athletes (convergent and discriminant validity data); and 762 male or female high school athletes, representing 6 sports and 13 high schools, and 104 professional minor league baseball players (predictive validity).

**Availability: Contact Ronald E. Smith, Department of Psychology, Box 351525, University of Washington, Seattle, WA 98195-1525. (Phone # 206-543-8817; FAX 206-685-3157; E-mail: resmith@u.washington.edu). Items are also listed in the *Source.*

References

*Christensen, D. S., & Smith, R. E. (1995). Psychological and physical skills as predictors of survival in professional baseball [Abstract]. *Journal of Applied Sport Psychology, 7* (Suppl.), S48.

Krane, V., & Leibold, B. (1994). Psychological factors related to the incidence of injury in collegiate soccer [Abstract]. *Journal of Sport & Exercise Psychology, 16* (Suppl.), S74.

*Petrie, T. A. (1993). Coping skills, competitive trait anxiety, and playing status: Moderating effects on the life stress-injury relationship. *Journal of Sport & Exercise Psychology, 15,* 261-274.

*Smith, R. E., & Christensen, D. S. (1995). Psychological skills as predictors of performance and survival in professional baseball. *Journal of Sport & Exercise Psychology, 17,* 399-415.

470

*Smith, R. E., Smoll, F. L., & Ptacek, J. T. (1990). Conjunctive moderator variables in vulnerability and resiliency research: Life stress, social support and coping skills, and adolescent sport injuries. *Journal of Personality and Social Psychology, 58,* 360-370.

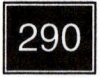

Athletic Motivation Inventory (AMI)
Bruce Ogilvie, Leland Lyon, and Thomas Tutko

Source: Hammer, W. M., & Tutko, T. A. (1974). Validation of the Athletic Motivation Inventory. *International Journal of Sport Psychology, 5,*3-12.

Purpose: To assess personality traits relevant to athletic performance.

Description: The AMI contains subscales designed to assess Drive, Aggression, Determination, Guilt-Proneness, Leadership, Self-Confidence, Emotional Control, Mental Toughness, Conscientiousness, Coachability, and Trust, plus accuracy and honesty scales.

Construction: Not discussed.

Reliability: Reliability coefficients ranged from .78 (Determination) to .93 (Mental Toughness)-- based on secondary reporting of data.

Validity: Correlation coefficients with relevant scales of Cattell's 16 PF among 112 collegiate football players indicated a number of significant but low relationships. However, there was evidence that responses to many of the AMI scales also correlated with the Honesty scale.

Norms: Not reported. Psychometric data were cited for 112 collegiate football players.

Availability: Contact Thomas Tutko, Department of Psychology, San Jose State University, San Jose, CA 95192. (Phone # 408-924-5600)

References
*Davis IV, Henry (1991). Criterion validity of the Athletic Motivation Inventory: Issues in professional sport. *Journal of Applied Sport Psychology, 3,* 176-182.

Jones, H. B. (1975). Athletic Motivation Inventory of sportwomen and nonathletes. In D. M. Landers (Ed.), *Psychology of sport and motor behavior II* (Penn State HPER Series No. 10) (pp. 153-164). State College, PA.

*Lyon, L. P. (1971). *A method for assessing personality characteristics in athletics: The Athletic Motivation Inventory.* Unpublished master's thesis, San Jose State College, San Jose, CA. (This thesis was used to summarize existing psychometric data on the AMI.)

*Morris, L. D. (1975). A socio-psychological study of highly skilled women field hockey players. *International Journal of Sport Psychology, 6,* 134-147.

Thomas, G. C., & Sinclair, G. D. (1977). The relationship between personality and performance of Canadian women intercollegiate basketball players. *In Human performance and behavior: Proceedings of the 9th Canadian Psycho-motor Learning and Sport Psychology Symposium* (pp.205-214). Banff, Alberta, Canada.

*Tutko, T. A. (1969, October). *A method of assessing athletic motivation: The Athletic Motivation Inventory.* Presentation made at the First Canadian Psycho-motor Learning and Sport Psychology symposium, University of Alberta, Edmonton, Alberta, Canada.

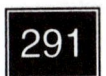 Belastungs-Symptom-Test (BST)
R. Frester

Source: Cited by Rieder, H. (1979). Measurement of precompetitive conditions with different sport groups. In G. C. Roberts & K. M. Newell (Eds.), *Psychology of motor behavior and sport-1978* (pp. 90-97). Champaign, IL: Human Kinetics Publishers.

Purpose: To determine precompetitive psychological conditions that the athlete views as activating or inhibiting to his or her performance.

Description: The BST contains 21 items that describe conditions the athlete must overcome in a competitive situation. The athlete responds to these items using a 9-point ordinal scale. Each point on the scale denotes how the athlete would respond to that particular condition.

Construction: Not discussed.

Reliability: A reliability coefficient of .88 was reported.

Validity: A factor analysis of the responses of 200 athletes resulted in three factors: psychological consistency, social/personal stability, and state anxiety.

Norms: Not cited.

Availability: Contact Hermann Rieder, Institut fur Sport U. Sportwissenschaft, Universitat Heidelberg, Germany.

292 *Coaching Sucess Questionnaire (CSQ)
Damon Burton and Tom Raedeke

Source: Burton, D., & Raedeke, T. (1993). Identifying successful coaches: The development and initial validation of the Coaching Success Questionnaire (CSQ) [Abstract]. *Journal of Sport & Exercise Psychology, 15* (Suppl.), S10.

Purpose: To identify critical psychosocial factors related to coaching success.

Description: The CSQ contains 32 items and eight subscales: Winning, Sport Skills/Strategies, Poise/Concentration, Conditioning/Wellness, Motivation/Responsibility, Social/Cooperation, Sport Values, and Fun/Self-Confidence.

Construction: The CSQ was initially conceptualized based on five dimensions of coaching success: winning, having fun, and developing physically, psychologically, and socially. The authors then developed 15 subdimensions of coaching success and created 10-12 items per subdimension. A panel of experts evaluated the items for face validity. The remaining 112 items were then administered to 139 high school athletes. Item analyses led to the retention of four items per subdimension. The revised questionnaire was then administered to 690 high school athletes. Confirmatory factor analyses led to the retention of eight factors.

Reliability: Cronbach alpha reliability coefficients averaged .76 across the eight subscales.

Validity: Discriminant validity was supported in that coaches with better win/loss records scored higher on coaching success than did coaches with poorer records.

Norms: Not cited. Psychometric data were reported for 690 high school athletes participating in seven sports.

Availability: Contact Damon Burton, Department of Physical Education, University of Idaho, 107 PEB, Moscow, ID 83843. (Phone #208-885-2186; FAX # 208-885-5929; E-mail: dburton@raven.csrv.uidaho.edu)

293 *[Costs/Benefits of Coaching Questionnaire] [CBCQ]
Maureen R. Weiss and Candie Stevens

Source: Weiss, M. R., & Stevens, C. (1993). Motivation and attrition of female coaches: An application of social exchange theory. *The Sport Psychologist*, 7, 244-261.

Purpose: "...to identify the positive and negative aspects of coaching, the resulting satisfaction or dissatisfaction associated with the coaching experience, and the costs, benefits, and satisfaction levels with potential professional options" (p. 248).

Description: The CBCQ contains 28 benefit items and 24 cost items. Two additional items assess overall satisfaction with coaching and satisfaction with alternative activities. Categories of benefits include positive team atmosphere, program success, feelings of competence, continue athletic experiences, external rewards, and financial gains. Categories of costs include time demands, low perceived competence, stress, external pressures, lack of support, and inadequate professional compensation. Coaches respond to these costs/benefits items using a Likert-type scale with the anchorings *not at all important* to *extremely important*.

Construction: Items were generated from the open-ended responses of 20 coaches and administrators with youth sport, high school, and/or collegiate coaching experience; these individuals were asked to identify factors influencing their decision to coach or discontinue coaching. The researchers and an independent rater assigned these items to five general areas pertaining to the benefits and five general areas pertaining to the costs of coaching. Subsequently, multiple items were developed reflective of these areas and placed in questionnaire format. Five experts in the field of coaching and physical education evaluated the items for accuracy, clarity, and relevance leading to the retention of 28 benefit items and 24 cost items.

Principal components and principal axis factor analyses (orthogonal and oblique rotations) produced six interpretable factors for the benefit items (49.5% accountable variance) and six interpretable factors for the cost items (59.8% accountable variance). The test description section above identifies the labels assigned to each of these twelve factors.

Reliability: Cronbach alpha reliability coefficients (N=153) ranged from .56 (Financial Gains) to .76 (Feelings of Competence) for the benefit factors, and from .62 (Inadequate Professional Compensation) to .88 (Stress) for the cost factors. The authors eliminated the Financial Gains and Inadequate Professional Compensation factors from further analyses because of the low internal consistency coefficients obtained.

Validity: Discriminant validity was supported in that current coaches (n=99) rated Program Success and Continue Athletic Experience (benefits) and Time Demands and Low Perceived Competence (costs) as higher in importance than did former coaches (n=54). Further, a classification analysis indicated that 74.4% of current coaches and 75.6% of former coaches were classified accurately according to group membership based on their responses to the CBCQ.

Norms: Not cited. Psychometric data were reported for 99 current high school female coaches (M age= 32.0 years) and 54 former high school female coaches (M age= 36.8 years) from Montana.

Availability: Items are identified in the *Source*. Contact Maureen R. Weiss, Department of Exercise and Movement Science, 1240 Esslinger Hall, University of Oregon, Eugene, OR 97403-1240. (Phone # 503-346-4108; FAX # 503-346-2841; E-mail: mrw@oregon.uoregon.edu)

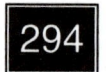

294 Daily Analyses of Life Demands for Athletes (DALDA)
Brent S. Rushall

Source: Rushall, B. S. (1990). A tool for measuring stress tolerance in elite athletes. *Journal of Applied Sport Psychology, 2,* 51-66.

Purpose: To assess sources of stress in sport, as well as external to sport, that affect the training and/or competitive performances of elite athletes.

Description: The first part of the DALDA asks the athlete to respond to general stress sources that occur in everyday life including diet, home-life, school/work, friends, training, climate, sleep, recreation, and health. The second part of the DALDA asks the athlete to respond to a list of 25 stress-reaction symptoms that he or she may be experiencing, such as muscle pains, tiredness, irritability, skin rashes, running nose, and boredom. Individuals respond to each item using one of three categories: "worse than normal," "normal," and "better than normal."

Construction: The author identified 12 areas of life stress and 42 symptoms of stress reaction, which were then subject to content validation using nine experts familiar with stress evaluation and high-level sports. On the basis of these experts' analyses, one further life stress and two symptoms were added. "It was deemed that this accumulation of factors represented the scope of sources of stress and symptoms of stress reactions that were associated with sporting environments" (p. 53).

A readability check was made using pupils in an elementary school sixth grade. They were asked to read the test booklet and indicate words they could not understand. As a result, seven definitions and four labels were changed.

Reliability: The DALDA was administered five times, 14 days apart, to 22 swimmers of the Nova Scotia Scientific Training Squad (ranging in age from 11 to 19 years). The criterion for reliability was that a stress source or symptom had to be responded to in exactly the same manner across 80% of the testing sessions by 80% of the participants. This analysis led to the retention of nine sources of life stress and 25 symptoms.

Validity: See discussion of content validity above.

Norms: Not indicated.

Availability: Contact Brent S. Rushall, Department of Exercise and Nutritional Sciences, San Diego State University, San Diego, CA 92182-0171. (Phone # 619-594-4094; FAX # 619-594-6553; E-mail: brushall@mail.sdsu.edu)

295	*Diagnostic Inventory of Psychological Competitive Ability for Athletes (DIPCA)

Mikio Tokunaga and Kimio Hashimoto

Source: Hashimoto, K., Tokunaga, M., & Takayanagi, S. (1993, June). *Diagnostic Inventory of Psychological Competitive Ability for Athletes (DIPCA) for predicting sport performance.* Paper presented at the 8th World Congress of Sport Psychology, Lisbon, Portugal.

Purpose: To assess "...the psychological-competitive ability, the mental power needed in a competitive situation" (p. 2).

Description: The DIPCA is a 52-item inventory and contains five factors: Competitive Motivation, Mental Stability and Concentration, Confidence, Strategy, and Cooperation. Participants respond to items such as "I am tough during a competition" or "I can make accurate decisions at crucial moments" using a 5-point ordinal scale with the anchorings 1 (*almost never*) to 5 (*always*)

Construction: Not discussed.

Reliability: Not discussed.

Validity: Multiple regression analysis supported the predicted, inverse relationship between participants' (N=284) DIPCA scores and their scores on the State Anxiety Inventory for Sports (1993). In addition, a positive relationship between participants' (N= 603) DIPCA scores and their scores on the Diagnostic Inventory for Psychological Performance (DIPP) and the degree of performance at the best of one's ability were found (Tokunaga, M., Hashimoto, K., Isogai, H., & Takayanagi, S., 1994).

Norms: Not cited. Descriptitive and psychometric data were reported for 284 high school baseball players who participated in the finals of the 72nd Japanese Senior High School Baseball Championship in the summer of 1990.

**Availability: Contact Mikio Tokunaga or Kimio Hashimoto, Institute of Health Science, Kyushu University, 6-1, Kasuga kouen, Kasuga city,

Fukuoka, Japan 816. (Phone/FAX #'s 011-81-92-583-7846; E-mail: tokunaga@ihs.kyushu-u.ac.jp)

References

*Kozuma, Y., & Okada, R., & Singer, R. N. (1994). A mental training program for a national collegiate top level judo team in Japan [Abstract]. *Journal of Sport & Exercise Psychology 16* (Suppl.), S74.

*Tokunaga, M., & Hashimoto, K. (1988). A study on the training of psychological-competitive ability for athletes (4): On making the diagnostic inventory. *Journal of Health Science, 10*, 73-84.

*Tokunaga, M., Hashimoto, K., Isogai, H., & Takayanagi, S. (1994). Relationship between psychological-competitive ability and competitive performance in Japanese athletes. *Journal of Health Science, 16*, 83-90.

[Environment Specific Behavior Inventories] [ESBI]

Brent S. Rushall

Source: Rushall, B. S. (1978). Environment specific behavior inventories: Developmental procedures. *International Journal of Sport Psychology, 9*, 97-110.

Purpose: To assess behavior unique to and consistent within a given sport.

Description: These sport-specific behavioral inventories contain items focusing on social, attitudinal, training, pre/post competitive behaviors, reactions to difficulties, rewards, and goals, and reactions to precompetitive stress. Behavioral inventories have been developed for such sports as swimming, soccer, rowing, and basketball. The majority of items on each inventory contain three response alternatives.

Construction: Item pools for each sport were generated from open-ended interviews with coaches, observations of coach and athlete behaviors in competitive and training situations, reviews of existing psychological tests, and reviews of sport science textbooks. Content validity of items was established by a panel of experts including national and provincial coaches.

Reliability: All items had a minimum percent of agreement value of 64% between test and retest.

Validity: Not discussed

Norms: Not cited. Sampling procedures for deriving reliability data were not discussed.

Availability: Contact Brent S. Rushall, Department of Exercise and Nutritional Sciences, San Diego State University, San Diego, CA 92182 0171. (Phone # 619-594-4094; FAX # 619-594-6553; E-mail: brushall@mail.sdsu.edu)

References

*Rushall, B. S., & Frey, D. C. (1980). Behaviour variables in superior swimmers. *Canadian Journal of Applied Sport Sciences, 5,* 177-182.

*Rushall, B. S., & Jamieson, J. (1979). The prediction of swimming performance from behavioral information: A further note. *Canadian Journal of Applied Sport Sciences, 4,* 154-157.

297 Family Sports Environment Interview Schedule (FSE)
Terry D. Orlick

Source: Orlick, T. D. (1974). An interview schedule designed to assess family sports environment. *International Journal of Sport Psychology, 5,* 13-27.

Purpose: To assess factors related to the family sports environment such as parental expectancies and encouragement of the child's participation.

Description: The FSE contains 27 questions used in interview format that describe five parts of the family sports environment including primary and secondary sports involvement of family, parental expectancies and athletic aspirations for child, encouragement for participation by parents, and general sports information. A 5-point ordinal scale is used to respond to the majority of items.

Construction: Items were derived from theoretical and empirical work on socialization, child development, psychology, and physical education. The items were reviewed by a psychologist and a sport psychologist. A pilot study contributed to the final refinement of the items.

Reliability: Interrater reliability coefficients ranged from .82 to .97 between a male physical education graduate student and a female teacher based on an analysis of taped interviews of four subjects.

Validity: The FSE discriminated between 8- and 9-year-old boys ($n=16$) in organized sports from those boys ($n=16$) who were not participants, based on interviews conducted with the boys' mothers.

Norms: Not cited.

Availability: Contact Terry Orlick, School of Human Kinetics, University of Ottawa, 125 University, Ottawa, Canada K1N 6N5. (Phone # 613-562-5800, Ext. 4272; FAX # 613-564-7689)

 ***Fitness Class Climate Questionnaire (FCCQ)**
Albert V. Carron, Lawrence R. Brawley, and W. Neil Widmeyer

Source: Carron, A. V., Brawley, L. R., & Widmeyer, W. N. (1990). The impact of group size in an exercise setting. *Journal of Sport & Exercise Psychology, 12*, 376-387.

Purpose: To assess perceptions of exercise program participants concerning various social psychological aspects of their exercise class.

Description: The FCCQ is a 28-item inventory that addresses (a) the nature of the instructor (6 items); (b) opportunities available for social interaction with other members (7 items); (c) perceptions of crowding and density (4 items); (e) feelings of conspicuousness (5 items); and (e) satisfaction (5 items). For example, exercise participants are asked to respond to "I feel like others are always evaluating me in exercise class" (feelings of conspicuousness). Participants' perceptions are assessed on a 9-point Likert scale with the anchorings *strongly disagree* and *strongly agree*.

Construction: Not discussed.

Reliability: Cronbach alpha reliability coefficients (N=192) ranged from .62 (Conspicuousness) to .77 (Crowding and Density) after items were removed to maximize internal consistency estimates.

Validity: Not discussed.

Norms: Not cited. Psychometric data were reported for 192 exercise participants (undergraduate and graduate students, faculty, and staff) involved in a university exercise program.

Availability: Contact Albert V. Carron, Faculty of Physical Education, University of Western Ontario, London, Ontario, Canada N6A 3K7. (Phone # 519-679-2111, Ext. 5475; FAX # 519-661-2008; E-mail: bert.carron@uwo.ca)

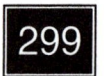 ***Golf Performance Survey** [GPS]
Patrick R. Thomas and Ray Over

Source: Thomas, P. R., & Over, R. (1994). Psychological and psychomotor skills associated with performance in golf. *The Sport Psychologist, 8,* 73 86.

Purpose: To evaluate psychological skills underlying successful golf performance, as well as psychomotor competencies and commitment in golf.

Description: The GPS assesses players' concentration levels, use of imagery, mental preparation, strategies and tactics, self-control, emotions and cognitions, psychomotor skills, commitment, and competitiveness. Participants respond to each of 95 items (e.g., "I am a mentally tough competitor in golf") using a 5-point Likert scale with anchorings ranging from *strongly disagree* to *strongly agree.*

Construction: Most of the items were original, although some items were borrowed from existing sport-specific psychological tests. Ten university staff members who were members of golf clubs responded to an initial version of the GPS. Their input led to some revisions in the items and instructions.

Exploratory principal axis factor analyses (oblique rotation) of the items concerned with psychological skills (n=165) produced five factors accounting for 43% of the variance. These factors were labeled as follows: (a) Negative Emotions and Cognitions, (b) Mental Preparation, (c) Conservative Approach, (d) Concentration, and (e) Striving for Maximum Distance.

Reliability: Cronbach alpha coefficients (N=165) and test-retest reliabilities (n=36) across a 3-month interval were as follows: (a) Negative Emotions and Cognitions=.81, .90; (b) Mental Preparation=.78, .90; (c) Conservative Approach=.67, .74; (d) Concentration=.74, .78); and (e) Striving for Maximum Distance=.69, .72.

Validity: The psychological skills portion of the GPS distinguished between low-handicap golfers (n=34) and high-handicap golfers (n=34). It was found that the low-handicap (more skilled golfers) scored higher on Mental Preparation and on Concentration. They were also less prone to negative emotions and cognitions.

Norms: Not cited. Psychometric data were reported for 165 male golfers (M age=48.15, SD=12.03) participating in competitive golf in Brisbane, Australia.

**Availability: Contact Patrick R. Thomas, Faculty of Education, Griffith University, Nathan, Australia 4111. [Phone # (61-7) 3875 5634; FAX # (61-7) 3875 5910; E-mail: pthomas@edn.gu.edu.au]

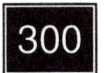 [Health Belief Questionnaire for Joggers] [HBQJ]

Suzanne E. Slenker, James H. Price, Stephen M. Roberts, and Stephen G. Jurs

Source: Slenker, S. E., Price, J. H., Roberts, S. M., & Jurs, S. G. (1984). Joggers versus nonexercisers: An analysis of knowledge, attitudes and beliefs about jogging. *Research Quarterly for Exercise and Sport, 55,* 371-378.

Purpose: To assess the knowledge, attitudes, and beliefs individuals have about jogging based on the Health Belief Model.

482

Description: The questionnaire contains 49 items designed to measure the Health Belief dimensions including Barriers, Motivation, Benefits, Complexity, Severity, Susceptibility, and Cues. Individuals respond to each item using a 5-point Likert scale.

Construction: An open-ended questionnaire based on the Health Belief Model was developed to elicit beliefs about jogging from a group of 40 joggers and 39 nonexercisers. All responses were accepted for the questionnaire until a cutoff point of 75% of total responses was reached.

Reliability: Kuder-Richardson Formula 20 internal consistency coefficients (n=124 joggers and 96 nonexercisers) were, for the majority of subscales, above .75.

Validity: Factor analysis supported, for the most part, the hypothesized constructs of perceived susceptibility, severity, benefits, barriers, health motivation, support, complexity, and cues. Barriers to action, such as lack of time, job, or family was the most potent predictor of nonexercising versus jogging behavior, accounting for approximately 40% of the variance.

Norms: Not cited. Psychometric data were cited for 124 joggers present at an organized race and 96 nonexercisers employed at a major corporation.

**Availability: Contact James H. Price, Department of Human Performance, University of Toledo, 2801 W. Bancroft, Toledo, OH 43606. (Phone # 419-530-2743; FAX # 419-530-4759; E-mail: jprice@utnet.utoledo.edu)

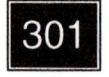 **[Jackson Personality Inventory--Wrestling] (JPI-W)**
John J. Dwyer and Albert V. Carron

Source: Dwyer, J. J., & Carron, A. V. (1986). Personality status of wrestlers of varying abilities as measured by a sport specific version of a personality inventory. *Canadian Journal of Applied Sport Science, 11,* 19-30.

Purpose: To examine personality traits considered to be desirable or undesirable in wrestling.

Description: The JPI-W contains the following personality scales with items worded specifically for wrestling: Anxiety, Energy Level, Interpersonal Affect, Organization, Risk Taking, Self-Esteem, Social Participation, Tolerance, and Infrequency (validity). The inventory contains 20 items per scale. Participants respond true or false to each item.

Construction: Six experts (one psychologist, two sport psychologists, two wrestling coaches, and one wrestler) converted the Jackson Personality Inventory items to JPI-W items. Three of the scales were conceptually altered: the Risk-Taking scale emphasized physical risks, the Self-Esteem scale focused on performance self-esteem, and the Tolerance scale emphasized openness to ideas and behaviors pertaining to wrestling. Item analyses (n=98 freestyle wrestlers) indicated that the items within a scale correlated favorably with the derived total score of that scale.

Reliability: Kuder-Richardson formula 20 internal consistency coefficients(n=87 freestyle wrestlers) ranged from .43 (Tolerance) to .81 (Energy Level). Test-retest reliability coefficients (n=21 freestyle wrestlers) ranged from .65 (Organization) to .93 (Interpersonal Affect) across an average time interval of 43 days.

Validity: Intercorrelation coefficients with corresponding JPI scales (n=87 freestyle wrestlers) were statistically significant supporting convergent validity. Discriminant function analyses yielded JPI-W self-esteem differences between wrestlers categorized as qualifiers (n=40) or nonqualifiers (n=47), based on whether these individuals were represented or had placed at specified wrestling tournaments.

Norms: Not cited. Descriptive and psychometric data were based on the responses of 98 freestyle wrestlers, ages 17-21+, who had competed in Ontario, Canada, in 1982-83.

Availability: Contact Albert V. Carron, Faculty of Kinesiology, University of Western Ontario, London, Ontario, Canada N6A 3K7. (Phone 519-679-2111, ext. 5475; FAX # 519-661-2008; E-mail: bert.carron@uwo.ca)

302 Motivational Rating Scale (MRS)
Thomas A. Tutko and Jack W. Richards

Source: Reviewed by Corbin, C. B. (1977). The reliability and internal consistency of the Motivational Rating Scale and the General Trait Rating Scale. *Medicine and Science in Sports, 9,* 208-211.

Purpose: To identify personality traits appropriate for success at high levels of athletic competition.

Description: The MRS is a 55-item test containing 11 subscales (and five items per subscale). Subscales include Aggression, Coachability, Emotional Control, Mental Toughness, Drive, Self-Confidence, Determination, Leadership, Responsibility, Trust, and Conscience Development. Athletes respond to each subscale on a 5-point Likert scale.

Construction: Not discussed. These traits are the same as evaluated on the original Athletic Motivation Inventory (AMI).

Reliability: Alpha internal consistency coefficients (n=74 male high school basketball players) ranged from .05 (Trust) to .76 (Leadership). Among 75 female high school basketball players, alpha internal consistency coefficients ranged from -.02 (Trust) to .67 (Coachability).

Test-retest reliability coefficients among these male athletes across a 7- to 10-day interval ranged from .49 (Emotional Control) to .80 (Leadership). For the female sample, test-retest reliabilities (7- to 10- day interval) ranged from .55 (Conscience Development) to .83 (Drive).

Validity: Concurrent validity was examined by correlating these athletes' scores on the MRS with their respective coaches' ratings of these individuals on these traits. The correlation coefficients ranged from -.01 (Mental Toughness) to .36 (Self-Confidence).

Norms: Not reported.

Availability: Contact Thomas A. Tutko, Department of Psychology, San Jose State University, San Jose, CA 95192. (Phone # 408-924-5600)

Reference

Dennis, P. W. (1978). Mental toughness and performance success and failure. *Perceptual and Motor Skills, 46,* 385-386.

*Ottawa Mental Skills Assessment Tool (OMSAT)

Natalie Durand-Bush and John H. Salmela

Source: Durand-Bush, N., & Salmela, J. H. (1995). Validity and reliability of the Ottawa Mental Skills Assessment Tool (OMSAT) [Abstract]. *Journal of Applied Sport Psychology, 7* (Suppl.), S46.

Purpose: "To assess a broad range of athletes' mental skills" (S46) and perspectives.

*Description: The OMSAT includes 12 mental skills scales regrouped under the following three broader conceptual components: (a) *Foundation Skills* (Goal Setting, Belief/Self-Confidence, Commitment), (b) *Affective/Arousal Skills* (Stress Control, Fear Control, Relaxation, Energizing), and (c) *Cognitive Skills* (Imagery, Mental Practice, Focusing, Refocusing, and Competition Planning). The inventory comprises 79 items. Participants respond to each item using a 7-point Likert scale.

*Construction: The OMSAT was devised by Salmela (1992) to measure athletes' perceived abilities and uses of a wide range of mental skills. Bota (1993) empirically tested the first and second versions of the OMSAT and recommended that the instrument be further revised. An enhanced version of the OMSAT (OMSAT-3) was thus created.

Items were initially devised based on (a) an extensive review of the literature on mental skills training and assessment, (b) expert opinions, and (c) results of pilot tests conducted with researchers, consultants, competitive athletes, and graduate/undergraduate students. The OMSAT is presently undergoing its fourth revision. Throughout these revisions, items were reconstructed or eliminated based on clarity, content/face validity, redundancy, item-total score correlations, and discriminant analysis.

*Note: Natalie Durand-Bush, personal communication, April 19, 1996.

*Reliability: Cronbach alpha reliability coefficients ($N=335$) ranged from .68 to .86 for the 12 OMSAT-3 scales, with a mean alpha reliability coefficient of .80. Test-retest reliability coefficients across a 2-week interval ranged from .61 to .89, with a mean test-retest reliability coefficient of .68

*Validity: A confirmatory factor analysis performed on the conceptual structure of the OMSAT revealed it was adequate. LISREL produced a chi square value of 11.5 with 41 degrees of freedom ($p=1.00$). The goodness of fit and adjusted goodness of fit indices were .996 and.994, respectively. The root mean square residual was .5311. A discriminant analysis revealed that the OMSAT discriminated between elite and competitive level athletes, with Commitment, Stress Control, and Refocusing being the best discriminating scales.

*Norms: Not reported. Psychometric data were based on the responses of 147 elite athletes (77 males and 70 females) competing at national and international levels and 188 competitive athletes (98 males and 90 females) enrolled in local and provincial sport clubs and schools or performing on university/college teams. Participants ranged in age from 9 to 42 years (M age= 19.6 years). Athletes came from 35 different sports with hockey ($n=56$), soccer ($n=39$), water polo ($n=37$), basketball ($n=34$), swimming ($n=33$), baseball ($n=23$), rowing ($n=17$), fencing ($n=13$), and karate ($n=10$) being the most predominant.

**Availability: Contact Natalie Durand-Bush or John H. Salmela, School of Human Kinetics, University of Ottawa, Ottawa, Ontario, Canada K1N 6N5. Phone 613-562-5600, ext. 4261; FAX 613-562-5149; E-mail: s540930@aix1.uottawa.ca)

References

*Bota, J. D. (1993). *Development of the Ottawa Mental Skills Assessment Tool* (OMSAT). Unpublished master's thesis, University of Ottawa, Ottawa, Canada.

*Draper, S., P., Salmela, J. H., & Durand-Bush, N. (1995). The Ottawa Mental Skills Assessment Tool: A confirmatory factor analysis. In R. Vanfraechem-Raway & Y. Vanden Auweele (Eds.), *Proceedings of the IXth European Congress on Sport Psychology* (pp. 82-89). Brussels: Free University of Brussels.

*Durand-Bush, N. (1995). *Validity and reliability of the Ottawa Mental Skills Assessment Tool* (OMSAT-3). Unpublished master's thesis, University of Ottawa, Ottawa, Canada.

*Salmela, J. H. (1992). *The Ottawa Mental Skills Assessment Tool* (OMSAT). Unpublished manuscript, University of Ottawa, Ottawa, Canada.

*Note: Natalie Durand-Bush, personal communication, April 19, 1996.

304 | *Personality Questionnaire for Sportsmen [QPS]
Edgar E. Thill

Source: Thill, E., & Brenot, J. (1982). Procédures d'analyse de la consistance d'un questionnaire de personnalité. *Le Travail humain, 45,* 268-283.*

Purpose: To assess personality traits to make decisions in sport and exercise domains, including selection and classification of sportsmen.

Description: The QPS contains 340 items and 16 scales: Intrinsic Motivation (DR 1), Extrinsic Motivation (DR 2), Psychological Endurance (EP), Speed-Intensity (VI), Competitiveness (CP), Control of Activity (CA), Risk Taking (PR), Emotional Control (CE), Psychological Stress (RP), Introversion-Extroversion (IE), Dominance (DO), Aggressivity (AG), Sociability (SO), Cooperation (CO), Acquiescence, (AQ), and Social Desirability (DS).

Construction: All scales (other than CP, AQ and DS scales) were developed according to the "a priori content validation method." This included a review by eight sport psychologists of an initial pool of 1,080 items, the selection of items by 10 judges, and exploratory factor analyses.

Reliability: Cronbach alpha coefficients ($N=309$) ranged from .92 to .97. Test-retest reliability coefficients across a 4-week interval, obtained for a second sample ($N=107$) of athletes, ranged from .42 (AQ) to .74 (DR 2).

Validity: Concurrent validity of the QPS was supported in that participants' responses correlated positively with their scores on various psychological tests, trainers' ($N=114$) evaluations, levels of practice in gun ($n=107$) and pistol shooting, and three levels in sport practice ($n=220$). Predictive validity was supported in that scores on the QPS were positively correlated with athletes' performances 2 years later in swimming ($r=.20$; $n=186$), rowing ($r=.57$; $n=44$), and sailing ($r=.60$; $n=80$). Construct validity was supported in that psychological endurance (EP) scores positively correlated with oxygen consumption (VO2) in liters per

*Note: The English translation of the material in the source and the summation of test information were provided by the test author (E. Thill, personal communication, October 18, 1993).

minute and negatively correlated with explosive strength (e.g., Sargent test) among fencers ($N=34$), swimmers ($N=211$), and volleyball participants ($N=27$). Further, participants' risk taking (PR) or speed intensity (VI) were positively correlated with tests of explosive strength (see Thill & Brenot, 1985).

Norms: Psychometric data were reported for 537 girls (ages 14 to 17 years old), 324 women, 736 boys (ages 14 to 17 years old), and 727 men.

**Availability: Contact Les Editions du Centre de Psychologie Appliquée, 25 rue de la Plaine, F-75980 Paris Cedex 20, France or Edgar E. Thill, Departement de Psychologie, Université Blaise Pascal, 34, boulevard Carnot, F-63.000-Clermont Ferrand, France. [Phone # (33) 73 40 64 73; FAX # (33) 73 40 64 82]

References

Thill, E. (1988). Evaluation longitudinale de traits de personnalité de sportifs et de non sportifs. *International Journal of Sport Psychology, 19*, 107-118.

Thill, E. (1988). Validations concourantes et conceptuelles du questionnaire de personnalité pour sportifs: des procédures symétriques. In *Proceedings VIIth Congress of the European Federation of Sport Psychology* (pp. 158-167). Leipzig, DDR: Wissenschaftlicher Rat.

Thill, E., & Brenot, J. (1985). Le modele de mesure des traits reconsidéré. Validité des interpretations descriptives et prédictives d'un questionnaire de personnalité. *Revue de Psychologie Appliquée, 35*, 175-200.

Thill, E., Chauvier, R., Leveque, M., Missoum, G., & Thomas, R. (1982). Validité de pronostic de la réussite sportive à partir de critères psychologiques. In T. Orlick, J. T., Partington, & J. Salmela (Eds.), *Proceedings of the Fifth World Sport Psychology Congress: Mental training for coaches and athletes* (pp. 102-104). Ottawa: Sport in Perspective, Inc.

Vanfraechem-Raway, R. (1993). Research concerning motivation level, efficiency and player/trainer relations in volleyball teams. In J. R. Nitsch & R. Seiler (Eds.), *Motivation, emotion, and stress* (pp. 293-297). Sankt Augustin, Germany: Academia Verlag.

305 Projective Sport Test (PST)
Michel A. Bouet

Source: Bouet, M. A. (1970). A projective test for sport participants. In G. S. Kenyon (Ed.), *Contemporary psychology of sport* (pp. 747-752). Chicago: Athletic Institute.

Purpose: To describe the motivation of sport participants in terms of the importance attributed to competition, reactions to success and failure, aggressiveness, personal conflicts, emotional maturity, and other factors.

Description: The PST is a sport-specific version of the projective technique titled the Thematic Apperception Test. The PST contains 16 photographs of action scenes from events in different sports. Participants are asked to examine each photo and respond by creating a story to what they see occurring in the photo. Responses are evaluated clinically in terms of the participant's depiction of the main character and his or her motivation, the participant's description of the obstacles the main character overcomes, and so forth.

Construction: Not discussed.

Reliability: Not presented.

Validity: Convergent validity was supported in that participants' ($n=40$ approx.) responses to the PST were related to their responses to the Rorschach Ink Blot Test and two projective techniques (Machover and Koch) that involve drawing.

Norms: Not presented.

Availability: Last known address: Michel A. Bouet, Section de Psychologie et Sciences Sociales, Universite de Rennes, Avenue Gaston-Berger, 35 Rennes, France.

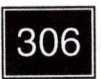

Psychological Preparation in Wrestling Questionnaire [PPWQ]
Daniel Gould, Maureen Weiss, and Robert Weinberg

Source: Gould, D., Weiss, M., & Weinberg, R. (1981). Psychological characteristics of successful and nonsuccessful Big Ten wrestlers. *Journal of Sport Psychology, 3,* 69-81.

Purpose: To assess the cognitive and behavioral strategies employed by wrestlers as they prepare for or engage in competition.

Description: This 107-item questionnaire contains 15 demographic and background information items and 92 items requiring wrestlers to respond on a 11-point Likert scale. The latter items center on eight scales plus 13 individual items. These eight scales include Kinds of Thoughts, Quantity of Thoughts, Imagery, Best Performance Attributions, Poor Performance Attributions, Cope With Anxiety, Anxiety, and Self-Talk.

Construction: The majority of items used in the questionnaire were adopted from an inventory developed by Highlen and Bennett based on personal communication and discussed in Highlen and Bennett (1979). In addition, a smaller number of items assessing preperformance mental preparation techniques and self-efficacy were included in the questionnaire.

Reliability: Alpha reliability coefficients (49 collegiate wrestlers) ranged from .60 (Quantity of Thoughts) to .83 (Anxiety).

Validity: Self-confidence, maximum potential, and use of attentional focusing were the most important variables discriminating successful from less successful wrestlers based on tournament placements and seasonal won-loss records.

Norms: None available. Psychometric data are cited for 49 wrestlers who participated in the Big Ten Conference Wrestling championships at Michigan State University.

**Availability: Contact Daniel Gould, Department of Exercise and Sport Science, University of North Carolina, 250 HHP Building Greensboro, NC 27412-5001. (Phone # 910-334-3037; FAX # 910-334-3238; E-mail: gouldd@iris.uncg.edu)

Reference

*Highlen, P. S., & Bennett, B. B. (1979). Psychological characteristics of successful and nonsuccessful elite wrestlers: An exploratory study. *Journal of Sport Psychology, 1,* 123-137.

307 *Psychological Profiles for the Selection of Talented Youth to Competitive Sport [PPSTYC]

Gershon Tenenbaum, Michael Bar-Eli, Noa Levy-Kolker, and Shraga Sade

Source: Tenenbaum, G., Bar-Eli, M., Levy-Kolker, N., & Sade, S. (1992). Psychological selection of young talented children for sport. In G. Tenenbaum, T. Raz-Liebermann, & Z. Artzi (Eds.), *Proceedings of the International Conference on Computer Applications in Sport and Physical Education* (pp. 268-274). Netanya: Gil Publications.

Purpose: To assess the necessary psychological traits for coping with competitive sport situations among physically talented children who are being considered for participation in elite competitive sport.

Description: The PPSTYC contains 84 items and 10 subscales that measure (a) behaviors following an unsuccessful action (i.e., cognitive anxiety, emotional involvement, positive thinking); (b) behaviors during stressful situations (i.e., self-efficacy, somatic arousal, positive feelings); (c) attributions following unexpected situations/unfulfilled expectations during competition; (d) attributions in expected situations/fulfilled expectations during competition; (e) behaviors during competition (i.e., control and self-regulation); (f) social interactions; (g) communications with the coach; (h) behaviors during practice; (i) cognitions in stressful situations; and (j) motives for competitive participation (8 motives). Participants respond to each item using a 4-point Likert scale.

Construction: The items were initially developed by three sport psychologists based on a review of the psychological literature pertaining to traits that are common characteristics in elite athletes.

Reliability: Cronbach alpha internal consistency coefficients ranged from .70 to .90, and test-retest correlation coefficients ranged from .75 to .92 (one-week interval) across the scales ($N=601$).

Validity: Exploratory and confirmatory factor analyses ($N=601$) supported the retention of the 10 scales. A 5-year longitudinal study is in

492

progress to determine the predictive validity of the PPSTYC to assessing adherence and skill acquisition among young, talented athletes.

Norms: Descriptive statistics for each scale (including percentile scores) are presented for 601 male or female athletes, ages 13-14 years, representing 12 competitive sports.

**Availability: Contact Gershon Tenenbaum, Department of Psychology, University of Southern Queensland, Toowoomba, Queensland 4350, Australia. (Phone # 76-31-1703; FAX # 76-31-2721; E-mail: tenenbau@zeus.usq.edu.au)

 # *[Psychological Skills in Sport Questionnaire] [PSSQ]
David Nelson and Lew Hardy

Source: Nelson, D., & Hardy, L. (1990). The development of an empirically validated tool for measuring psychological skill in sport [Abstract]. *Journal of Sports Sciences, 8,* 71.

Purpose: To assess a wide range of psychological skills thought to be required to enhance sport performance and coping in competitive and stressful situations.

Description: The PSSQ assesses Imaginal Skill, Mental Preparation, Self Efficacy, Cognitive Anxiety, Concentration Skill, Relaxation Skill, and Motivation using Likert-scale type items.

Construction: Not discussed.

Reliability: Cronbach alpha reliability coefficients exceeded .78 for each of the seven scales.

Validity: Not discussed

Norms: Not provided

Availability: Contact Lew Hardy, Division of Health and Human Performance, University College of North Wales, Victoria Drive,

Bangor, Gwyneed LL57 2EN, United Kingdom. (Phone # +44 1248-382823; FAX # +44 1248-371053)

Reference
Kingston, K., & Hardy, L. (1994). When are some goals more beneficial than others? [Abstract]. *Journal of Sports Sciences, 12*, 198-199.

Psychological Skills Inventory for Sports (PSIS)
Michael J. Mahoney, Tyler J. Gabriel, and T. Scott Perkins

Source: Mahoney, M.J., Gabriel, T. J., & Perkins, T. S. (1987). Psychological skills and exceptional athletic performance. *The Sport Psychologist, 1*, 181-199.

Purpose: The PSIS is designed to assess psychological skills that are relevant to elite athletic performance.

Description: The PSIS (Form R-5) contains 45 items and assesses Anxiety, Concentration, Self-Confidence, Mental Preparation, and Team Orientation. For example, athletes are asked to respond (on a 5-point Likert scale) to items such as "I sometimes feel intense anxiety while I am actually performing" (anxiety scale).

Construction: The PSIS was rationally derived and constrained by the use of a true-false format. The test was then modified to a 5-point Likert format, and nondifferentiating items have been replaced.

Reliability: Internal consistency coefficients of .72 (Spearman-Brown), .70 (Guttman-Rulon), and .64 (Cronbach alpha) were reported (Mahoney, 1989).

Validity: Construct validity was evidenced by support of the hypothesized discrimination of elite athletes from nonelite athletes on the five subscales using item analyses, stepwise discriminant and regression analyses, and factor and cluster analyses. The authors cautioned that the PSIS is a pilot instrument awaiting formal and extensive psychometric evaluation.

494

Norms: Not available. Psychometric data were reported for elite athletes ($n=126$), preelite athletes ($n=141$), and nonelite athletes ($n=446$) representing nationally a total of 23 sports. Average ages of the elite, preelite, and nonelite athletes sampled were 24.1, 18.6, and 19.8 years, respectively.

Availability: Contact Michael J. Mahoney, Department of Psychology, 258 Terrill Hall, P. O. Box 13587, University of North Texas, Denton, TX 76203 6587. (Phone # 817-565-3289; FAX # 817-565-4682)

References

*Bahner, K. R., & Kubitz, K. A. (1992). An examination of the relationship between perceived competitive skill levels and psychological skills in race car drivers using Tamen et al.'s revision of the PSIS R-5 [Abstract]. *Proceedings of the North American Society for the Psychology of Sport and Physical Activity annual convention* (p. 132). Pittsburgh, PA.

Bryant, F., Mahoney, M., & Meyers, A. (1989). Removing performance feedback to assess strength of psychological skills [Abstract]. *Proceedings of the annual conference of the Association for the Advancement for Applied Sport Psychology* (p. 33). Seattle, WA.

Bull, S. J. (1991). Personal and situational influences on adherence to mental skills training. *Journal of Sport & Exercise Psychology, 13,* 121-132.

*Chartrand, J. M., Jowdy, D. P., & Danish, S. J. (1992). The Psychological Skills Inventory for Sports: Psychometric characteristics and applied applications. *Journal of Sport & Exercise Psychology, 14,* 405-413.

Clark, R. A., & Sachs, M. L. (1991). Challenges and opportunities in psychological skills training in deaf athletes. *The Sport Psychologist, 5,* 392-398.

*Cox, R. H. (1989). A comparison of disabled and able-bodied athletes relative to psychological skills [Abstract]. *Psychology of motor behavior and sport Proceedings of the North American Society for the Psychology of Sport and Physical Activity annual convention* (p. 116). Kent, OH.

*Cox, R. H. (1994). Psychological skills of elite Chinese athletes [Abstract]. *Journal of Sport & Exercise Psychology, 16* (Suppl.), S43.

*Cox, R. H., & Liu, Z. (1993). Psychological skills: A cross-cultural investigation. *International Journal of Sport Psychology, 24,* 326-340.

Cox, R. H., & Yoo, H. S. (1995). Playing position and psychological skill in American football, *Journal of Sport Behavior, 18,* 183-194.

*Greenspan, M., Murphy, S. M., Tammen, V., & Jowdy, D. (1989). Effects of athlete achievement level and test administration instructions on the Psychological Skills Inventory for Sport (PSIS) [Abstract]. *Proceedings of the annual conference of the Association for the Advancement for Applied Sport Psychology* (p. 55). Seattle, WA.

Hardy, L., & Parfitt, G. (1994). The development of a model for provision of psychological support to a national squad. *The Sport Psychologist, 8,* 126-142.

*Johnson, J., & Camburn, C. (1992). Cultural differences in the psychological characteristics of ultraendurance triathletes [Abstract]. *Proceedings of the Association for the Advancement of Applied Sport Psychology annual convention* (p. 75). Savannah, GA.

*Johnson, J., Wong, V., & Wainwright, T. (1993). Psychological characteristics of American, German and Japanese ironman triathletes. *Proceedings of the Eighth World Congress of Sport Psychology* (pp. 928-932). Lisbon, Portugal.

*Mahoney, M. J. (1989). Psychological predictions of elite and non-elite performance in Olympic weightlifting. *International Journal of Sport Psychology, 20,* 1-12.

*Meyers, M. C., LeUnes, A., & Bourgeois, A. E. (1995). Comparison of psychological skills across event, gender, nature of competition, and athletic skill level in collegiate rodeo athletes [Abstract]. *Journal of Applied Sport Psychology, 7* (Suppl.), S92.

*Meyers, M. C., Sterling, J. C., Treadwell, S., Bourgeois, A. E., & LeUnes, A. (1994). Mood and psychological skills of world-ranked female tennis players. *Journal of Sport Behavior, 17,* 156-165.

*Millhouse, J. I., Willis, J. D., & Layne, B. H. (1989). The clinical utility of three recent psychological instruments with advanced female gymnasts: A preliminary study [Abstract]. *Proceedings of the annual conference of the Association for the Advancement for Applied Sport Psychology* (p. 79). Seattle, WA.

Murphy, S. M., Fleck, S. J., Dudley, G., & Callister, R. (1990).Psychological and performance concomitants of increased volume training in elite athletes. *Journal of Applied Sport Psychology, 2,* 34-50.

*Tammen, V. V., & Murphy, S. M. (1991). Reevaluating the Psychological Skills Inventory for Sports [Abstract]. *Proceedings of the North American Society for the Psychology of Sport and Physical Activity annual convention* (p. 197). Pacific Grove, CA.

*White. S. A. (1993). The relationship between psychological skills, experience, and practice commitment among collegiate male and female skiers. *The Sport Psychologist, 7,* 49-57.

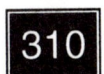

*Psychological Skills Test for Golfers (PSTG)

Tamotsu Nishida and Eiichi Kato

Source: Nishida, T., & Kato, E. (1994). Psychological Skills Test for Golfers [Abstract]. *Proceedings of the World Scientific Congress of Golf.* St. Andrews, Scotland.

Purpose: To assess psychological skills employed by golfers.

Description: The PSTG contains 25 items and five subscales: (a) Persistence and Concentration, (b) Ability to Change Thinking or Feelings, (c) Self-Confidence, (d) Positive Thinking, and (e) Anxiety about Mistakes. Participants respond to each item on a four-point scale with anchorings ranging from *always* to *seldom*.

Construction: Items were extracted from an analysis of psychological research investigations on golf.

Reliability: Cronbach alpha coefficients (n=225) ranged from .61 to .82.

Validity: Participants' (*n*=225) responses on the PSTG were related to such golf performance measures as their official handicap, mean golf score, number of putts, number of out of bounds, and number of birdies.

Norms: Not cited. Psychometric data were reported for 225 male professional or amateur golfer ranging in age from 16 to 70 years who were residing in Japan.

**Availability: Contact Tamotsu Nishida, Research Center of Health, Fitness and Sports, Nagoya University, Furo-cho, Chikusa-ku, Nagoya, 464 01 Japan. (Phone # 052-789-3952; FAX # 052-789-3957; E-mail: a40453a@nucc.cc.nagoya-u.ac.jp)

311 [Running Addiction Scales] [RAD]
Jeffrey J. Summers and Elizabeth R. Hinton

Source: Summers, J. J., & Hinton, E. R. (1986). Development of scales to measure participation in running. In L.-E. Unestahl (Ed.), *Contemporary sport psychology* (pp. 73-84). Oreboro, Sweden: VEJE.

Purpose: To assess (a) addiction and commitment to running, (b) withdrawal symptoms associated with nonrunning periods, and (c) mood states during a run.

Description: The RAD contains eight scales: (a) Addiction to Running, (b) Commitment to Running, (c) Exercise Running, (d) Runner's High, (e) Psychophysiological Well-Being During Running, (f) Psychophysiological Uneasiness During Running, (g) Withdrawal Effects For Addicted Runners, and (h) Withdrawal Effects For Exercise Runners. Runners respond to all items using a 5-point Likert scale.

Construction: Items were either empirically or rationally generated.

Reliability*: Cronbach alpha internal consistency coefficients (*n*=220 runners) ranged from .77 (Withdrawal Effects For Exercise Runners) to .95 (Withdrawal Effects For Addicted Runners). Test-retest reliability coefficients (*n*=49 runners) ranged from .48 (Withdrawal Effects For

*J. J. Summers, personal communication, March 9, 1990

Exercise Runners) to .89 (Addiction to Running; Commitment to Running).

Validity: Principal components factor analysis with iteration and varimax rotations (n=179 runners) supported the construct validity of the RAD. Multiple regression analyses indicated that the scales were useful in predicting addiction to running. Multivariate analyses of variance indicated that runners high on addiction and low on commitment could be differentiated on the basis of frequency of running, number of breaks from running taken, and number of fun races run.

Norms: Not cited. Psychometric data were reported for 154 male and 24 female runners recruited in Australia from the University of Melbourne and Lincoln Institute of Technology, from three fun/run races, and from two private companies. Runners ranged in age from 18 to 60 years.

Availability: Contact Jeffery J. Summers, Department of Psychology, University of Southern Queensland, Toowoomba, Queensland, Australia 4350. [Phone # 61 (076) 31 2712; E-mail: summers@zeus.usq.edu.au]

Reference

*Summers, J. J., Machin, V. J., & Sargent, G. I. (1983). Psychosocial factors related to marathon running. *Journal of Sport Psychology, 5*, 314-331.

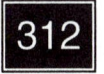

312 Sport Motivation Scales [SMS]
D. Susan Butt

Source: Butt, D. S. (1995). On the measurement of competence motivation. In P. E. Shrout (Ed.), *Personality research, methods, and theory: A festschrift honoring Donald W. Fiske* (pp. 313-331). Hillsdale, NJ: Lawrence Erlbaum.

Purpose: To evaluate three psychological motivations (aggression, conflict, and competence) and two social motivations (competition and cooperation) germane to sport participation.

Description: The SMS assess Aggression, Conflict, Competence,

Competition, and Cooperation in athletics. Each construct is measured by 10-item self-report scales. Items are presented in the following format: "During the last month while participating (training or competing) in _____ (fill in activity) did you ever feel...?" Participants respond to each item using a yes-no format.

Construction: Twenty items were written to assess each of the five constructs resulting in a pool of 100 items. Item analyses led to the retention of 50 items.

Reliability: Internal consistency coefficients (n=55 male students; n= 90 female students) ranged from .56 (Aggression-female sample) to .87 (Cooperation-female sample). The author also reported test stability coefficients for an earlier, shortened version of the SMS.

Validity: The author cited unpublished data documenting the convergent validity of the Competence scale. Further, extensive data are cited documenting the validity of an earlier, shortened version of the SMS.

Norms: Not cited. Descriptive and psychometric data were based on the responses of 145 undergraduate students.

Availability: Contact Susan Butt, Department of Psychology, University of British Columbia, 2136 West Mall, Vancouver, British Columbia, Canada V6T 1Z4. (Phone # 604-228-3269; FAX # 604-822-6923)

References

*Butt, D. S. (1973). Aggression, neuroticism and competence: Theoretical models for the study of sports motivation. *International Journal of Sport Psychology, 4,* 3-15.

*Butt, D. S. (1979). Short scales for the measurement of sport motivations. *International Journal of Sport Psychology, 10,* 203-216.

*Butt, D. S. (1985). Psychological motivation and sports performance in world class women field hockey players. *International Journal of Women's Studies, 8,* 328-337.

*Butt, D. S. (1987). *Psychology of sport: The behavior, motivation, personality and performance of athletes.* New York: Van Nostrand Reinhold.

*Butt, D. S. (1990). The sexual response as exercise: A brief review and theoretical proposal. *Sports Medicine, 9,* 330-343.

*Butt, D. S. (1991). Motivation in sports, exercise, and fitness. In L. Diamant (Ed.), *Mind-body maturity: The psychology of sports, exercise and fitness* (pp. 213-226). Washington, DC: Hemisphere Publishing.

*Butt, D. S., & Cox, D. N. (1992). Motivational patterns in Davis Cup, university, and recreational tennis players. *International Journal of Sport Psychology, 23,* 1-13.

*Wrisberg, C. A., Donovan, T. J., Birtton, S. E., & Ewing, S. J. (1984). Assessing the motivations of athletes: Further tests of Butt's theory. *Proceedings of the 1984 Olympic Scientific Congress* (p. 90). Eugene, OR: College of Human Development and Performance Microform publications.

313 | *Sports Injury Survey [SIS]
Lydia Ievleva and Terry Orlick

Source: Ievleva, L., & Orlick, T. (1991). Mental links to enhanced healing: An exploratory study. *The Sport Psychologist, 5,* 25-40.

Purpose: To identify psychological characteristics, conditions, or practices related to the sport injury healing process.

Description: The SIS contains 25 questions that focus on attitude, outlook, level of stress, social support, self-talk, goal setting, and mental imagery. Questions requiring a numerical responses are rated on a 0 to 10 scale.

Construction: Items for the SIS were derived from previous research on the relationship of mental factors to human performance and injury rehabilitation.

Reliability: Not cited.

Validity: The SIS successfully discriminated between individuals (*N*=32) identified as having fast or slow recovery times from ankle or knee injuries. Goal setting, positive self-talk, and imagery were most related to rapid recovery times from injury.

Norms: Not cited. Psychometric data were based on the responses of 32 athletes who were former patients at a major sports medicine clinic in Canada.

Availability: Contact Lydia Ievleva, Physical Education Department, University of Western Sydney, MacArthur, Campelltown, NSW, Australia 2550. [Phone: 61 (046) 20 6349; E-mail: aali@musica.macarthur.uws.edu.au or l.ievleva@uws.edu.au]

314 *Team Psychology Questionnaire [TSQ]
John T. Partington and Giselle M. Shangi

Source: Partington, J. T., & Shangi, G. M. (1992). Developing and understanding of team psychology. *International Journal of Sport Psychology, 23,* 28-47.

Purpose: To identify key psychosocial elements in successful team performance.

Description: The TSQ contains 53 items and seven scales: (a) Player Talent and Attitude, (b) Technical Coach Leadership, (c) Task Integration, (d) Social Cohesion, (e) Team Identity, (f) Style of Team Play, and (g) Interpersonal Coach Leadership. Individuals respond to each item on a 0- to 10-point rating scale with the anchors 0 (*not at all like my team*) and 10 (*exactly like my team*).

Construction: Seven psychosocial dimensions were derived from a review of the sport psychology literature on team psychology and written (or audiotaped) comments from coaches of seven Canadian national teams, a coach of a Canadian professional soccer team, and other coaches of elite teams. Item analyses of 15 experienced athletes' responses to 96 preliminary items was conducted. A total of 48 items were retained based on the ability of these items to discriminate between successful and unsuccessful athletic team experience. Five additional items were included based on the comments of these 15 athletes, resulting in the 53-item TSQ.

Reliability: Cronbach alpha reliability coefficients of .90 (Technical Coach Leadership), .85 (Interpersonal Coach Leadership), .77 (Player Talent and Attitude), .62 (Task Integration), .85 (Social Cohesion), .77 (Team Identity), and .84 (Style of Team Play) were reported ($N=171$).

Validity: Each of the seven scales discriminated between successful and unsuccessful teams supporting the discriminant validity of the TSQ. A factor analysis (varimax rotation) of participants' ($N=171$) responses to the TSQ extracted eight factors accounting for 84% of the variance. Examination of the item loadings indicated support for the seven subscales.

Norms: Not cited. Psychometric data were reported for 171 university and senior high school students (n=102 males; n=69 females) playing in interactive sports in competitive leagues.

Availability: Contact John Partington, Department of Psychology, Carleton University, Ottawa, Canada K1S 5B6. (Phone # 613-520-2600, ext. 2695).

Subject Index*

*Note: Numbers refer to test numbers and not to page numbers.

Test Title Index*

*Note: Numbers refer to test numbers and not to page numbers.

Test Acronym Index*

*Note: Numbers refer to test numbers and not to page numbers.

524

Test Author Index*

*Note: Numbers refer to test numbers and not to page numbers.